Birth
Settings
in America

OUTCOMES, QUALITY, ACCESS, AND CHOICE

Committee on Assessing Health Outcomes by Birth Settings

Susan C. Scrimshaw and Emily P. Backes, *Editors*

Board on Children, Youth, and Families

Division of Behavioral and Social Sciences and Education

Health and Medicine Division

A Consensus Study Report of

The National Academies of
SCIENCES · ENGINEERING · MEDICINE

THE NATIONAL ACADEMIES PRESS
Washington, DC
www.nap.edu

THE NATIONAL ACADEMIES PRESS   500 Fifth Street, NW   Washington, DC 20001

This activity was supported by contracts between the National Academy of Sciences and National Institutes of Health (#HHSN26300013). Support for the work of the Board on Children, Youth and Families is provided primarily by grants from the Heising-Simons Foundation (award number 2016-210), Jacobs Foundation (award number 2015-1168), and the Marguerite Casey Foundation (award number 2018-245). Any opinions, findings, conclusions, or recommendations expressed in this publication do not necessarily reflect the views of any organization or agency that provided support for the project.

International Standard Book Number-13: 978-0-309-66982-5
International Standard Book Number-10: 0-309-66982-0
Digital Object Identifier: https://doi.org/10.17226/25636
Library of Congress Control Number: 2020934621

Additional copies of this publication are available from the National Academies Press, 500 Fifth Street, NW, Keck 360, Washington, DC 20001; (800) 624-6242 or (202) 334-3313; http://www.nap.edu.

Suggested citation: National Academies of Sciences, Engineering, and Medicine. (2020). *Birth Settings in America: Improving Outcomes, Quality, Access, and Choice.* Washington, DC: The National Academies Press. https://doi.org/10.17226/25636.

The National Academies of
SCIENCES · ENGINEERING · MEDICINE

The **National Academy of Sciences** was established in 1863 by an Act of Congress, signed by President Lincoln, as a private, nongovernmental institution to advise the nation on issues related to science and technology. Members are elected by their peers for outstanding contributions to research. Dr. Marcia McNutt is president.

The **National Academy of Engineering** was established in 1964 under the charter of the National Academy of Sciences to bring the practices of engineering to advising the nation. Members are elected by their peers for extraordinary contributions to engineering. Dr. John L. Anderson is president.

The **National Academy of Medicine** (formerly the Institute of Medicine) was established in 1970 under the charter of the National Academy of Sciences to advise the nation on medical and health issues. Members are elected by their peers for distinguished contributions to medicine and health. Dr. Victor J. Dzau is president.

The three Academies work together as the **National Academies of Sciences, Engineering, and Medicine** to provide independent, objective analysis and advice to the nation and conduct other activities to solve complex problems and inform public policy decisions. The National Academies also encourage education and research, recognize outstanding contributions to knowledge, and increase public understanding in matters of science, engineering, and medicine.

Learn more about the **National Academies of Sciences, Engineering, and Medicine** at www.nationalacademies.org.

The National Academies of
SCIENCES · ENGINEERING · MEDICINE

Consensus Study Reports published by the National Academies of Sciences, Engineering, and Medicine document the evidence-based consensus on the study's statement of task by an authoring committee of experts. Reports typically include findings, conclusions, and recommendations based on information gathered by the committee and the committee's deliberations. Each report has been subjected to a rigorous and independent peer-review process and it represents the position of the National Academies on the statement of task.

Proceedings published by the National Academies of Sciences, Engineering, and Medicine chronicle the presentations and discussions at a workshop, symposium, or other event convened by the National Academies. The statements and opinions contained in proceedings are those of the participants and are not endorsed by other participants, the planning committee, or the National Academies.

For information about other products and activities of the National Academies, please visit www.nationalacademies.org/about/whatwedo.

COMMITTEE ON ASSESSING HEALTH OUTCOMES BY BIRTH SETTINGS

SUSAN C. SCRIMSHAW (*Chair*), The Sage Colleges
JILL ALLIMAN, Frontier Nursing University
WANDA BARFIELD, Centers for Disease Control and Prevention (*resigned March 2019*)
MELISSA CHEYNEY, Oregon State University
MICHELLE R. COLLINS, Rush University College of Nursing
BROWNSYNE TUCKER EDMONDS, Indiana University School of Medicine
WENDY GORDON, Bastyr University
MARIAN FRANCES MACDORMAN, Maryland Population Research Center
M. KATHRYN MENARD, University of North Carolina
KAREN MILGATE, Karen Milgate Health Policy Consulting
JOCHEN PROFIT, Stanford University
CAROL SAKALA, National Partnership for Women & Families
NEEL SHAH, Harvard Medical School and Ariadne Labs
KATHLEEN RICE SIMPSON, Mercy Hospital St. Louis
RUTH E. ZAMBRANA, University of Maryland, College Park

EMILY P. BACKES, *Study Director*
ELIZABETH S. HOWE-HUIST, *Associate Program Officer*
DARA SHEFSKA, *Associate Program Officer*
MARY GHITELMAN, *Senior Program Assistant*
LESLEY WEBB, *Senior Program Assistant (through October 2019)*
LORI TREGO, *NAM Distinguished Nurse Scholar-in-Residence (through August 2019)*

BRIDGET B. KELLY, *Consultant*
ERIN HAMMERS FORSTAG, *Technical Writer*

Preface

The United States spends more on childbirth than any other country in the world, with worse outcomes than other high-resource countries, and even worse outcomes for women of color. Our committee was charged with finding ways to improve these outcomes. We regarded this as an extraordinary opportunity to make recommendations to reverse a trend of increasing negative birth outcomes, do so more economically, and improve the childbirth experience for women and their families.

For me, this assignment circled back over three decades to a series of multicultural research projects on childbirth, notably with colleagues Christine Dunkel-Schetter and Ruth Zambrana along with many others. Among other things, we did early work associating the experience of racism and low birthweight for Black women and established the importance of social support. During that time, I lost a newborn daughter to unavoidable complications, and this strengthened my determination to prevent such outcomes whenever possible. Chairing this committee provided an opportunity to continue that work.

The committee composition reflected the range of health professionals who care for pregnant and birthing women and their babies, and those who look at data, policy, and wider social contextual factors affecting birth outcomes. Committee members included those with expertise in midwifery, obstetrics, nursing, pediatrics, demography, public health, health services research, health care policy, economics, sociology, and anthropology. There was a wide range of experience in different birth settings and with different economic and ethnic groups. This led to rigorous examination of the great variety of evidence, and vigorous debate around what that evidence could and could not support. The range of experience on the committee also necessitated working to understand settings and experiences of disciplines not well known to each other and a willingness to listen to each other and respect the evidence. Working together across such diverse experience and disciplines underscored for us the vital importance of interprofessional understanding, respect, and cooperation in order to improve birth outcomes within and across settings.

Looking through the lens of birth settings and multiple disciplines allowed us to examine childbirth with fresh eyes. The complexity of factors affecting childbirth was an important part of our discussion. In particular, the role of social determinants such as income, educational levels, access to care, financing, transportation, structural racism, and geographic variability in birth settings is clear, taking needed improvements far beyond the traditional clinical environments where nearly 98 percent of women in the United States give birth. Possible improvements both within and outside of specific birth settings ranged from easily achieved to extremely difficult, and near term to long term. Committee members decided to include all improvements supported by the evidence. While some improvements would take longer and be more difficult to achieve than others, we felt it was important to go on the record with recommendations we believed would benefit all mothers and babies in all settings.

As we weighed the competing economic access issues, professional values and mandates, economic and managerial pressures within settings, and professional boundaries, we established that our priority must always be the best possible pregnancy, birth, and postnatal experience and outcomes for mothers and babies. It is our expectation and our hope that childbirth in America can be both reframed and reformed to achieve the improved outcomes that we know are possible at less economic cost and at great gain for families and communities, as well as for our nation.

Susan C. Scrimshaw, *Chair*
Committee on Assessing Health
Outcomes by Birth Settings

Acknowledgments

This Consensus Study Report would not have been possible without the contributions of many people. First, we thank Congresswoman Lucille Roybal-Allard (D-CA) and Congresswoman Jaime Herrera Beutler (R-WA) for requesting this study and the study's sponsor the *Eunice Kennedy Shriver* National Institute of Child Health and Human Development at the National Institutes of Health for funding the project.

Special thanks go to the members of the study committee, who dedicated extensive time, thought, and energy to the project. Thanks are also due to NAM Distinguished Nurse Scholar-in-Residence Lori Trego (University of Colorado, Denver), who contributed her time and expertise throughout the report process.

In addition to its own research and deliberations, the committee received input from several outside sources, whose willingness to share their perspectives and experiences was essential to the committee's work. We thank Abigail Aiyepola (National Association to Advance Black Birth), Tanya Alteras (MITRE), Melissa Avery (University of Minnesota), Haywood L. Brown (University of South Florida), Steve Calvin (Minnesota Birth Center), Joia Crear-Perry (Black Mamas Matter), Susan Dentzer (Duke-Margolis Center for Health Policy), Jennie Joe (Native American Research and Training Center, University of Arizona), Diana Jolles (Frontier Nursing University), Jennie Joseph (Commonsense Childbirth, Inc.), Ebony Marcelle (Community of Hope), Mary Faith Marshall (University of Virginia), Peter Nielsen (Baylor College of Medicine), and Saraswathi Vedam (University of British Columbia, Canada).

The committee also gathered information through a commissioned paper. We thank the authors Holly Powell Kennedy (Yale University), Marie-Clare Balaam (University of Central Lancashire), Hannah Dahlen (Western Sydney University, Australia), Eugene Declercq (Boston University), Ank de Jong (Amsterdam University Medical Center, The Netherlands), Soo Downe (University of Central Lancashire, UK), David Ellwood (Griffith University School of Medicine, Australia), Caroline S.E. Homer (Burnet Institute, Australia), Jane Sandall (Kings College London, UK), Saraswathi Vedam (University of British Columbia, Canada), and Ingrid Wolfe (King's College London, UK) for "International Insights for Maternity Care in the United States." In addition, we thank Kylee Barnes and Leah Houtman for their commissioned analysis.

This Consensus Study Report was reviewed in draft form by individuals chosen for their diverse perspectives and technical expertise. The purpose of this independent review is to provide candid and critical comments that will assist the National Academies of Sciences, Engineering, and Medicine in making each published report as sound as possible and to ensure that it meets the institutional standards for quality, objectivity, evidence, and responsiveness to the study charge. The review comments and draft manuscript remain confidential to protect the integrity of the deliberative process.

We thank the following individuals for their review of this report: Claire D. Brindis (Philip R. Lee Institute for Health Policy Studies, University of California, San Francisco), Ana Delgado (Zuckerberg San Francisco General, Department of Obstetrics and Gynecology and Inpatient Midwifery Services, University of California, San Francisco), Joyce K. Edmonds (W.F. Connell School of Nursing, Boston College), Alan R. Fleischman (Albert Einstein College of Medicine, New York Academy of Medicine), Sandra D. Lane (Public Health and Anthropology, Syracuse University and Obstetrics and Gynecology, Upstate Medical University), Mary Lawlor (Office of the Executive Director, National Association of Certified Professional Midwives and Monadnock Birth Center, Swanzey, New Hampshire), Scott A. Lorch (Perelman School of Medicine, University of Pennsylvania and Neonatal-Perinatal Fellowship Program, The Children's Hospital of Philadelphia), Monica R. McLemore (Family Health Care Nursing Department and Advancing New Standards in Reproductive Health, University of California, San Francisco), Jennifer Moore (Office of the Executive Director, Institute for Medicaid Innovation and Department of Obstetrics and Gynecology, University of Michigan Medical School), and Jonathan M. Snowden (School of Public Health, Department of Obstetrics and Gynecology, Oregon Health and Science University).

Although the reviewers listed above provided many constructive comments and suggestions, they were not asked to endorse the conclusions or recommendations of this report nor did they see the final draft before its release. The review of this report was overseen by Elena Fuentes-Afflick (Pediatrics, Zuckerberg San Francisco General and Vice Dean for Academic Affairs, University of California, San Francisco) and Maxine Hayes (Pediatrics, School of Medicine and Health Services, School of Public Health, University of Washington). They were responsible for making certain that an independent examination of this report was carried out in accordance with the standards of the National Academies and that all review comments were carefully considered. Responsibility for the final content rests entirely with the authoring committee and the National Academies.

The committee also wishes to extend its gratitude to the staff of the National Academies, in particular to Elizabeth Howe-Huist and Dara Shefska, who contributed research and writing assistance to the committee's work and played an important role in editing portions of the report. Lesley Webb provided key administrative and logistical support and made sure that committee meetings ran efficiently and smoothly. Mary Ghitelman also provided administrative support in the final stages of the project and assisted with report production. Thanks are also due to consultant Bridget B. Kelly for her contributions to the formation of the committee and guidance throughout the study process, as well as consulting technical writer Erin Hammers Forstag, who provided invaluable writing assistance.

Throughout the project, Natacha Blain, director of the Board on Children, Youth, and Families, provided helpful oversight. The committee is also grateful to Anthony Bryant and Pamella Atayi for their financial and administrative assistance on the project. From the Division of Behavioral and Social Sciences and Education Office of Reports and Communication, we thank Kirsten Sampson-Snyder, Douglas Sprunger, and Yvonne Wise, who shepherded the report through the review and production process and assisted with its communication and dissemination. We also thank Rona Briere for her skillful editing.

Susan C. Scrimshaw, *Chair*
Emily P. Backes, *Study Director*
Committee on Assessing Health
Outcomes by Birth Settings

Contents

Summary

Childbirth services play a critical role in the provision of U.S. health care. The current U.S. maternity care system, however, is fraught with inequities in access and quality and high costs, and there is growing recognition of the mismatch between the collective expectations of the care and support women[1] deserve and what they actually receive. Moreover, the United States has among the highest rates of maternal and neonatal mortality and morbidity of any high-resource country, particularly among Black and Native American women. It is clear, then, that the systems supporting childbirth in the United States are in need of improvement. This report focuses on opportunities for improvement in one crucial component of U.S. maternity care: the settings in which childbirth occurs. While the vast majority of U.S. women experience childbirth in hospital settings, there is wide variation in the geographic availability of maternity hospitals and in hospital capabilities, types of maternity care providers available, and access to minimal-intervention birth options. In addition, a small (but growing) percentage of women give birth in birth centers or at home (0.52% and 0.99%, respectively). Yet not all women are able to access these options should they desire them, nor is it easy to transfer to a higher level of care when a transfer is indicated. In this context, and given the current state

---

[1]For the purposes of this report, the term "pregnant women" is used to describe pregnant individuals. The committee recognizes that intersex people and people of various gender identities, including transgender, nonbinary, and cisgender individuals, give birth and receive maternity care. Because we understand the term "woman" may be isolating and not reflective of how some individuals choose to identify, we periodically use the terms "pregnant people" or "pregnant individuals" in place of "pregnant women." See Box 1-1 in this report.

1

of U.S. maternity care, two urgent questions for women, families, policy makers, and researchers arise: How can an evidence-informed maternity care system be designed that allows multiple safe and supportive options for childbearing families? How can birth outcomes be improved across and within all birth settings?

To address these questions, congressional representatives asked the *Eunice Kennedy Shriver* National Institute of Child Health and Human Development (NICHD) to task the National Academies of Sciences, Engineering, and Medicine with convening an ad hoc committee of experts to provide an evidence-based analysis of the complex findings in the research on birth settings, focusing particularly on health outcomes experienced by subpopulations of women.

CONCEPTUAL MODEL

In conducting this study, the committee developed a conceptual model (see Figure S-1) identifying key opportunities that can be leveraged to improve policy and practice across birth settings. The triangle at the center indicates three elements that contribute to the ultimate goal of positive outcomes in maternity care: access to care, quality of care, and informed choice and risk assessment. The pregnant person and infant are at the center of this triad, surrounded by the maternity care team; the systems and settings in which care takes place; and collaboration and integration among providers and systems. The physical setting in which a birth takes place is one part of this overall picture, but it is nested among other elements that are relevant regardless of setting and that can be optimized for positive outcomes across and within different birth settings. All of these elements are embedded within the complex sociocultural environment that shapes health outcomes at the individual level and can affect whether these elements are optimally achieved. The components of this environment—the social, clinical, financial, and structural factors that contribute to access, informed choice, quality of care, and outcomes—represent opportunities for interventions to improve individual and population health, well-being, and health equity.

UNDERSTANDING BIRTH SETTINGS

As noted above, women in the United States give birth at home, in birth centers, and in hospitals. Across and even within these categories, the resources and services available differ significantly.[2] Women also are cared for

---

[2]For the purposes of this report, the committee defines a birth center as a freestanding health facility not attached to a hospital. Home births are those that occur at a woman's residence and can be either planned or unplanned.

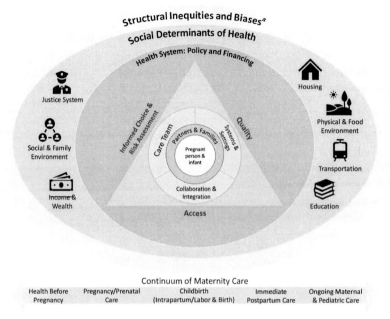

FIGURE S-1 Interactive continuum of maternity care: A conceptual framework.
ᵃStructural inequities and biases include systemic and institutional racism. Interpersonal racism and implicit and explicit bias underlie the social determinants of health for women of color.

by a number of different providers during their pregnancy and when giving birth, and these providers differ in how they are educated, trained, licensed, and credentialed. Moreover, women pay for maternity care through a variety of mechanisms, including private insurance (both individually purchased and employer-sponsored), Medicaid, Medicare, and self-pay; and the payment mechanism can affect what services, providers, and settings are available. State policies and regulations, too, can influence a woman's birth experience, through laws as to which providers can practice, their scope of practice, and the legal status of birth settings. Contextual factors (e.g., the social determinants of health, structural inequities and biases, medical risk factors) also influence where care is delivered and the content of care.

CLINICAL RISK AND SYSTEMIC INFLUENCES ON OUTCOMES IN PREGNANCY AND CHILDBIRTH

Although pregnancy and birth unfold without complication in most cases, neither is devoid of risk, and some groups of women enter pregnancy and birth with more risk than others. Risk during pregnancy—which the committee defines as the increased likelihood of an adverse maternal, fetal, or neonatal outcome—is conferred by four main sources: individual medical and obstetrical factors; health system–related factors, such as policy and financing decisions; the social determinants of health; and structural inequities and biases in the health system and in society at large. At a population level, these risk factors reflect the pattern of inequities in maternity care observed along racial/ethnic, geographic, and economic lines. For an individual woman, these sources of risk can interact and intersect, in some cases amplifying each other. For example, women with substance use disorders, a medical risk factor, are also less likely to receive adequate prenatal care and more likely to experience intimate partner violence than are pregnant women without substance use disorders, thereby increasing their risk in pregnancy and childbirth. Moreover, these risk factors affect both the pregnant individual's and the health care provider's decision making, shaping which birth settings have the capacity to offer safe, risk-appropriate care.

Women, however, may conceive of, tolerate, or understand risk differently from their health care providers, or may simply have competing priorities and values (e.g., control, respect, faith) that they prioritize over and above medical risks. There is broad consensus that women capable of doing so have the right to make informed decisions about their care, including decisions about their choice of care provider and place of birth (American College of Nurse-Midwives, 2017b; American College of Obstetricians and Gynecologists, 2017a). Informed choice, however, requires a set of real options, accurate and accessible information about the risks and benefits of those options, appropriate and ongoing medical/obstetrical risk assessment, respect for women's informed decisions (including informed refusals), and recognition that those choices may change over the course of care.

Such choice is often constrained by systemic factors that limit access. In its conceptual model, for example, the committee recognizes that structural inequities and biases are historically rooted and deeply embedded in policies, laws, governance, and culture such that power and resources are distributed differentially across characteristics of identity (race, ethnicity, gender, class, sexual orientation, and others), all of which influence health outcomes. For example, any discussion of risk assessment, choice, and equity in birth settings and birth outcomes must encompass the historical problem of disparate outcomes influenced by structural racism. Racism and discrimination—both in the health care system and in everyday life—have a well-documented impact on the health of marginalized communities. The adverse impacts of racism can be manifested in lower-quality health care; residential segregation and lack of affordable housing; or the accumulation of daily stressors resulting from micro- and macro-level aggressions, unconscious and conscious bias, and discrimination. They can thereby influence the health outcomes of pregnant people and their infants, causing considerable racial/ethnic disparities in pregnancy-related outcomes.

Moreover, birthing facilities and maternity care providers are unevenly distributed across the United States, leaving many women without access to prenatal, birthing, and postpartum care and choices among options near home. Women living in rural communities and underserved urban areas also have greater risks of such poor outcomes as preterm birth and maternal and infant mortality, in part because of a lack of access to maternity and prenatal care in their local area. In addition, some areas may lack access to midwifery care because certain types of midwives are not licensed in some states and do not have admitting privileges in some medical facilities, a factor that varies across the country. Indeed, the wide variation in regulation, certification, and licensing of maternity care professionals across the United States is an impediment to access across all birth settings. Moreover, access to all types of birth settings and providers is limited because of the lack of universal coverage of the cost of care for all women, for all types of providers, and at all levels. Taken together, system-level factors and social determinants of health such as structural racism, lack of financial resources, availability of transportation, housing instability, lack of social support, stress, limited availability of healthy and nutritious foods, lower level of education, and lack of access to health care (including mental health care) are correlated with higher risk for poor pregnancy outcomes and inequity in care and outcomes.

MATERNAL AND NEWBORN OUTCOMES BY BIRTH SETTING

Data and methodological limitations make the study of outcomes by birth setting challenging. Both vital statistics and birth registry data have limitations for evaluating birth outcomes by setting, provider type, and intentionality. In addition to these data deficiencies, the literature on birth settings compares a wide array of beneficial and nonbeneficial outcomes across and within settings. Studies often use differing definitions and terminology and report differing outcomes, making it difficult to conduct assessments or draw useful conclusions. In addition, the overall small number of women giving birth in home and birth center settings in the United States leads to unstable estimates with wide confidence intervals for outcomes of such rare events as maternal and fetal death. Furthermore, the literature on health outcomes by birth setting largely does not address difference by race/ethnicity or other subpopulations.

With these caveats in mind, the committee reviewed the available evidence and concluded that each birth setting—home, birth center, and hospital—has both risks and benefits for either the pregnant woman or the newborn. "Too little, too late" (TLTL) and "too much, too soon" (TMTS) patterns in the provision of maternity care contribute to excess morbidity and mortality, and in the context of inequality, these extremes often coexist within a single health care system. While the evidence suggests that no setting can fully eliminate risk from birth, many risks are modifiable at the level of systems, policies, processes, and providers.

Based on its review of the evidence, the committee found the following regarding outcomes comparing birth settings:

- Statistically significant increases in the relative risk of neonatal death in the home compared with the hospital setting have been reported in most U.S. studies of low-risk births using vital statistics data. However, the precise magnitude of the difference is difficult to assess given flaws in the underlying data. Regarding serious neonatal morbidity, studies report a wide range of risk for low-risk home versus hospital birth and by provider type. Given the importance of understanding these severe morbidities, the differing results among studies are of concern and require further study.

- Vital statistics studies of low-risk births in freestanding birth centers show an increased risk of poor neonatal outcomes, while studies conducted in the United States using models indicating intended place of birth have demonstrated that low-risk births in birth centers and hospitals have similar to slightly elevated rates of neonatal mortality. Findings of studies of the comparative risk of neonatal morbidity between low-risk birth center and hospital births are mixed, with variation across studies by outcome and provider type.

- In the United States, low-risk women choosing home or birth center birth compared with women choosing hospital birth have lower rates of intervention, including cesarean birth, operative vaginal delivery, induction of labor, augmentation of labor, and episiotomy, and lower rates of intervention-related maternal morbidity, such as infection, postpartum hemorrhage, and genital tract tearing. These findings are consistent across studies. The fact that women choosing home and birth center births tend to select these settings because of their desire for fewer interventions contributes to these lower rates.

- Some women experience a gap between the care they expect and want and the care they receive. Women want safety, freedom of choice in birth setting and provider, choice among care practices, and respectful treatment. Individual expectations, the amount of support received from caregivers, the quality of the caregiver–patient relationship, and involvement in decision making appear to be the greatest influences on women's satisfaction with the experience of childbirth.

- International studies suggest that home and birth center births may be as safe as hospital births for low-risk women and infants when (1) they are part of an integrated, regulated system; (2) multiple provider options across the continuum of care are covered; (3) providers are well-qualified and have the knowledge and training to manage first-line complications; (4) transfer is seamless across settings; and (5) appropriate risk assessment and risk selection occur across settings and throughout pregnancy. Such systems are currently not widespread in the United States.
- A lack of data and the relatively small number of home and birth center births prevent exploration of the relationship between birth settings and maternal mortality and severe maternal morbidity.

In summary, given both the acute and downstream risks of unnecessary interventions and the risks associated with potentially delayed access to lifesaving obstetric and neonatal interventions, there is no risk-free option for giving birth.

FRAMEWORK FOR IMPROVING BIRTH OUTCOMES ACROSS BIRTH SETTINGS

The system-level factors that influence outcomes across birth settings are responsive to intervention, yet these interventions are largely outside the scope of the health care system. Housing instability, limited transportation, and intimate partner violence (i.e., social determinants of health) fall into this category. Given the committee's charge, we focus on factors that can be influenced within the health care system, through changes to either service delivery or the services themselves. Of course, the committee acknowledges that while many disparities in outcomes accrue within the health care system, drivers of inequities in these outcomes begin outside the health care system. This reality undergirds our framework for maternal and newborn care in the United States—recognizing the need to build a culture of health equity; ensuring that pregnant people and infants receive the right amount of care at the right time; and delivering care in a respectful way, regardless of circumstance—but there is a critical need for more research on how these factors affect birth outcomes.

Because the committee recognizes that no birth setting is risk free and supports a woman's right to choose where and with whom she gives birth, we focus on opportunities for addressing the question of how each setting can improve outcomes and make birth safer. With the goal of building respect for pregnant people, their infants, their partners, and their families regardless of their circumstances (race, ethnic origin or immigration status, gender identity, sexual orientation, marital status, family composition, religion, income, or education) or birth or health choices, the committee suggests opportunities for practice, policy, and systems change that reduce barriers to the exercise of those choices.

Hospital Settings

The committee recognizes that many interventions are overused in U.S. hospital settings today. There are promising strategies and approaches for lowering the rates of nonmedically indicated and morbidity-related interventions, such as the primary cesarean rate in hospital settings. Evidence from promising models in the United States points to performance measurement, support for continuous quality improvement (QI), and mechanisms for accountability as key strategies for improving outcomes for pregnant women and infants while potentially yielding high-value care through cost savings as well. Emerging literature points to four core components of successful QI initiatives: engagement of multiple disciplines and partner organizations, mobilization of low-burden and rapid-cycle data, provision of up-to-date guidance for implementation using safety bundles and toolkits, and availability of coaching and peer learning. While many QI initiatives have shown promising results, many current QI initiatives are underfunded. To build on these promising findings and effectively implement QI at all levels of health care, QI initiatives will need to receive sufficient and sustainable financing from both government and private entities.

> **CONCLUSION 7-1:** Quality improvement initiatives—such as the Alliance on Innovation in Maternal Health and the National Network of Perinatal Quality Collaboratives—and adoption of national standards and guidelines—such as the Maternal Levels of Care of the American College of Obstetricians and Gynecologists and Society for Maternal-Fetal Medicine; the American Academy of Pediatrics' Neonatal Levels of Care; and guidelines for care in hospital settings developed by the Association of Women's Health, Obstetric, and Neonatal Nurses, the Society for Obstetric Anesthesia and Perinatology, and the American College of Nurse-Midwives—have been shown to improve outcomes for pregnant people and newborns in hospital settings.

Women's ability to exercise choice with regard to birth setting is also limited by a lack of access-to-care options in hospital settings.

> **CONCLUSION 7-2:** Providing currently underutilized nonsurgical maternity care services that some women have difficulty obtaining, including vaginal birth after cesarean, external cephalic version, planned

vaginal breech, and planned vaginal twin birth, according to the best evidence available, can help hospitals and hospital systems ensure that all pregnant people receive care that is respectful, appropriate for their condition, timely, and responsive to individual choices. Developing in-hospital low-risk midwifery-led units or adopting these practices within existing maternity units, enabling greater collaboration among mater-nity care providers (including midwives, physicians, and nurses), and ensuring cultivation of skills in obstetric residency and maternal-fetal medicine fellowship programs can help support such care.

High-value payment models with measures, performance targets, and value-based payment are also mechanisms for accountability. While maternity care costs have risen, performance has routinely fallen short and is worsening for some indicators. Payment tied to value, whether or not optimal care occurred or an optimal outcome was achieved, can incentivize quality, create conditions for innovative systems, improve care and out-comes, and reduce costs, among other favorable improvements.

CONCLUSION 7-3: Efforts are needed to pilot and evaluate high-value payment models in maternity care and identify and develop effective strategies for value-based care.

Home and Birth Center Settings

Examples from international experience demonstrate that positive out-comes for pregnant women and infants can be achieved across birth settings in the context of a system that promotes coverage for all women and types of providers, collaboration, seamless transfer, and coordination among providers and settings. Moreover, a recent U.S. study suggests that greater integration of midwifery professionals within a state's maternal care system may be related to improved maternal and newborn health outcomes. This evidence indicates that key components of integration and collaboration include shared care and access to safe and timely consultation, seam-less transfer across settings, appropriate risk assessment and risk selection across settings and throughout the episode of care, well-qualified maternity care providers with the knowledge and training to manage first-line compli-cations, collaborative QI initiatives, and the use of multidisciplinary model guidelines for transfer between settings.

CONCLUSION 7-4: Integrating home and birth center settings into a regulated maternity and newborn care system that provides shared care and access to safe and timely consultation; written plans for dis-cussion, consultation, and referral that ensure seamless transfer across settings; appropriate risk assessment and risk selection across settings and throughout the episode of care; and well-qualified maternity care providers with the knowledge and training to manage first-line complications may improve maternal and neonatal outcomes in these settings.

Key to this integration is the appropriate education and training of all maternal and newborn care providers, reflecting the setting and the risk level of those they serve. Appropriate education, training, and certification coupled with licensing statutes, generally written with great specificity, can ensure that planned home and birth center births are limited, to the extent feasible, to healthy, low-risk women and that midwives and other providers working in those settings continually assess and monitor risks and complications so they can be properly and promptly addressed. Such risk assessment would need to consider not only medical and obstetric risk, but also social risk and the contextual lives of pregnant people. When assessing medical risk and monitoring for medical and obstetric complications among women of color, it is critically important that membership in a racial/ethnic group not overdetermine the assessment and constrain the birth setting or maternity care provider options made available to a given woman.

Currently, as noted above, certain types of midwives cannot be licensed in some states or obtain admitting privileges to some medical facilities, and this wide variation in regulation, certification, and licensing of maternity care professionals is an impediment not only to integration but also to access to high-quality care across all birth settings. Therefore, the committee endorses efforts to license certified nurse midwives, certified midwives, and certified professional midwives whose education meets International Confederation of Midwives (ICM) Global Standards for midwifery education, who have completed an accredited midwifery education program, and who are nationally certified in all jurisdictions in the United States.

CONCLUSION 7-5: The availability of mechanisms for all freestanding birth centers to access licensure at the state level and requirements for obtaining and maintaining accreditation could improve access to and quality of care in these settings. Additional research is needed to understand variation in outcomes for birth centers that follow accreditation standards and those that do not.

CONCLUSION 7-6: The inability of all certified nurse midwives, certified midwives, and certified professional midwives whose education meets International Confederation of Midwives Global Standards, who have completed an accredited midwifery education program, and who are nationally certified to access licensure and practice to the full extent of their scope and areas of competence in all jurisdictions in the United States is an impediment to access across all birth settings.

Informed Choice and Risk Selection

Women have the right to informed choice of the birth setting they desire, but to exercise that choice, they must have access to options for birth settings. As discussed above, therefore, informed choice requires a set of real options, accurate information about the risks and benefits of each option, respect for women's informed decisions, and recognition that choices may change over the course of care. Decision aids have been found to be useful and effective in helping health care consumers access and understand treatment options and their risks and benefits and in facilitating shared decision making. Counseling can also help women make an informed choice of birth setting, and risk assessment is a vital component of determining the optimal approach to providing such counseling.

CONCLUSION 7-7: Ongoing risk assessment to ensure that a pregnant person is an appropriate candidate for home or birth center birth is integral to safety and optimal outcomes. Mechanisms for monitoring adherence to best-practice guidelines for risk assessment and associated birth outcomes by provider type and settings is needed to improve birth outcomes and inform policy.

CONCLUSION 7-8: To foster informed decision making in choice of birth settings, high-quality, evidence-based online decision aids and risk-assessment tools that incorporate medical, obstetrical, and social factors that influence birth outcomes are needed. Effective aids and tools incorporate clinical risk assessment, as well as a culturally appropriate assessment of risk preferences and tolerance, and enable pregnant people, in concert with their providers, to make decisions related to risk, settings, providers, and specific care practices.

Access to Care and Birth Settings

The committee's review of the current financing mechanisms and costs associated with maternity care in the United States revealed that access to care is often limited by a woman's ability to pay, as only a limited number of insurance payers offer coverage for care in home or birth center settings or for certain provider types, and some women are unable to access insurance coverage at all. Moreover, many beneficial maternity care services and supports are not covered. For instance, doula support across birth settings—a model associated with better outcomes for women and infants, as well as cost savings—is covered by Medicaid in only three states.

> CONCLUSION 7-9: Access to choice in birth settings is curtailed by a pregnant person's ability to pay. Models for increasing access to birth settings for low-risk women that have been implemented at the state level include expanding Medicaid, Medicare, and commercial payer coverage to cover care provided at home and birth centers within their accreditation and licensure guidelines; cover care provided by certified nurse midwives, certified midwives, and certified professional midwives whose education meets International Confederation of Midwives Global Standards, who have completed an accredited midwifery education program, and who are nationally certified; and cover care provided by community-based doulas. Additional research, demonstration, and evaluation to determine the potential impact of these state-level models is needed to inform consideration of nationwide expansion, particularly with regard to effects on reduction of racial/ethnic disparities in access, quality, and outcomes of care.

It is also important that reimbursement levels be adequate to support quality care and allow providers across settings to sustain services. Currently, payment to providers through Medicaid and Medicare may not cover the full cost of care and prevents some providers from accepting more women with Medicaid coverage.

> CONCLUSION 7-10: Ensuring that levels of payment for maternity and newborn care across birth settings are adequate to support maternity care options across the nation is critical to improving access.

Access is also limited by the availability of a range of birth settings, including hospital maternity units, in a woman's locality. Because birthing facilities and maternity care providers are unevenly distributed across the United States, many women cannot access prenatal, birthing, and postpartum care options near their homes. In particular, women living in rural communities and underserved urban areas face greater risks of such poor outcomes as preterm birth and maternal and infant mortality. Rural and urban maternity care deserts present unique challenges to improving maternal and newborn care in the United States, and efforts are urgently needed to resolve disparities in outcomes by geographic location.

> CONCLUSION 7-11: Research is needed to study and develop sustainable models for safe, effective, and adequately resourced maternity care in underserved rural and urban areas, including establishment of

sustainably financed demonstration model birth centers and hospital services. Such research could explore options for using a variety of maternity care professionals—including nurse practitioners, certified nurse midwives, certified professional midwives, certified midwives, public health nurses, home visiting nurses, and community health workers—in underserved communities to increase access to maternal and newborn care, including prenatal and postpartum care. These programs would need to be adequately funded for evaluation, particularly with regard to effects on reduction of racial/ethnic and geographic disparities in access, quality, and outcomes of care.

Analyses of the current composition of the maternity and newborn care workforce in the United States show a mismatch between the care needs of the population as a whole and the proportion of providers best equipped to meet those needs. While the system at present relies primarily on a surgical specialty to provide front-line care, most childbearing women are largely healthy and do not need that type of care in first-line providers. The composition of the maternity care workforce in the United States stands in great contrast to that in a number of other countries where the ratio of midwives to obstetricians is much higher. The growing shortage of obstetricians in the United States, due to such factors as early retirement and job dissatisfaction, offers an opportunity to rectify this situation by focusing resources on growing the cadre of providers with nationally recognized credentials who are especially prepared to provide care to healthy low-risk women. As part of these efforts and to address racial/ethnic inequities in outcomes, attention is needed to ensure that the maternity and newborn care workforce resembles the racial/ethnic composition of the population of childbearing women, as well as its linguistic, geographic, and socioeconomic diversity. A large body of literature demonstrates the benefits of a diverse workforce, ranging from providing culturally concordant care to fostering trust in providers and improving outcomes.

CONCLUSION 7-12: To improve access and reduce racial/ethnic disparities in quality of care and treatment, investments are needed to grow the pipeline for the maternity and newborn care workforce— including community health workers, doulas, maternity nurses, nurse practitioners and physicians' assistants, public health nurses, family medicine physicians, pediatricians, midwives, and obstetricians—with the goal of increasing its diversity, distribution, and size. Greater opportunities for interprofessional education, collaboration, and research across all birth settings are also critical to improving quality of care.

Research, Evaluation, and Data Collection

Despite decades of advancement in medical science and technology, much remains unknown about perinatal health. The scientific challenge is to better understand the science of childbirth—from biology to policy—to improve outcomes for mothers, infants, and families. The committee offers a number of priority areas for future research in this report. In addition, the committee emphasizes that strengthening data collection, in particular, improving the usefulness of birth certificate records for birth settings research, is key to advancing understanding of outcomes across birth settings.

CONCLUSION

The challenges facing the current U.S. maternity care system, while urgent, are not insurmountable, and opportunities for improving the systems that support childbirth exist. To improve maternal and infant outcomes in the United States, it is necessary to provide economic and geographic access to maternity care in all settings, from conception through the first year postpartum; to provide high-quality and respectful treatment; to ensure informed choices about medical interventions when appropriate for risk status in all birth settings; and to facilitate integrated and coordinated care across all maternity care providers and all birth settings. Achieving these objectives will require coordination and collaboration among multiple actors—professional organizations, third-party payers, governments at all levels, educators, and accreditation bodies, among others—to ensure systemwide improvements for the betterment of all women, newborns, and families.

1

Introduction

The U.S. maternity system is fraught with uneven access and quality, stark inequities, and exorbitant costs, particularly in comparison with other peer countries. At the same time, the United States has among the highest rates of maternal and neonatal mortality and morbidity of any high-resource country, particularly among Black and Native American women[1] (Organisation for Economic Co-operation and Development, 2019; Centers for Disease Control and Prevention, 2019a; Petersen et al., 2019). There is also growing recognition of a mismatch between the collective expectations of the care and support women deserve and what they actually receive (Vedam et al., 2019).

Childbirth services play a critical role in the provision of American health care. Childbirth is the most common reason U.S. women are hospitalized, and one of every four persons discharged from U.S. hospitals is either a childbearing woman or a newborn (Sun et al., 2018). As a result, childbirth is the single largest category of hospital-based expenditures for public payers in the country, and among the highest investments by large employers in the well-being of their employees (Podulka et al., 2011).

---

[1]For the purposes of this report, the committee uses the term "women" throughout to describe pregnant individuals. However, we recognize that people of various gender identities, including transgender, nonbinary, and cisgender individuals, give birth and receive maternity care. See Box 1-1 for a more detailed discussion. In addition, the committee recognizes that multiple terms may be used to describe different cultural and ethnic groups, and that "race" is a social construct. For the purposes of this report, we use Black, White, Native American, and Latino (women) throughout. Box 1-2 provides additional context for the committee's use of terminology in reference to ethnicity, race, and racism.

BOX 1-1
A Note on Terminology: Pregnant Individuals

Gender-neutral language across different fields and in research is ever-evolving. Various stakeholders interested in birth settings and maternity care more generally use a variety of terms when reporting results for sex-specific findings. The *Journal of Midwifery and Women's Health*, for example, uses the terms *woman* and *women* when reporting results (Likis et al., 2018). The National Institutes of Health recognizes sex as a biological component and suggests the terms *female* or *male* be used when reporting on the sex of participants (National Institutes of Health, n.d.). The American Medical Association advises the use of "*woman* or *women* when referring to a special woman or a group of women" (Young, 2009, p. 2). For the purpose of this report, the term "pregnant women" is used to describe pregnant individuals. The committee recognizes that intersex people and people of various gender identities, including transgender, nonbinary, and cisgender individuals, give birth and receive maternity care. Because we understand the term women may be isolating and not reflective of how some individuals choose to identify, we periodically use the terms "pregnant people" or "pregnant individuals" in place of "pregnant woman" (see, e.g., Likis et al., 2018).

In addition, the committee was careful to use language that is supportive and inclusive to all women and pregnant people. The individuals discussed in this report are more than the risks and conditions they carry with them before, during, and after pregnancy, and thus the committee adopts people-centered language where possible. We use "women in labor" or "women with obesity," for example, to denote that women are the focal point, not the conditions they exhibit.

BOX 1-2
A Note on Terminology: Ethnicity, Race, and Racism

The question of how to refer to different racial/ethnic groups is complex. First, "race" is a social construct that has no biological meaning (Lemelle et al., 2011). Ethnic group refers to either self-identified groups or groups identified by others who share common characteristics such as language and culture. Descriptions such as "Black," "Latino," or "Native American" may be useful for data analytic and broad-brush comparative purposes, but conceal the heterogeneity within such groups. "Black" can include, for example, people of African origin brought to the United States generations ago against their will, as well as recent immigrants; descendants of immigrants from Africa and people from regions that received willing or unwilling immigration from Africa, such as the Caribbean, Latin America, and Great Britain. "Hispanic" refers to individuals who themselves are and/or

BOX 1-2 Continued

have ancestors from a country where Spanish is spoken, meaning "Hispanic" denotes Spain's influence in a country's history. To people from Latin America, the Caribbean (Puerto Rico, Cuba, Dominican Republic), South America (Ecuador, Bolivia, Colombia, Peru, etc.), and Central America (Honduras, Costa Rica, etc.), "Latino" is more broadly defined as denoting individuals from 22 countries throughout the world who may be White, Black, Mestizo, or Indigenous. "Hispanic" and "Latino" are disputed terms because not all people from or descended from populations in Spanish-speaking countries come directly from Spain (Hispanic); they can include people from a wide range of countries and a wide range of populations, including Native, African-origin, and European-origin populations in Spanish-speaking countries (see, e.g., González Burchard et al., 2005). The term "Native American," along with such terms as "American Indian" and "First People," conceals the heterogeneity within this population category, which includes many distinct tribal groups with strict criteria for membership.

For the purposes of this report, we use the terms "Black," "Hispanic/Latino," and "Native American" to best capture the available data classifications, fully understanding the complexities underlying each term. These terms refer specifically to traditionally and historically underrepresented groups that via land takeover, slavery/colonization, and systemic oppression are denied access to the nation's social and economic opportunity structure. These groups have been and continue to be historically underserved and disproportionately impacted by racial discrimination and limited economic opportunity and continue to experience the most adverse outcomes (National Academies of Sciences, Engineering, and Medicine, 2017).

It should also be noted that even though "race" is a social construct with no clear genetic basis, "racism" is a powerful and negative force in U.S. society. This report examines the impact of racism on women's lives, on access to health care related to pregnancy and birth, and on how women are perceived and treated within the health care system in order to help better understand and address discrepancies in birth outcomes.

Racism has been described as interpersonal, internalized, and structural. Interpersonal racism includes social distancing, stigmatization, and discrimination, as well as threats and harassment and even physical violence. Internalized racism occurs when negative feelings and stereotypes are turned inward, both in the form of low self-esteem and in racist attitudes toward oneself and others in one's ethnic group. Structural inequities are historically rooted and deeply embedded in policies, laws, governance, and culture, such that power and resources are distributed differentially across characteristics of identity (perceived race, ethnicity, gender, class, sexual orientation, and others) (National Academies of Sciences, Engineering, and Medicine, 2017). Racism has been described as an "underlying determinant" of many structural inequities (Prather et al., 2016; Hardeman et al., 2018; Ford et al., 2019).

Cumulatively, this spending accounts for 0.6 percent of the nation's entire gross domestic product (Rosenthal, 2013), roughly one-half of which is paid for by state Medicaid programs (MacDorman and Declercq, 2019).

For most American women, childbirth is also the first memorable time they are hospitalized, an episode that can frame their future engagement with the broader health system. Particularly for otherwise young and healthy women, pregnancy often serves as an initial entry point to receiving sustained health services as an adult. It is also common for some women to newly acquire health insurance during the months leading up to the birth of a child (The Medicaid and CHIP Payment and Access Commission, 2014). As a result, pregnancy can unmask existing chronic diseases, such as diabetes and hypertension, which require ongoing management. It can also reveal high-risk behaviors such as excessive drug or alcohol use, and high-risk situations, such as no or poor housing, issues with food availability, exposure to racism, stress, and negative family dynamics that can be mitigated by behavioral interventions, social support, and community support.

Despite their vital role in U.S. health care and in the lives of individual women, it is clear that the systems supporting childbirth in the United States are in need of improvement, and several examples of promising approaches to that end have shown reductions in cesarean and preterm births (see, e.g., Schneider et al., 2017). This report focuses on opportunities for improvement in one crucial component of U.S. maternity care: the settings in which childbirth occurs. It is important to note that this report recognizes variation among and within birth settings. Broadly speaking, possible intended birth settings include hospitals, birth centers, and home. There is extensive variation among hospitals and in the management of labor and birth and related staffing within any given hospital. Birth centers can be adjacent to or even within hospitals or can be freestanding, with varied transfer and backup arrangements. And home births vary by type of birth attendant and transfer and backup options. These and many more variations in models of care and resources are explored in this report, along with available evidence on birth outcomes in each setting.

While the vast majority of U.S. women—nearly 98.4 percent (MacDorman and Declercq, 2019)—experience childbirth in hospital settings, a small (but growing) percentage give birth in birth centers or at home. Not all women are able to access these options should they desire them, and within hospitals, not all women are able to access models of care that minimize interventions and allow for social support and informed decision making. In this context, and given the issues of cost, access, and content that characterize current U.S. maternity care, two urgent questions for women, families, policy makers, and researchers arise: How can an evidence-informed maternity care system be designed that allows multiple safe and supportive options for childbearing families? How can birth outcomes be improved across and within all birth settings?

PURPOSE AND SCOPE OF THIS STUDY

In 2018, the Congressional Caucus on Maternity Care, led by Congresswoman Lucille Roybal-Allard (D-CA) and Congresswoman Jaime Herrera Beutler (R-WA), recognized the great need for policy solutions to better the health of mothers and children. The March 2018 omnibus appropriations bill included language calling on the *Eunice Kennedy Shriver* National Institute of Child Health and Human Development (NICHD) to request that the National Academies of Sciences, Engineering, and Medicine conduct the study that resulted in this report. In response, the National Academies convened an ad hoc committee of experts that was tasked with examining the evidence on health outcomes across birth settings, particularly with regard to subpopulations of women. (See Box 1-3 for the committee's full statement of task.)

This study served as an update to two previous activities of the National Academies (see Box 1-4). In examining the research on birth settings, the committee was asked to analyze the current state of the science on six topics:

BOX 1-3
Statement of Task

An ad hoc committee will provide an evidence-based analysis of the complex findings in the research on birth settings, focusing particularly on health outcomes experienced by subpopulations of women. It will bring together key stakeholders in a public workshop to further inform this analysis, including representatives from government, academia, health care provider organizations, third-party payers, and women's health organizations.

The ad hoc committee will explore and analyze the current state of science on the following topics, identifying those questions that cannot be answered given available findings.

1. Risk factors that affect maternal mortality and morbidity
2. Access to and choice in birth settings
3. Social determinants that influence risk and outcomes in varying birth settings
4. Financing models for childbirth across settings
5. Licensing, training, and accreditation issues pertaining to professionals providing maternity care across all settings
6. Learning from international experiences

BOX 1-4
Previous Activities of the National Academies on Birth Settings

This committee's work served as an update to a 1982 report on *Research Issues in the Assessment of Birth Settings* and a 2013 workshop on the same topic.

The 1982 report, produced by the Institute of Medicine and National Research Council, identified a number of trends in birth settings emerging in the literature, including a new focus on the psychosocial components of the birth experience, an increasing interest in births occurring at home and in birth centers, concerns over rising health care costs, and a desire for deliveries with fewer interventions. The 1982 committee noted that while the data were unreliable for determining the number of planned home births, the number of freestanding birth centers had increased from 3 in 1975 to 130 in 1982, suggesting a significant upswing in women choosing to give birth outside the hospital setting. The report also highlighted differences in birth practices across settings. For example, hospital settings were more likely to have protocols for care of high-risk mothers and infants, while home and birth center settings were more likely to serve healthy, low-risk women and to include the participation of the entire family in the birth. They were also less likely to use technology and medication during birth.

The 1982 committee concluded that reliable information was lacking in several areas: the safety of different birth settings, the benefits and risks of various birth practices, and the economic costs associated with different settings and practices. The committee made the following recommendations:

- Research should be conducted on the safety and efficacy of different birth settings, using randomized clinical trials or other robust study designs whenever possible.
- Birth and fetal death certificates should include an area for routine recording of the intended and actual site of delivery, as well as the specific type of provider.
- Risk assessment tools should be made more reliable; accurate screening would minimize the need to transfer women and babies to a hospital.
- Sound empirical data were needed on the psychological benefits of different birth settings (e.g., whether one particular setting fosters a closer relationship between parent and child than another).
- Research on birth settings should be designed and conducted using a multidisciplinary team approach that includes a variety of investigators, as well as experts in research design.

As a follow-up to the 1982 report, the Institute of Medicine held a 2013 workshop titled "An Update on Research Issues in the Assessment of Birth Settings." While the workshop produced no consensus statements or recommendations, speakers and participants highlighted a number of recurring themes. First, participants identified an ongoing need to improve the quality of data on birth settings and birth outcomes, both by improving the collection of vital statistics data and by conducting controlled research studies. Second, participants noted the need for a more nuanced discussion of the risks and benefits of various birth settings and practices, and for acknowledgment that people's perceptions of risk and safety vary. Finally, participants expressed concern about women lacking the information and resources necessary to make an informed choice of birth settings, providers, and practices.

1. What risk factors affect maternal mortality and morbidity overall? (See Chapters 3 and 4.)
2. What factors affect the choice of and access to birth settings? (See Chapters 3 and 4.)
3. What are the social determinants of health that influence risk and outcomes in varying birth settings? (See Chapter 4.)
4. What are the financing models for childbirth across settings? (See Chapters 2 and 7.)
5. What are the licensing, training, and accreditation issues pertaining to professionals providing maternity care across all settings? (See Chapters 2 and 7.)
6. What lessons are learned from international experiences? (See Chapters 6 and 7.)

During its first meeting, the committee had the opportunity to discuss the objectives of the study with congressional staff and representatives from NICHD. In the course of these discussions, the sponsors made clear that they hoped the committee's report would be used "to create policies to better the health of mothers and children" and "to find policy solutions to save lives." They highlighted the need for a synthesis of evidence to inform decision making by members of congress and other policy makers, regulators and payers, practitioners, pregnant women, and the research community.

To carry out its task, the committee needed to define the continuum of care at the core of its scope of interest. While the committee's charge (refer to Box 1-3) was to focus on the childbirth experience, we elected to focus on the period from conception through the first year postpartum. The effects of the longitudinal, multifaceted, socially determined health inputs a woman brings to her pregnancy influence outcomes for both mother and newborn. Moreover, prenatal care plays a pivotal role in birth outcomes, and these outcomes are reflected throughout the first postpartum year. Prenatal care settings and provider types also can influence maternal choice of birth setting, as, for example, when a woman chooses to give birth in the hospital where her prenatal care provider has admitting privileges or chooses in-home care with a midwife because she lives in a rural community and lacks reliable transportation. The committee understands that broader societal forces and the life circumstances of preceding generations affect birth outcomes, which in turn are modified far beyond the first year of life.[2]

The committee also recognizes that the model of prenatal and postpartum care varies by birth setting and within types of settings, that pre-

---

[2]For further information on how critical neurobiological systems develop in the prenatal through early childhood periods and how social, economic, cultural, and environmental factors significantly affect a woman's and child's health ecosystem and ability to thrive, see National Academies of Sciences, Engineering, and Medicine (2019).

natal care plays a role in intrapartum care, and that both prenatal and postpartum care influence birth outcomes. For these reasons, we review the evidence on birth settings across the childbearing year, from preconception to the postpartum period, but dedicate the majority of our analysis to the intrapartum period.

The study's charge also asked the committee to focus on "subpopulations of women." In discussions with the sponsors, it became clear that "subpopulations of women" referred to groups of women experiencing higher pregnancy- and birth-related maternal morbidity and mortality. U.S. data indicate that these are Black and Native American women in particular, as well as women in underserved areas, such as certain rural and urban populations.

THE PROBLEM

Maternal and newborn care is critical to the nation's health. Equitable access to such care and the best possible outcomes for all racial/ethnic and socioeconomic groups are also essential. For women, maternal exposures during pregnancy can have profound long-term consequences for health later in life, such as risk of cardiovascular disease and hypertension (Arabin and Baschat, 2017; Oliveira et al., 2014). As will be discussed in further detail in this report, U.S. levels of maternal mortality and morbidity exceed those of many other countries, even as more is spent on maternity care.[3] To make matters worse, the morbidity and mortality outcomes are worse for Black and Native American women, and the trend is not encouraging.

For children, the appropriate care of newborns is crucial during a window of rapid growth and development at the beginning of life. The effects of exposures to factors that shape the health trajectories of newborns start before conception; thus, the preconception and prenatal periods are

---

[3]This report uses the terms "maternal mortality" or "pregnancy-related deaths," and "maternal morbidity" or "severe maternal morbidity." The World Health Organization (WHO) defines maternal mortality as "the death of a woman while pregnant or within 42 days of termination of pregnancy, irrespective of the duration and site of the pregnancy, from any cause related to or aggravated by the pregnancy or its management but not from accidental or incidental causes" (World Health Organization, 2019). The Centers for Disease Control and Prevention (CDC) defines pregnancy-related deaths as "the death of a woman while pregnant or within 1 year of the end of a pregnancy—regardless of the outcome, duration, or site of the pregnancy—from any cause related to or aggravated by the pregnancy or its management, but not from accidental or incidental causes" (Centers for Disease Control and Prevention, 2019a). WHO defines maternal morbidity as "any health condition attributed to and/or aggravated by pregnancy and childbirth that has a negative impact on the woman's wellbeing" (Firoz et al., 2013, p. 795). The CDC defines severe maternal morbidity as including "unexpected outcomes of labor and delivery that result in significant short- or long-term consequences to a woman's health" (Centers for Disease Control and Prevention, 2019b).

vital to setting the odds for lifelong health (National Academies of Sciences, Engineering, and Medicine, 2019). Growing scientific understanding of the early determinants of health (Hanson and Gluckman, 2014) in the fields of the microbiome (Mueller et al., 2015), epigenetics (Dahlen et al., 2013), life-course health development (Halfon et al., 2018), and the hormonal physiology of childbearing (Buckley, 2015) increasingly shows that exposures to such factors during sensitive periods of rapid fetal and neonatal development have the potential for long-term and even lifelong positive or negative effects on the health of the child.

Despite the importance of high-quality maternal and newborn care to the nation's health, however, access to services essential to such care is a concern for many U.S. women. In 2016, more than 5 million women lived in counties (rural or urban) with neither an obstetrician/gynecologist nor a nurse midwife, nor a hospital with a maternity unit (March of Dimes, 2018a). Among the 42 percent of childbearing women who rely on Medicaid for maternity care coverage (Martin et al., 2019), many live in states that have not expanded eligibility for Medicaid, meaning that some women can gain Medicaid coverage only after becoming pregnant.[4] These women then lose Medicaid coverage about 2 months after giving birth (Daw et al., 2017), despite growing recognition of the considerable postpartum health needs and vulnerabilities that persist through at least the first year following birth (American College of Obstetricians and Gynecologists, 2018a; Ranji et al., 2019). Of additional concern is the fact that some women are not eligible for Medicaid because they lack documentation that they are legal residents of the United States. This means that they do not have access to prenatal care and that postpartum care for the woman and infant will be extremely limited, but that hospital deliveries will be covered even though, paradoxically, such births may be complicated by the lack of prenatal care.

Regardless of the type of coverage, moreover, many childbearing women and newborns do not reliably receive quality care that is safe, evidence based, and appropriate for their health needs and preferences. Maternal and newborn care in the United States is characterized by broad variations in practice, with considerable overuse of nonmedically indicated care, underuse of beneficial care, and gaps between practice and evidence (Glantz, 2012; Miller et al., 2016; Shaw et al., 2016; Fingar et al., 2018). For example, access to prenatal care varies greatly across racial/ethnic groups, and many U.S. women lack access to essential maternity care services. Prenatal care provides risk assessment and treatment of some conditions, monitoring of the health of mother and baby, and vital health

---

[4]As of 2019, 33 states and the District of Columbia had adopted and implemented Medicaid expansion, and 14 states had not. Three states had adopted Medicaid expansion and hoped to have it implemented by 2020 (Kaiser Family Foundation, 2019a).

information and education for the pregnant woman. In 2018, more than 77.5 percent of all women who gave birth initiated prenatal care in the first trimester. Yet this was the case for only 67.1 percent of Black, 72.7 percent of Hispanic, 62.6 of American Indian/Alaska Native, and 51.0 percent of Native Hawaiian or other Pacific Islander women, compared with 82.5 percent of non-Hispanic White women (Martin et al., 2019).

In addition to the problem of "too little" care is that of "too much" care. Healthy women and newborns are often subject to costly care practices that are better suited for those at higher risk or with complications, even though many of these practices can have harmful side effects (Avery et al., 2018; Kennedy et al., 2018; Miller et al., 2016). For example, the United States has one of the highest rates of caesarean birth among high-resource countries (Organisation for Economic Co-operation and Development, 2019)—31.9 percent of all births (Hamilton et al., 2019). While there is no evidence-based number for the ideal cesarean birth rate, most experts agree that this rate is too high (American College of Obstetricians and Gynecologists, 2019a; World Health Organization, 2015).[5] Cesarean births generally carry greater risks to the mother than do vaginal births, including a longer recovery time (Gregory et al., 2012), and data from several countries show lower rates of cesarean birth along with better outcomes for infants and pregnant women (Kennedy et al., 2019).

In addition to the problems of too little and too much care, the quality of care is uneven. Substandard care results in poor maternal and fetal outcomes that are largely preventable (Ozimek et al., 2015; Howell, 2018; Review to Action, 2018). Moreover, structural racism, implicit and explicit bias, and discrimination underlie large and persistent racial/ethnic disparities in the quality of care received by childbearing women and infants (Howell, 2018; McLemore, 2019; Sigurdson et al., 2018).

These issues of access and quality—driven by such system-level factors as racism and discrimination and unequal allocation of resources, among others (discussed below and in Chapter 4)—are reflected in trends in maternal and infant mortality and morbidity. Childbearing women and newborns in the United States have worse outcomes than their peers internationally. Unlike other high-resource countries, the United States has seen a rise in pregnancy-related mortality (see Figure 1-1). After decades of decline, the U.S. pregnancy-related mortality rate was recorded at about 7.2 maternal deaths per 100,000 live births in 1987. The rate then began to increase, and at its height in 2014, there were 18 pregnancy-related deaths per 100,000 live births (Centers for Disease Control and Prevention,

[5] According to WHO, "the international healthcare community has considered the ideal rate for cesarean birth to be between 10 percent and 15 percent" (World Health Organization, 2015, p. 1).

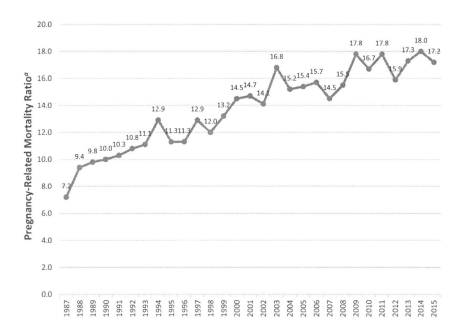

FIGURE 1-1 Trends in pregnancy-related mortality in the United States, 1987–2015.
[a]Number of pregnancy-related deaths per 100,000 live births per year.
SOURCE: Centers for Disease Control and Prevention (2019a).

2019a). In contrast, the rate of maternal mortality has consistently dropped in most high-resource countries over the past 25 years (Geller et al., 2018).

Severe maternal morbidity has been increasing in the United States as well (Centers for Disease Control and Prevention, 2017a). It is estimated that for every woman who dies in childbirth, 70 more come close to dying (Montagne, 2018). All told, more than 50,000 U.S. women each year suffer severe maternal morbidity or "near miss" mortality, and roughly 700 die (Centers for Disease Control and Prevention, 2019b), leaving partners and families to raise children while coping with a devastating loss. Like the rates of maternal mortality, U.S. rates of severe maternal morbidity are high relative to those in other high-resource countries (Geller et al., 2018). In this context, it is notable that some local efforts in the United States have shown progress in reducing rates of maternal mortality and morbidity. In California, for example, the California Maternal Quality Care Collaborative led an initiative that reduced rates of maternal mortality by 55 percent (from 2006 and 2013) (Main et al., 2018; see also Chapter 7).

As will be discussed in detail in Chapters 3 and 4, maternal mortality and morbidity rates are not the same for all ethnic groups. Higher rates persist and have even increased for Black and Native American women. Even such successes as the California Maternal Quality Care Collaborative show ethnic group differences in improvements (Main et al., 2018). In 2005, the maternal mortality rate for White individuals was 11.8 per 100,000 live births, increasing to 19.0 per 100,000 in 2014, while the corresponding rates for non-Hispanic Black individuals were 39.2 and 48.7 per 100,000, respectively. Native American and Alaska Native individuals also saw large increases in maternal mortality rates from 2005 to 2014, from 11.1 per 100,000 to 37.8 per 100,000. Increases were seen for Hispanic women as well, increasing from 9.6 per 100,000 to 12.5 per 100,000 between 2005 and 2014 (McLemore, 2019). Figure 1-2 shows the U.S. maternal mortality rate over time, by race and ethnicity. Disparities are also present in maternal mortality rates by geographic location. According to the CDC, in 2015 the maternal mortality rate in large metropolitan areas was 18.2 per 100,000 live births, while in the most rural areas it was 29.4 per 100,000 (Centers for Disease Control and Prevention, 2017a).

In contrast to maternal mortality, infant mortality in the United States has been declining over the past 20 years (see Figure 1-3), and there are expanded opportunities for survival at increasing levels of prematurity and illness complexity. However, large disparities persist among racial/ethnic groups and between rural and urban populations. In 2017, infant mortality rates per 1,000 live births by race and ethnicity were as follows: non-Hispanic Black, 10.97 per 1,000; American Indian/Alaska Native, 9.21 per 1,000; Native Hawaiian or Other Pacific Islander, 7.64 per 1,000; Hispanic, 5.1 per 1,000; non-Hispanic White, 4.67 per 1,000; and Asian, 3.78 per 1,000 (Ely and Driscoll, 2019; see Figure 1-4).

Mirroring these disparities, in 2014 infant mortality in rural counties was 6.55 deaths per 1,000 births, 6 percent higher than in small and medium urban counties and 20 percent higher than in large urban counties (Ely et al., 2017). Neonatal mortality was 8 percent higher in both rural (4.11 per 1,000 births) and small and medium (4.12 per 1,000 births) urban counties than in large urban counties (Ely et al., 2017, p. 4). Mortality for infants of non-Hispanic White mothers in rural counties (5.95 per 1,000) was 41 percent higher than in large urban counties and 13 percent higher than in small and medium urban counties (Ely et al., 2017, p. 4). For infants of non-Hispanic Black mothers, mortality was 16 percent higher in rural counties (12.08) and 15 percent higher in small and medium urban counties than in large urban counties (Ely et al., 2017).

Rates of preterm birth and low birthweight have increased since 2014, and as with other outcomes, show large disparities by race and ethnicity (Ely and Driscoll, 2019; Hamilton et al., 2019). Low-birthweight (less than 5.5 pounds at birth) and preterm babies are more at risk for many short- and long-term health problems, such as infections, delayed motor and social

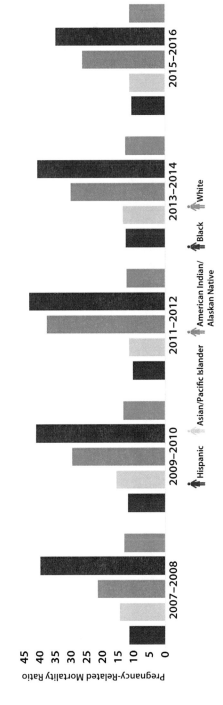

FIGURE 1-2 Trends in pregnancy-related mortality ratio: United States, 2005–2016.
SOURCE: Centers for Disease Control and Prevention (2019g).

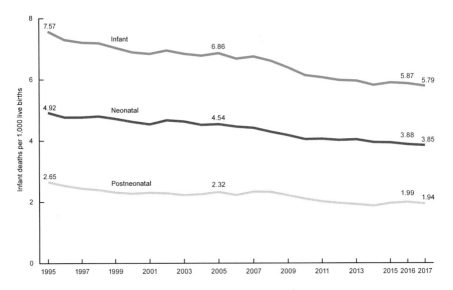

FIGURE 1-3 Infant, neonatal, and postneonatal mortality rates: United States, 1995–2017.
SOURCE: Ely and Driscoll (2019).

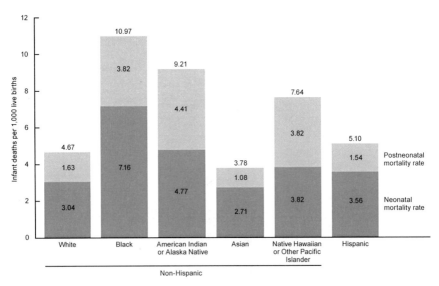

FIGURE 1-4 Infant, neonatal, and postneonatal mortality rates, by race and Hispanic origin:
United States, 2017.
NOTE: Neonatal and postneonatal rates may not add to total infant mortality rate due to
rounding.
SOURCE: Ely and Driscoll (2019).

development, and learning disabilities (March of Dimes, 2018b). About one-third of infant deaths in the United States are related to preterm birth; in 2017, the rate of preterm-related infant death was 199.1 per 100,000 births (Ely and Driscoll, 2019). However, the rate of preterm-related infant mortality for non-Hispanic Black women (454.1) was more than three times the rate for non-Hispanic White women (135.1) (Ely and Driscoll, 2019). Rates of low birthweight by race/ethnicity in 2018 ranged from 6.91 percent for births to non-Hispanic White women to 14.07 percent for births to non-Hispanic Black women, with rates of 8.58 percent for Asian women, 8.0 percent for American Indian/Alaska Native women, and 7.40 percent for Hispanic women. Black infants are also more than twice as likely as other infants to have very low birthweight—less than 3 pounds, 5 ounces—at 2.92 percent in 2018 compared with 1.02 to 1.24 percent for White and Hispanic infants, respectively (Martin et al., 2019). Low birthweight is associated with such social and economic factors as low income, low parental education level, maternal stress, racism, and domestic violence or other abuse, as well as maternal smoking, use of alcohol, or low weight gain (Institute of Medicine, 2007).

While the United States lags behind other high-resource nations in terms of maternal and some newborn outcomes, moreover, it continues to outpace its peer countries in the costs of maternity care. Together, maternal and newborn care are the most expensive hospital conditions for Medicaid, private insurance, and all payers (Wier and Andrews, 2011). Just as the United States' overall health care cost per capita and health care cost as a proportion of gross domestic product far exceed those of any other nation (Organisation for Economic Co-operation and Development, 2018), maternity care costs also are generally higher than those of other countries (International Federation of Health Plans, 2015). According to the International Federation of Health Plans (2015), the average cost of services for a spontaneous vaginal birth in the private sector is approximately five times higher in the United States than in Spain. While this higher cost is due to a combination of factors, much of it is driven by considerable variation in cost for healthy low-risk births (Xu et al., 2015). Institutional factors—but not quality—are associated with higher costs for low-risk births (Xu et al., 2018). In short, the U.S. maternity care system currently incurs extraordinary costs to produce among the poorest outcomes among high-income nations, while simultaneously failing to effectively redress racially and ethnically driven inequities.

THE OPPORTUNITY

Given the current state of maternity care in the United States as reviewed above, further study of the birth settings chosen by or assigned to women and the factors that go into those choices is warranted, and examining variation in the outcomes experienced in different types of settings is a priority. Moreover, unprecedented maternity-related developments (described in Box 1-5) have occurred in the 6-year period between the 2013 National Academies workshop and the work of this committee. This report builds upon ongoing efforts toward greater integration of the nation's maternity care system across care teams and birth settings, major

---

BOX 1-5
Birth Settings: Key Changes Since 2013

Many maternity-related developments occurred in the 6-year period between the 2013 National Academies workshop and this report. Examples of these developments in the areas of integration across care teams and birth settings and maternity care quality improvement are detailed below. Additionally, research expanded knowledge of physiologic childbearing (see, e.g., Buckley, 2015).

The field took steps toward greater *integration across care teams and birth settings*:

- **Consensus team-based care report:** The American College of Obstetricians and Gynecologists (ACOG) led a multistakeholder Task Force on Collaborative Practice in preparing *Collaboration in Practice: Implementing Team-Based Care*. This report defines and provides guiding principles for team-based care, supports the transition to team-based care, discusses regulatory frameworks that support such care, and identifies opportunities for its implementation (Jennings et al., 2016).
- **Consensus on levels of maternal care:** ACOG and the Society for Maternal-Fetal Medicine (SMFM) published an obstetric care consensus document that established guidelines for levels of maternity care. These guidelines, call for "the growth and maturation of systems for the provision of risk-appropriate care specific to maternal health needs" in order to reduce maternal morbidity and mortality (Menard et al., 2015, p.1).
- **Licensure requirements for certified professional midwives:** The United States Midwifery Education, Regulation, and Association (U.S. MERA), a collaboration of eight national midwifery organizations, with input from ACOG, created a process to ensure in future state statutes that the holders of the certified professional midwife (CPM) credential meet standards of the International Confederation of Midwives (U.S. Midwifery Education, Regulation, and Association Professional Regulation Committee, 2015a).
- **Guidelines for home-to-hospital transport of childbearing individuals and newborns:** *Best Practices Guidelines: Transfer from Planned Home Birth to Hospital* was created by a multidisciplinary Home Birth Summit Collaboration Task Force for the seamless transfer of women and newborns from home to hospital birth when needed. The guidelines

steps toward responding to the maternal health crisis, the great potential for quality improvement in maternity care, and increased knowledge of and support for women's and newborns' experience of perinatal care with a maximum of informed choice based on careful risk assessment and a minimum of interventions unless and until needed. Other important trends include a heightened awareness of disparities, institutional racism, and rural and urban inequities in health outcomes/health resource distribution.

are accompanied by model transfer forms for the woman, newborn, and nurse to foster optimal communication, collaboration, and other protocol processes (Home Birth Summit, n.d.).

The field took steps toward recognizing the great potential for *maternity care quality improvement*:

- **Professional organizations' development of focused quality improvement care bundles:** The Alliance for Innovation on Maternal Health (AIM) is a national program focused on maternal safety and quality improvement initiatives. In partnership with more than 25 clinical professional societies and other associations, AIM develops and implements Maternal Safety Bundles of care practices for readiness, recognition and prevention, and response to address leading causes of maternal mortality and severe maternal morbidity (American College of Obstetricians and Gynecologists, 2018b).
- **National Network of Perinatal Quality Collaboratives:** The Centers for Disease Control and Prevention fostered the establishment of the National Network of Perinatal Quality Collaboratives (NNPQC). NNPQC supports state Perinatal Quality Collaboratives (PQCs) by providing tools and resources and fostering shared learning through annual meetings, webinars, and an online forum (Henderson et al., 2018).
- **Obstetric Data Definitions Project:** ACOG led the multidisciplinary consensus reVITALize project to precisely define essential terms relating to mode of birth, hypertension, labor, rupture of membranes, gestational age, and parity. It is intended that the definitions will be incorporated into clinical practice and will serve as standards for electronic health records, coding, and clinical practice guidelines and policy statements (Menard et al., 2014).
- **Paying for value and incentivizing delivery system transformation:** The Health Care Payment Learning & Action Network (LAN) developed a white paper outlining recommended parameters for a maternity care episode alternative payment model (Health Care Payment Learning and Action Network, 2016), and subsequently carried out a Maternity Multistakeholder Action Collaborative. An online maternity episode payment resource bank was created to support implementation of maternity care episode alternative payment models (Health Care Payment Learning and Action Network, n.d.).

In addition, there is greater recognition of a preconceptual window for assessing women's desire for pregnancy and their health status, including detecting diabetes and hypertension, as well as behavioral health issues such as use of opioids and other harmful substances. Current trends also focus on postnatal care for the first year, patient engagement, and patient-centered care.

Thus this report coincides with a period of significant efforts to improve the quality, experiences, outcomes, and costs of maternity care in the United States. It provides a path forward for continued improvements to ensure that all women and children have access to quality, affordable, safe, and supportive care across all birth settings.

STATISTICS AND TRENDS IN BIRTH SETTINGS

As noted earlier, the vast majority of women in the United States give birth in a hospital, but rates of home and birth center births are increasing, particularly in certain states and among certain populations (see Figure 1-5). At the turn of the 20th century, nearly all births occurred at home. By 1969, only 1 percent of births occurred outside a hospital; this rate remained steady throughout the 1970s and 1980s (Institute of Medicine, 2013). The rate of out-of-hospital births gradually declined during the 1990s and early 2000s, but then began to reverse course. Between 2004 and 2017, the percentage of out-of-hospital births increased 85 percent, from 0.87 percent of all births (35,578 births) to 1.61 percent (62,228 births) (MacDorman and Declercq, 2019); the rate of home births increased by 77 percent, rising to 0.99 percent of all births; and the rate of birth center births more than doubled, rising to 0.52 percent of all births (MacDorman and Declercq, 2019). About 85 percent of home births were planned, while 15 percent were unplanned (MacDorman and Declercq, 2019). Rates of out-of-hospital births vary considerably among states, with higher rates in the Pacific Northwest and lower rates in the South (MacDorman and Declercq, 2019).

The data in this section are from a 2019 study by MacDorman and Declerq, "Trends and State Variations in Out-of-Hospital Births," for which national birth certificate data from 2004 to 2017, as well as national data on method of payment for delivery, were used. While these data are quite comprehensive, including information on the entire population of around 3.9 million births in the United States each year, there are limitations. These limitations include less than national coverage for some variables; for example, two states that account for 15 percent of births do not report on smoking rates. Further, California does not report whether a home birth was planned or unplanned, making it impossible to ascertain the planning status for 12 percent of births nationally. While the other 49 states and the District of Columbia do report planning status, there is no way to differ-

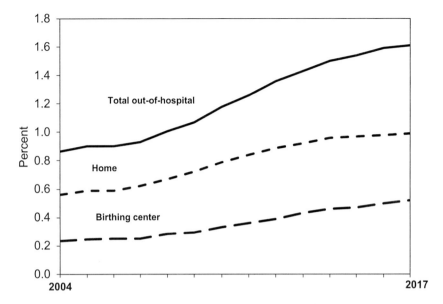

FIGURE 1-5 Trends in home and birth center births in the United States, 2004–2017.
NOTE: Out-of-hospital births include those occurring in a home, birthing center, clinic, or doctor's office, or other location.
SOURCE: MacDorman and Declercq (2019, p. 11), based on birth certificate data from the National Vital Statistics System.

entiate between planned hospital births and births that were planned for home but transferred to the hospital. Therefore, the number of planned home births reported in the study is an underestimate of the actual number of births that began as planned home births. Finally, births reported as "out-of-hospital" include home and birth center births as well as births that occurred at a doctor's office, clinic, or other location (MacDorman and Declercq, 2019).

By Race and Ethnicity[6]

The percentage of out-of-hospital births has increased among all racial/ethnic groups over the past decade, but the most dramatic increase has been among non-Hispanic White women, whose rate more than doubled from 2004 to 2017, from 1.2 percent to 2.43 percent (MacDorman and Declercq, 2019). In 2017, 1 of every 41 births in the United States to a non-Hispanic

---

[6]Recent changes to race classification data allow for the reporting of multiple race data in vital statistics; however, to ensure consistency of categories over time, multiple race data were bridged back to single race categories for this trend analysis (Martin et al., 2019).

White woman occurred out of hospital (MacDorman and Declercq, 2019). Out-of-hospital births also increased for all other racial/ethnic groups, but with a smaller rate of growth and a lower overall rate (see Figure 1-6). The percentage of home births that were planned varied widely by race and ethnicity, from a low of 39.5 percent for non-Hispanic Black women to a high of 90.9 percent for non-Hispanic White women in 2017 (MacDorman and Declercq, 2019).

By Age and Education

A higher proportion of planned home births (23.5%) were to individuals ages 35 and older compared with birth center (18.1%) and hospital (17.5%) births; see Table 1-1. Conversely, among teens, a higher proportion of births were in a hospital (5.2%) compared with planned home births (<1%). Regarding woman's education, more planned home (36.3%) and birth center (47.8%) births were to women with a bachelor's degree or higher, compared with hospital (32.2%) births. And a higher proportion of planned home births (23.9%) were to people with less than a high school

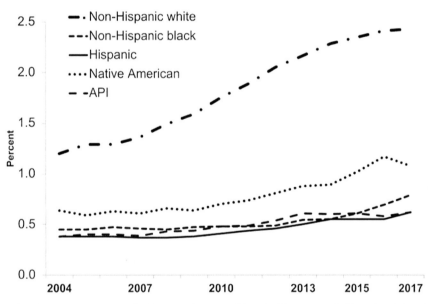

FIGURE 1-6 Percentage of births occurring out of hospital by race and Hispanic origin of childbearing woman, United States, 2004–2017.
NOTE: API = Asian or Pacific Islander.
SOURCE: MacDorman and Declercq (2019, p. 4), based on birth certificate data from the National Vital Statistics System.

TABLE 1-1 Percentage of Births by Level of Education and Place of Birth

Education of Mother (%)	All Births (n = 3,855,500)	Hospital (n = 3,793,272)	Out of Hospital[a] (n = 62,228)	Birth Center (n = 19,878)	Home[b] (n = 38,343)	Planned Home[b,c] (n = 28,994)
Less than high school	13.3	13.2	19.9	12.8	21.9	23.9
High school graduate	25.6	25.7	14.7	11.7	15.5	13.0
Some college	28.8	28.8	26.8	27.7	26.9	26.8
Bachelor's degree or higher	32.3	32.2	38.6	47.8	35.6	36.3

NOTES: Column percentage computed per 100 women in specified group. Not-stated responses (<4% for all variables) were dropped before percentages were computed.

[a] Category includes 3,273 "other," 553 "clinic or doctor's office," and 181 "unknown" location.

[b] Does not include planned home births that were transferred to hospitals.

[c] Excludes data from California, which did not report planning status of home births.

SOURCE: MacDorman and Declercq (2019).

education, compared with birth center (12.8%) and hospital (13.2%) births (MacDorman and Declercq, 2019).

By Financing

Compared with hospital births, women with planned home and birth center births are far more likely to pay for birth out of pocket rather than through Medicaid or private insurance (employer-sponsored or individually purchased) coverage. In 2017, 43.4 percent of hospital births were paid for by Medicaid, compared with 17.9 percent of birth center births and only 8.6 percent of planned home births. People with planned home births were also less likely to be covered by private insurance. Only 19.0 percent of planned home births were paid for by private insurance, compared with 47.5 percent of birth center and 49.4 percent of hospital births. More than two-thirds (67.9%) of planned home births were paid for out of pocket. Almost one-third of birth center births were paid for out of pocket, but this was the case for only a small percentage (3.4%) of hospital births. A small percentage of births in each birth setting category were reported as paid for by some "other" payment method (MacDorman and Declercq, 2019, p. 5). Table 1-2 shows the distribution of type of financing by birth setting.

THE COMMITTEE'S CONCEPTUAL MODEL

The committee's conceptual model (see Figure 1-7) aims to identify key areas for improving the knowledge base around birth settings and levers for improving policy and practice across settings. The triangle at the center indicates three elements that contribute to the ultimate goal of positive outcomes in maternity care: access to care, encompassing both medical insurance and coverage and affordable care options; quality of care; and informed choice about care. The childbearing woman and infant are at the center of that triad (and of the entire graphic), surrounded by the maternity care team; the systems and settings in which the team cares for mothers and infants; and collaboration and coordination, as well as integration, among providers and systems. The maternity care team includes partners, family members, and friends directly involved with support and care during pregnancy and birth, in addition to the clinicians and other professionally prepared members of the team. All of these elements are embedded in the broader social support a woman has or is provided as part of maternity care. The physical setting in which a birth takes place is one part of this overall picture, but it is nested among other elements that are relevant re-gardless of setting and that can be optimized for positive outcomes across and within different birth settings. As noted in the above discussion of the scope of this study, this triad is equally important along the entire con-

TABLE 1-2 Percentage of Births by Type of Financing and Birth Setting, United States, 2017

Method of Payment for Delivery (%)	All Births (n = 3,855,500)	Hospital (n = 3,793,272)	Out of Hospital[a] (n = 62,228)	Birth Center (n = 19,878)	Home[b] (n = 38,343)	Planned Home[c] (n = 28,994)
Medicaid	43.0	43.4	17.5	17.9	15.4	8.6
Private insurance	49.1	49.4	29.6	47.5	20.6	19.0
Self-pay	4.1	3.4	48.9	32.2	59.4	67.9
Other	3.8	3.8	4.0	2.4	4.7	4.6

NOTES: Column percentage computed per 100 women in specified group. Not-stated responses (<4% for all variables) were dropped before percentages were computed.
[a]Category includes 3,273 "other," 553 "clinic or doctor's office," and 181 "unknown" location.
[b]Does not include planned home births that were transferred to hospitals.
[c]Excludes data from California, which did not report planning status of home births.
SOURCE: MacDorman and Declercq (2019).

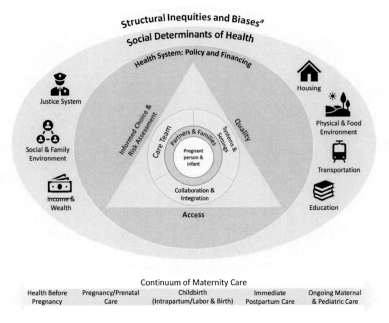

Continuum of Maternity Care

Health Before Pregnancy	Pregnancy/Prenatal Care	Childbirth (Intrapartum/Labor & Birth)	Immediate Postpartum Care	Ongoing Maternal & Pediatric Care

FIGURE 1-7 Interactive continuum of maternity care: A conceptual framework.

[a]Structural inequities and biases include systemic and institutional racism. Interpersonal racism and implicit and explicit bias underlie the social determinants of health for women of color.

tinuum of care, beginning with health before pregnancy and continuing through maternal and pediatric care during the first year postpartum.

Around the center triangle are the factors that can affect whether its elements are optimally achieved. These circles illustrate the complex socio-cultural environment that shapes health outcomes at the individual level and the opportunities for interventions to improve individual and population health, well-being, and health equity. This environment encompasses social, clinical, financial, and structural factors that contribute to access and informed choice, and to quality of care and outcomes. Of course, many of these factors overlap or interact, and the context and conditions illustrated continue to play an important role in health and well-being throughout the continuum of care. That is, structural inequalities and biases intersect with the social determinants of health as all the layers of the model interact in dynamic, complex ways.

Specifically, the outer circle, "structural inequities and biases," represents the structural inequities that are historically rooted and deeply embedded in policies, laws, governance, and culture, such that power and resources are distributed differentially across characteristics of identity (race, ethnicity, gender, class, sexual orientation, and others) (National Academies of Sciences, Engineering, and Medicine, 2017).[7] This unequal allocation of power and resources—including goods, services, and societal attention—manifests in unequal social, economic, and environmental conditions, represented in the figure as the "social determinants of health" (National Academies of Sciences, Engineering, and Medicine, 2017, p. 7). These factors include education, employment, nutrition and food, housing, income and wealth, physical environment, transportation, public safety, and social environment (National Academies of Sciences, Engineering, and Medicine, 2017, p. 7). It is important to note that although the term "social determinants of health" is widely used in the literature, it may incorrectly suggest that such factors are immutable. It may be more appropriate to say, for example, "social influences on health." Factors included among the social determinants of health are indeed modifiable, and can be influenced by social, economic, and political processes and policies (National Academies of Sciences, Engineering, and Medicine, 2017, p. 116). Thus, one advantage of adopting a social determinants of health lens in the analysis of maternal and newborn health is that it offers the possibility of identifying factors associated with health inequities that may be amenable to change through efforts aimed at prevention or intervention, as discussed further in Chapter 4.

KEY TERMS

The committee was charged with assessing health outcomes by birth setting. In general, we interpreted this task to mean assessing pregnancy, birth, and postpartum outcomes. Pregnancy outcomes are the results of pregnancy from preconception and conception through childbirth. They can include outcomes during pregnancy, such as spontaneous abortion,

---

[7]The National Academies of Sciences, Engineering, and Medicine recently summarized this large body of literature in its report *Communities in Action: Pathways to Health Equity*: "The dimensions of social identity and location that organize or 'structure' differential access to opportunities for health include race and ethnicity, gender, employment and socioeconomic status, disability and immigration status, geography, and more. Structural inequities are the personal, interpersonal, institutional, and systemic drivers—such as, racism, sexism, classism, able-ism, xenophobia, and homophobia—that make those identities salient to the fair distribution of health opportunities and outcomes. Policies that foster inequities at all levels (from organization to community to county, state, and nation) are critical drivers of structural inequities. The social, environmental, economic, and cultural determinants of health are the terrain on which structural inequities produce health inequities. These multiple determinants are the conditions in which people live, including access to good food, water, and housing; the quality of schools, workplaces, and neighborhoods; and the composition of social networks and nature of social relations" (National Academies of Sciences, Engineering, and Medicine, 2017, pp. 100–101).

induced abortion, fetal death, and maternal morbidity (illness) or death; they also include positive outcomes, such as a live birth of a healthy baby or patient satisfaction. Birth outcomes are the results of pregnancy, childbirth, and the postpartum period, and they may also be influenced by the woman's health status prior to pregnancy. They can be positive or negative and encompass the condition of both mother and infant following childbirth. For this report, birth outcomes are considered to be both clinical and psychosocial. As noted in the discussion of the scope of this study, moreover, while most of the literature focuses on birth outcomes that are measured early in the postpartum and newborn period, effects of childbearing are salient for this study through the first year postpartum. Limiting outcomes to those that can be measured before hospital discharge fails to include many outcomes that are of great interest to women, families, and society, including maternal–infant attachment, breastfeeding, maternal mood, and general maternal health status. While the committee recognizes that effects of childbearing can be important through the life course, that analysis is beyond the scope of this report. Additional key terms of relevance to this study are defined in Box 1-6.

BOX 1-6
Key Terms Used in This Report

Assisted vaginal birth: Refers to the use of forceps or a vacuum to assist with vaginal birth, wherein the woman pushes while the physician applies traction with either forceps or a vacuum extractor applied to the fetal head (Menard et al., 2014).

Cesarean birth: Birth of the fetus(es) from the uterus through abdominal incisions (Menard et al., 2014).

Early postpartum hemorrhage: Cumulative blood loss of ≥1000 ml accompanied by signs/symptoms of hypovolemia within 24 hours following the birth process (includes intrapartum loss) (Menard et al., 2014).

Gestational age: Expressed in both weeks and days (e.g., 39 weeks and 0 days), is calculated using the best obstetrical estimated date due (EDD) based on the following formula: gestational age = (280 − (EDD − reference date))/7 (Menard et al., 2014).

Intrapartum: The period from the onset of labor or of scheduled birth (planned cesarean or attempted labor induction) through the birth and the immediate transitions of the woman and newborn (Menard et al., 2014).

Labor: Uterine contractions resulting in cervical change (dilation and/or effacement) that in vaginal birth bring the fetus down through the cervical opening and vagina. Includes two phases: the latent phase, from the onset of labor to the onset

BOX 1-6 Continued

of the active phase; and the active phase, accelerated cervical dilation typically beginning at 6 cm (Menard et al., 2014).

Maternal mortality: "The death of a woman while pregnant or within 42 days of termination of pregnancy, irrespective of the duration and site of the pregnancy, from any cause related to or aggravated by the pregnancy or its management but not from accidental or incidental causes" (World Health Organization, 2019).

Maternal morbidity: "Any health condition attributed to and/or aggravated by pregnancy and childbirth that has a negative impact on the woman's wellbeing" (Firoz et al., 2013).

Nulliparous: Denotes a woman with a parity of zero (Menard et al., 2014).

Parity: The number of pregnancies reaching 20 weeks and 0 days of gestation or beyond, regardless of the number of fetuses or outcomes (Menard et al., 2014).

Perinatal: Literally "around the birth," the perinatal period extends from late pregnancy through the early postpartum and newborn period (Menard et al., 2014).

Physiologic birth: Spontaneous labor and birth at term without the use of pharmacologic and/or mechanical interventions for labor stimulation or pain management throughout labor and birth (Menard et al., 2014). A physiologic labor and birth is powered by the innate human capacity of the woman and fetus (American College of Nurse-Midwives, 2012).

Postpartum: Literally "after birth," the period from birth/loss through the first year afterward.

Pregnancy-related death: "The death of a woman while pregnant or within 1 year of the end of a pregnancy—regardless of the outcome, duration, or site of the pregnancy—from any cause related to or aggravated by the pregnancy or its management, but not from accidental or incidental causes" (Centers for Disease Control and Prevention, 2019a).

Prenatal: The period from conception to the onset of labor or scheduled birth (Menard et al., 2014).

Preterm: Less than 37 weeks and 0 days. Late preterm is 34 weeks and 0 days through 36 weeks and 6 days (Menard et al., 2014).

Severe maternal morbidity: Includes "unexpected outcomes of labor and delivery that result in significant short- or long-term consequences to a woman's health" (Centers for Disease Control and Prevention, 2017a).

Term: Greater than or equal to 37 weeks and 0 days using best EDD. It is divided into the following categories (Menard et al., 2014):

> Early term—37 weeks and 0 days through 38 weeks and 6 days
> Full term—39 weeks and 0 days through 40 weeks and 6 days
> Late term—41 weeks and 0 days through 41 weeks and 6 days
> Post term—greater than or equal to 42 weeks and 0 days

STUDY METHODS

The committee convened to conduct this study consisted of 14 prominent scholars and practitioners representing a broad array of disciplines, including health care, nursing, midwifery, obstetrics, neonatology, statistics, medical ethics, anthropology, sociology, and financing and public policy. The committee held four in-person meetings and conducted additional deliberations by teleconference and electronic communications during the course of the study. The first and second in-person meetings were information-gathering sessions during which the committee heard from a variety of stakeholders, including the study's sponsors and representatives from government, academia, health care provider organizations, third-party payers, and women's health organizations. The third and fourth meetings were closed to the public so the committee could deliberate and finalize its conclusions.

The information-gathering process revealed some strongly held values and goals in both the testimony provided and some of the literature. These values and goals served as important context for the committee's deliberations, and are reflected in our conclusions when justified by the evidence and models reviewed. The most salient of these values and goals emerging from public testimony and the literature are outlined below:

- *The need of women and their children for access to affordable, respectful, responsive, clinically and culturally safe, high-quality care from the prenatal period through at least 1 year postpartum.*
- *Women's right to informed choice in maternity care.* Informed choice includes having access to options for and choices among birth settings, care providers, and care practices whereby women are cared for with the highest level of respect, bodily autonomy, bodily integrity, quality care, safety, and protection from abuse, and respectful, culturally concordant care is provided in health systems that are actively addressing implicit bias and the pernicious legacy of racism.
- *Women's need for a continuum of health care.* Women's maternal care ideally involves a continuum within a health care and financing system in which affordable, accessible, integrated, risk-stratified, coordinated, comprehensive, and equitable care is delivered by interdisciplinary teams of health care professionals across multiple birth settings.
- *Recognition of midwives, obstetrician/gynecologists, family physicians, labor and delivery nurses, pediatricians, neonatologists, doulas, and laborists, among others, as critical contributors to the maternal and child health continuum of care team.* Interdisciplinary team col-

laboration among these personnel, supported by interprofessional education and communication within seamlessly integrated systems of care, can improve the quality of care as well as maternal and infant birth outcomes.

- *Community co-located, culturally matched, integrated, and comprehensive services provided by personnel who are knowledgeable about and responsive to that community and have connections and collaborations with a regionalized network of services.*

ORGANIZATION OF THE REPORT

This report is organized into seven chapters. Following this introduction, Chapter 2 describes the current landscape of maternal and newborn care in the United States, including the variety of providers and birth settings. Chapter 3 summarizes the epidemiology of clinical and social risks in pregnancy and childbirth at the individual level, such as medical and obstetric risk factors, and the relationship among choice, risk assessment, and informed decision making. Chapter 4 reviews system-level risks in pregnancy and childbirth, including structural inequities and biases, as well as the social determinants of health that influence psychosocial, medical, and obstetric risk. Next, Chapter 5 outlines the data sources and methodology typical of research on birth settings and describes the general strengths and limitations of this literature. Chapter 6 synthesizes and assesses the available literature on health outcomes for home, birth center, and hospital births. Finally, the report concludes with Chapter 7, which summarizes the committee's key findings and conclusions and presents a path forward for improving maternal and neonatal care for childbearing women and infants in the United States. The Appendix contains biographical sketches of the committee members and staff.

2

Maternal and Newborn Care
in the United States

As discussed in Chapter 1, women in the United States give birth at home, in birth centers, and in hospitals. Across and even within these categories, the resources and services available can vary significantly. Women are cared for by a number of different health care professionals during pregnancy and birth, and these professionals differ in how they are educated, trained, licensed, and credentialed. Women also pay for care through different mechanisms, and the payment mechanism can affect what services, providers, and settings are available to them. State policies and regulations can affect a woman's birth experience as well, through laws as to which providers can practice, their scope of practice, and the legal status of birth settings. This chapter provides a detailed look at the practices, resources, and services available in different birth settings; statistics and trends in birth settings; the education, training, credentialing, and practice of maternity care providers, as well as other clinicians and other members of the care team; and how policy and financing impact choices about birth experience.

It is important to note that the perinatal care system in the United States is unique as compared with the systems of other countries in a number of ways. For example, the United States utilizes a regionalized system of maternity care that involves the potential for transfers from one level to another (American College of Obstetricians and Gynecologists, 2019a). This type of system requires strong relationships and communication between facilities so that individuals receive the appropriate level of care (American College of Obstetricians and Gynecologists, 2019a). The way that medical care is paid for in the United States is also unique, with women relying on a variety of mechanisms, including private insurance (both purchased individually and employer-sponsored), Medicaid, Medicare, and self-pay. Each of these payers has different eligibility requirements, covers services and providers differently, and entails variable out-of-pocket costs. Finally, the United States has three distinct nationally credentialed types of midwives, each of which completes different education and training requirements and whose authority to practice varies by state. These traits make maternity care in the United States complex, can make it difficult for women and families to negotiate the care system, and can have consequences for access to care and health outcomes.

BIRTH SETTINGS

In the United States, the vast majority (98.4%) of women give birth in hospitals, with 0.99 percent giving birth at home and 0.52 percent giving birth in freestanding birth centers (MacDorman and Declercq, 2019; see Chapter 1). Both across and within these three settings, there are wide variations regarding approach to childbirth, available resources and services, birth attendants, and costs. Table 2-1 summarizes information on all three birth settings—home, birth center, and hospital—including the birth attendants that may be present and the services, supports, resources, and tools available to woman and newborns. This section provides further detail on these variations. See Chapter 6 for information about outcomes in each setting, and Chapter 7 for a discussion of initiatives to improve care and outcomes, such as the California Maternal Quality Care Collaborative.

Hospitals

Hospitals are the most common place of birth in the United States, with 98.4 percent of births taking place in a hospital in 2017 (MacDorman and Declercq, 2019). In this report, the committee considers hospital births to be those occurring in a hospital, whether a Level 1 community hospital or a Level 4 maternity unit. Among birth settings, hospitals provide the widest array of medical interventions for pregnant women and newborns. However, there is wide variation in provider types and practices among hospitals. Thus, the woman's experience may vary widely from hospital to hospital, depending on such factors as the hospital's level of care, staffing, maternal–fetal status, local values and culture, resources, and more. For example, a study of 88 hospitals in Michigan found that 43.2 percent of hospitals had no vaginal births after cesarean (VBACs) between 2009 and 2015, and among the hospitals that had at least one VBAC, rates ranged from 0.5 percent to 48.1 percent (Triebwasser et al., 2018). The study's authors concluded that the choice of hospital can significantly impact the individual's chances of VBAC. Another study in California found that low-performing and high-performing hospitals (as rated by the California Hospital Assessment and Reporting Taskforce) varied widely on measures including low-risk cesarean birth (56% vs. 19%), episiotomy (46% vs. 2%), and VBAC (1% vs. 27%) (California Health Care Foundation, 2014).

Care providers at hospital maternity care units may include nurses, obstetricians, family physicians, pediatricians, and midwives (although family physicians and midwives do not practice in all maternity care units). Some hospitals may also have specialists, such as anesthesiologists, maternal-fetal medicine specialists, and neonatologists, immediately available or on call. Despite their variation, the vast majority of hospital births are attended by physicians (90.6% of hospital births in 2017), while 8.7 percent were attended by certified nurse midwives (CNMs) or certified midwives (CMs) (MacDorman and Declercq, 2019).

All hospitals in the United States are accredited or certified, either through the state or through such organizations as The Joint Commission, which accredits about 81 percent of the hospitals accredited in the United States (The Joint Commission, 2018). The Joint Commission also offers a voluntary Perinatal Care Certification, which requires adherence to specific standards and clinical practice guidelines, as well as continuous data collection on such performance measures as rates of cesarean birth and exclusive breastfeeding (Isbey and Martin, 2017).

Maternal Levels of Care

In 2019, the American College of Obstetricians and Gynecologists (ACOG) and the Society for Maternal-Fetal Medicine (SMFM) published an Obstetric Care Consensus statement (American College of Obstetricians and Gynecologists, 2019a).[1] This statement, an update of a 2015 document, reaffirmed the need for clear, standardized levels of maternal care. The four levels identified are accredited birth centers, basic care (Level I), specialty care (Level II), subspecialty care (Level III), and regional perinatal health care centers (Level IV). Criteria for designation of each level are based on the availability of resources, including specialists for women with high-risk pregnancies. The statement is intended to improve maternal care, in part by facilitating admission or transfer of women with high-risk pregnancies to the perinatal centers, which have the appropriate resources and providers

---

[1]The statement was endorsed by the American Association of Birth Centers; the American College of Nurse-Midwives; the Association of Women's Health, Obstetric and Neonatal Nurses; the Commission for the Accreditation of Birth Centers; and the Society for Obstetric Anesthesia and Perinatology. The statement was supported by the American Academy of Family Physicians. The American Society of Anesthesiologists reviewed the statement (American College of Obstetricians and Gynecologists, 2019a).

TABLE 2-1 Description of Attendants and Care Across Birth Settings

	Home (Planned)
Prevalence	0.99% of U.S. births (85% of these were planned)
Attendant	Physician: 0.7% CNM/CM: 29.4% Other midwife: 50.7% Other: 19.1%
Prenatal care	Attendant provides 9–12 prenatal visits in the office or at home; variable based on practice
Birth	Attendant provides 1-to-1 continuous management of labor in the woman's home; a second attendant or birth assistant attends the birth along with the primary attendant
Fetal assessment	Fetal assessment usually occurs via intermittent auscultation
Availability of interventions	Licensed midwives carry oxygen, neonatal and adult resuscitation equipment, suturing equipment, and medications for preventing or managing postpartum hemorrhage; attendant may offer deep tubs for pain relief in labor
Transfers	In some situations, the mother is transferred to the hospital; the midwife may or may not be able to continue to provide care, depending on whether agreements are in place between the midwife and the hospital
Trainees	A midwife trainee may be in attendance under supervision
Post-birth care	Attendant generally stays 4–6 hours after the birth based on individual clinical situation

NOTE: CM = certified midwife; CNM = certified nurse midwife.
SOURCE: These data are from the 50 states and Washington, DC, in 2017 (MacDorman and Declercq, 2019).

Birth Center	Hospital
0.52% of U.S. births	98.4% of U.S. births
Physician: 2.7% CNM/CM: 56.6% Other midwife: 36.7% Other: 3.9%	Physician: 90.6% CNM/CM: 8.7% Other midwife: 0.1% Other: 0.5%
Pregnant woman attends 9–12 prenatal visits at the birth center or an affiliated outpatient clinic	Pregnant woman attends 9–12 prenatal visits at an outpatient clinic or provider office; generally, that provider has privileges to attend birth at the hospital or an arrangement for another provider to do so
Attendant provides 1-to-1 continuous management of labor in the birth center; a second attendant or birth assistant attends the birth along with the primary attendant	Majority of hands-on care is usually provided by a labor and delivery nurse; birth attendant may be midwife (CM or CNM), family medicine physician, obstetrician, or maternal–fetal medicine specialist
Fetal assessment usually occurs via intermittent auscultation; however, some birth centers may use periodic electronic fetal monitoring	Fetal assessment usually occurs via continuous electronic fetal monitoring; however, some hospitals offer periodic electronic fetal monitoring or intermittent auscultation
Birth centers supply oxygen, neonatal and adult resuscitation equipment, suturing equipment, and medications for preventing or managing postpartum hemorrhage; birth centers generally have deep tubs for pain relief in labor, and some also offer nitrous oxide	In addition to medications and operative interventions to prevent and manage postpartum hemorrhage, interventions and procedures that may be offered in the hospital setting that are generally not offered at home or in birth centers include medications to ripen the cervix (Cervidil or Misoprostol) or induce or augment labor (Pitocin), epidural anesthesia, and cesarean birth; some hospitals also have deep tubs for pain relief in labor, and some offer nitrous oxide
In some situations, the mother is transferred to the hospital; the midwife may or may not be able to continue to provide care, depending on whether agreements are in place between the midwife and the hospital	In some situations, the mother is transferred to a higher-level hospital; the provider usually does not continue to provide care after the patient has been transported
A midwife trainee may be in attendance under supervision	Trainees such as medical students, student midwives, and resident physicians may be in attendance under supervision
Women generally stay 4–6 hours after the birth based on individual clinical situation	Length of stay in hospital varies based on individual clinical situation; federal law mandates that insurers may not restrict benefits for stays of 48 hours (vaginal) or 96 hours (cesarean)

to care for them in a safe and timely manner. The standardization of levels of maternal care also allows states to map the geographic distribution of the various levels and to identify and address gaps in care (American College of Obstetricians and Gynecologists, 2019b). However, the exact resources that are available within hospitals of a specific level could vary by state, depending on whether state legislation mandates that a hospital of a certain level must have specific resources or personnel.

Currently, maternal care levels are unevenly distributed across the United States, leaving some women without access to appropriate resources and providers (see Chapter 4 for further detail). Just as women birthing at home or in birth centers may need to be transferred to a hospital for more intensive care, women birthing at lower-level hospitals may need to be transferred to a higher-level hospital with the appropriate resources. For example, if birth was expected to be low risk but complications develop, the individual may need to be transferred from a Level II to a Level III hospital for access to providers with experience in the management of the specific issue. See Table 2-2 for the full description of the ACOG/SMFM levels of care.

It should be noted that these are maternal levels of care only and do not include requirements about neonatal care. Neonatal levels of care have been developed by the American Academy of Pediatrics.[2]

Care Routine

Generally, when a pregnant woman presents for care in a hospital, she undergoes an obstetric (OB) triage process to determine whether she should be admitted and if so, to which unit. This process includes a federally mandated medical screening examination by a qualified provider, consisting of initial assessment and prioritization for evaluation (American Academy of Pediatrics and American College of Obstetricians and Gynecologists, 2017; Centers for Medicare & Medicaid Services, 2012). A hospital may also conduct triage by telephone in order to prevent unnecessary in-person visits and the potential for unnecessary admissions. Acuity and disposition are based in part on maternal condition, fetal heart rate tracing, uterine contractions, reason for presentation, labor status (presence of uterine contractions, vaginal bleeding, membrane status), estimated due date, woman's perception of fetal movement, and any high-risk medical or OB conditions identified by a review of history or the woman's report (American Academy of Pediatrics and American College of Obstetricians and Gynecologists, 2017). Some hospitals use a standard process, such as the Maternal-Fetal Triage Index, for evaluating women and prioritizing the order of and type

---

[2] See https://pediatrics.aappublications.org/content/130/3/587.

TABLE 2-2 Levels of Maternal Care: Definitions, Capabilities, and Health Care Providers

Accredited Birth Center	
Definition	Care for low-risk women with uncomplicated singleton term vertex pregnancies who are expected to have an uncomplicated birth.
Capabilities and health care providers	Refer to birthcenters.org for American Association of Birth Centers' Standards for Birth Centers.
Level I (Basic Care)	
Definition	Care of low- to moderate-risk pregnancies with the ability to detect, stabilize, and initiate management of unanticipated maternal–fetal or neonatal problems that occur during the antepartum, intrapartum, or postpartum period until the patient can be transferred to a facility at which specialty maternal care is available.
Capabilities	• Capability and equipment to provide low-risk and appropriate moderate-risk maternal care and a readiness at all times to initiate emergency procedures to meet unexpected needs of women and newborns within the center. This includes
	o Ability to begin emergency cesarean delivery within a time interval that best incorporates maternal and fetal risks and benefits.
	o Limited obstetric ultrasonography with interpretation readily available at all times.[a]
	o Support services readily available at all times,[a] including laboratory testing and blood bank.
	o Capability to implement patient safety bundles[b] for common causes of preventable maternal morbidity, such as management of maternal venous thromboembolism, obstetric hemorrhage, and maternal severe hypertension in pregnancy.[c]
	o Ability at all times[a] to initiate massive transfusion protocol, with process to obtain more blood and component therapy as needed.
	• Stabilization and the ability to facilitate transport to a higher-level hospital when necessary. This includes
	o Risk identification and determination of conditions necessitating consultation, referral, and transfer.
	o A mechanism and procedure for transfer/transport to a higher-level hospital available at all times.[a]
	o A reliable, accurate, and comprehensive communication system among participating hospitals, hospital personnel, and transport teams.
	• Ability, in collaboration with higher-level facility partners, to initiate and sustain education and quality improvement programs to maximize patient safety.

continued

TABLE 2-2 Continued

Health care providers	• Every birth attended by at least one qualified birthing professional (midwife,[d] family physician, or OB/GYN) and an appropriately trained and qualified registered nurse (RN) with level-appropriate competencies as demonstrated by nursing competency documentation. • Physician with privileges to perform emergency cesarean readily available at all times.[a] • Primary maternal care providers, including midwives,[d] family physicians, or OB/GYNs readily available at all times.[a] • Appropriately trained and qualified RNs with level-appropriate competencies as demonstrated by nursing competency documentation readily available at all times.[a] • Nursing leadership has level-appropriate formal training and experience in maternal care. • Anesthesia providers, such as anesthesiologists, nurse anesthetists, or anesthesiologist assistants working with an anesthesiologist,[e] for labor analgesia and surgical anesthesia readily available at all times.[a]

Level II (Specialty Care)

Definition	Level I facility plus care of appropriate moderate- to high-risk antepartum, intrapartum, or postpartum conditions.
Capabilities	Level I facility capabilities plus • Computed tomography scan, magnetic resonance imaging, nonobstetric ultrasound imaging, and maternal echocardiography with interpretation readily available daily (at all times not required). • Standard obstetric ultrasound imaging with interpretation readily available at all times.[a]

Health care providers	Level I facility health care providers plus
	• OB/GYN readily available at all times.[a]
	  o Based upon available resources and facility determination of most appropriate staffing, it may be acceptable for a family physician with obstetric fellowship training or equivalent training and skills in obstetrics and with surgical skill and privileges to perform cesarean delivery to meet the criteria for being readily available at all times.
	• Physician obstetric leadership is board-certified[f] OB/GYN with experience in obstetric care.
	  o Based upon available resources and facility determination of the most appropriate staffing, it may be acceptable for such leader to be board-certified in another specialty with privileges and expertise in obstetric care, including with surgical skill and privileges to perform cesarean delivery.
	• Maternal–fetal medicine (MFM) subspecialist readily available at all times[a] for consultation onsite, by phone, or by telemedicine, as needed.
	• Anesthesiologist readily available at all times.[a]
	• Internal or family medicine physicians and general surgeons readily available at all times[a] for obstetric patients.

TABLE 2-2 Continued

Level III (Subspecialty Care)

Definition	Level II facility plus care of more complex maternal medical conditions, obstetric complications, and fetal conditions.
Capabilities	Level II facility capabilities plus • In-house availability of all blood components. • Computed tomography scan, magnetic resonance imaging, maternal echocardiography, and nonobstetric ultrasound imaging services and interpretation readily available at all times.[a] • Specialized obstetric ultrasound and fetal assessment, including Doppler studies, with interpretation readily available at all times.[a] • Basic interventional radiology (capable of performing uterine artery embolization) readily available at all times.[a] • Appropriate equipment and personnel physically present at all times[g] onsite to ventilate and monitor women in labor and delivery until they can be safely transferred to intensive care unit (ICU). • Onsite medical and surgical ICUs that accept pregnant women and women in postpartum period. The ICUs have adult critical care providers physically present at all times.[g] An MFM subspecialist is readily available at all times[a] to actively communicate or consult for all obstetric patients in the ICU. • Documented mechanism to facilitate and accept maternal transfers/transports. • Provide outreach education and patient transfer feedback to Level I and Level II designated facilities to address maternal care quality issues. • Provide perinatal system leadership if acting as a regional center (e.g., in areas where Level IV facilities are not available, see Level IV).

continued

TABLE 2-2 Continued

Health care providers	Level II health care providers plus • Nursing leaders and adequate number of RNs who have special training and experience in the management of women with complex and critical maternal illnesses and obstetric complications. • Board-certified[f] OB/GYN physically present[g] at all times. • An MFM subspecialist with inpatient privileges readily available at all times,[a] either onsite, by phone, or by telemedicine. Timing of need to be onsite is directed by urgency of clinical situation. However, an MFM subspecialist must be able to be onsite to provide direct care within 24 hours. • Director of MFM service is a board-certified MFM subspecialist. • Director of obstetric service is a board-certified OB/GYN or MFM subspecialist. • Board-certified anesthesiologist[f] physically present[g] at all times. • Director of obstetric anesthesia services is board-certified anesthesiologist with obstetric anesthesia fellowship training or experience in obstetric anesthesia. • Full complement of subspecialists, such as subspecialists in critical care, general surgery, infectious disease, hematology, cardiology, nephrology, neurology, gastroenterology, internal medicine, behavioral health, neonatology, readily available for inpatient consultation at all times.[a]

Level IV (Regional Perinatal Health Care Centers)

Definition	Level III facility plus onsite medical and surgical care of the most complex maternal conditions and critically ill pregnant women and fetuses throughout antepartum, intrapartum, and postpartum care.
Capabilities	Level III facility capabilities plus • Onsite medical and surgical care of complex maternal conditions with the availability of critical care unit or ICU beds. • Onsite ICU care for obstetric patients with primary or co-management by MFM team. Co-management includes at least daily rounds by an MFM subspecialist, with interaction with the ICU team and other subspecialists with daily documentation. In some settings, the ICU is an adjoining or connected building, which is acceptable as long as MFM care is as noted above. If the woman must be transported by ambulance to the ICU, this is not considered onsite. • Perinatal system leadership, including facilitation of collaboration with facilities in the region, analysis and review of system perinatal outcome and quality data, provision of outreach education, and assistance with quality improvement as needed.

TABLE 2-2 Continued

Health care providers	Level III health care providers plus • MFM care team with expertise to manage highly complex, critically ill, or unstable maternal patients. A board-certified MFM subspecialist attending with full inpatient privileges is readily available at all times[a] for consultation and management. This includes co-management of ICU-admitted obstetric patients. • Nursing Service Line leadership with advanced degree and national certification. • Continuous availability of adequate numbers of RNs who have experience in the care of women with complex medical illnesses and obstetric complications, with close collaboration between critical care nurses and obstetric nurses with expertise in caring for critically ill women. • Board-certified anesthesiologist with obstetric anesthesia fellowship training or experience in obstetric anesthesia physically present at all times.[g] • At least one of the following adult subspecialties readily available at all times for consultation and treatment as needed onsite: neurosurgery, cardiac surgery, or transplant. If the facility does not have all three subspecialties available, there should be a process in place to transfer women to a facility that can provide the needed service.

NOTES: These guidelines are limited to maternal needs. Consideration of fetal or neonatal needs and the appropriate level of care should occur following existing guidelines. In fact, levels of maternal care and levels of neonatal care may not match within facilities. Additionally, these are guidelines, and local issues will affect systems of implementation for regionalized maternal care, perinatal care, or both.

[a]Readily available at all times: the specific person should be available 24 hours a day, 7 days a week for consultation and assistance, and able to be physically present onsite within a time-frame that incorporates maternal and fetal or neonatal risks and benefits with the provision of care. This timeframe should be further defined and individualized by facilities and regions, with input from their obstetric care providers. If referring to the availability of a service, the service should be available 24 hours a day, 7 days a week unless otherwise specified.

[b]See https://safehealthcareforeverywoman.org/patient-safety-bundles.

[c]See also American College of Obstetricians and Gynecologists (2017a).

[d]Midwives who meet International Confederation of Midwives standards, such as certified nurse midwives (CNMs) and certified midwives (CMs), and who are legally recognized to practice within the jurisdiction of the state.

[e]Scope of practice for nurse anesthetists and anesthesiologist assistants may vary by state.

[f]Also includes physicians who have completed residency training and are eligible for board certification according to applicable board policies.

[g]Physically present at all times: the specific person should be onsite in the location where the perinatal care is provided, 24 hours a day, 7 days a week.

SOURCE: Adapted from American College of Obstetricians and Gynecologists (2019d). Reprinted with permission from Levels of maternal care. Obstetric Care Consensus No. 9. American College of Obstetricians and Gynecologists. *Obstetrics and Gynecology* 134(4), pp. e41–e55.

of care (Association of Women's Health, Obstetric and Neonatal Nurses, 2015). OB triage may occur in a specialty unit or in the labor room. Specialty OB triage units are more common in high-volume perinatal facilities. If the triage process reveals that the woman is not in labor or that she is in very early stages of labor, she will likely be sent home, provided that there are no maternal or fetal conditions warranting admission (Angelini and Howard, 2014).

Once a decision has been made to admit a woman to the labor and delivery unit, a number of options are available based on whether the admission is due to spontaneous labor or planned, and if planned, whether the admission is elective or medically indicated. The woman's preferences, the labor nurse assigned to her, her choice of birth attendant, and the hospital are key influences on how labor and birth care proceed. Interventions and procedures that can occur in the hospital during labor and birth include insertion of an intravenous (IV) line, continuous electronic fetal monitoring, bed rest, limited oral intake during labor, cervical ripening, induction or augmentation of labor, artificial rupture of membranes, epidural analgesia, blood draws for laboratory studies, episiotomy, vacuum- or forceps-assisted birth, and cesarean birth. Rates of these procedures are highly variable across hospitals (Lundsberg et al., 2017). For example, Lundsberg and colleagues (2017) found significant differences among hospitals in use of routine IV lines, blood draws, and oral intake.

Nurse staffing during labor and birth differs among hospitals as well: in some hospitals, women will have one-to-one nursing care during labor and birth, while in others, nurses must devote their attention to more than one woman (Simpson et al., 2019). Also variable is the availability of labor support, birth and peanut balls for comfort and positioning, hydrotherapy in the shower or tub, telemetric electronic fetal monitoring (to allow continuous fetal assessment while ambulating or out of bed), intermittent auscultation, and doulas. Varying as well are hospital policies and routines for enabling other individuals to be in attendance to support the woman, from strict rules allowing one or two "visitors" to policies encouraging the woman to choose how many people and whom she would like to be with her during birth.

Hospital births vary in a number of other ways as well. Birthing positions vary, for example, with some women giving birth in the lithotomy position and others in an upright or side-lying position. Births can also occur in the labor room or in the operating room (OR). Examples of births in the OR include cesarean birth, vaginal birth of twins, or a woman at risk for complications. Recovery after birth lasts at least 2 hours, typically with one-to-one nursing care, and can occur in the labor room (vaginal birth and some cesarean births) or the postanesthesia recovery room (cesarean births) (American Academy of Pediatrics and American College of Obstetricians and Gynecologists, 2017; Association of Women's Health, Obstetric and Neonatal Nurses, 2010). After this immediate postpartum recovery period, the woman may be transferred to another unit in the hospital (mother–baby unit) within the perinatal service or remain in the room where she gave birth (labor–delivery–recovery–postpartum room). This placement is based on the configuration of the maternity unit. Generally, large-volume perinatal facilities have separate units for labor and birth care and woman–baby care postpartum. Also varying is the practice of rooming-in, whereby the newborn remains with the mother in her postpartum room, which may or may not be standard practice and is based on the mother's and newborn's condition and hospital routines. Likewise, support for breastfeeding, including access to lactation professionals, varies across hospitals.

Finally, length of stay postpartum differs significantly across birthing hospitals, and depends on length of labor, whether the birth was vaginal or cesarean, maternal–fetal complications, regional and hospital routines, and type of reimbursement the hospital receives. In the United States, women stay an average of 48 hours for a vaginal birth. Federal law requires that most insurance companies cover a postdelivery hospital stay of 48 hours for vaginal birth and 96 hours for cesarean birth (Centers for Medicare & Medicaid Services, n.d.), although women may opt to leave earlier if they and their babies are healthy. Before leaving the hospital, the woman and newborn are seen by a midwife or physician, pediatric provider, lactation consultant, and/or other providers. Some providers offer a checkup within the first week after discharge from the hospital; ACOG recommends contact between provider and woman within the first 3 weeks postpartum, followed by a comprehensive postpartum visit within 12 weeks after birth (American College of Obstetricians and Gynecologists, 2018a).

In-Hospital "Birth Centers"

Some hospitals in the United States have separate units within or associated with the labor and delivery unit that offer women a more home-like atmosphere. These units are often called "birth centers" by the hospital; however, the services they offer and the extent to which they resemble freestanding birth centers vary widely.

Some, like freestanding birth centers, use the midwifery model of care, are available only to low-risk mothers, and offer only physiologic birth without medical interventions. For example, the Midwifery Center at Tucson Medical Center in Arizona is located within the hospital but offers a low-intervention, midwife-led birth experience. If complications arise, or if the woman desires or needs an epidural, she can quickly be transferred to the hospital's standard labor and delivery unit (The Midwifery Center Healthcare, 2019). These types of units are called "alongside maternity centers" by the Commission for the Accreditation of Birth Centers (CABC). To receive CABC accreditation, an alongside maternity center must meet a number of requirements; for example, the center may not offer augmentation of labor, continuous electronic monitoring, epidurals, or assisted vaginal birth. As of November 2019, there were four such centers accredited by CABC (Commission for the Accreditation of Birth Centers, 2019); there are many similar centers across the nation that are either unaccredited at this time or in the process of accreditation.[3]

Other "birth centers" that are located within hospitals in the United States vary widely in the resources and care model that they offer. Some may essentially be standard labor and delivery units but with additional options such as tubs for hydrotherapy, birthing balls, and nitrous oxide for pain relief. Others may emphasize and encourage low-intervention birth, but also offer interventions as needed or desired (e.g., augmentation of labor, continuous fetal heart rate monitoring, and medication for pain management). Depending on the hospital, some interventions may be offered directly in the "birth center," while others require transfer to the hospital's standard labor and delivery unit. In the event that the mother requires more intensive care (e.g., a caesarean birth), the hospital usually has the capacity to provide that service immediately or to call in a specialist.

The fact that the term "birth center" is used to describe a wide variety of birth options can cause confusion. In the remainder of this report, the term "birth center" refers only to freestanding birth centers, not in-hospital units.

Freestanding Birth Centers

As noted above, for the purposes of this report, a birth center is defined as a freestanding health facility not attached to or inside a hospital. Birth centers are intended for low-risk women who desire less medical intervention during birth, a home-like atmosphere, and an emphasis on individually tailored care. Birth center numbers are increasing in the United States, with 375 such centers in operation as of November 2019.[4] In a review of birth centers in 33 states, Stapleton and colleagues (2013) found 23.8 percent of birth center participants were Medicaid enrollees, and 28.3 percent had equal to or less than a high school education.

Birth center care is typically led by midwives (CNMs, CMs, and certified professional midwives [CPMs]), sometimes with additional care

---

[3] These types of centers have also been expanding in the United Kingdom and Canada, where they are called "alongside maternity units" (AMUs). In the United Kingdom, the number of AMUs nearly doubled between 2010 and 2016, and about 12 percent of women gave birth in an AMU in 2016, compared with 3 percent in 2010 (Walsh et al., 2018).
[4] Personal communication, Kate Bauer, executive director AABC.

from other maternity care support staff, such as registered nurses (RNs), doulas, and birth assistants. In 2017, 56.6 percent of births at birth centers were attended by CNMs/CMs, 36.7 percent by CPMs, and 2.7 percent by physicians (MacDorman and Declercq, 2019; see Table 2-3). Midwives in birth centers provide the full scope of maternity care, from the prenatal through the intrapartum and postpartum periods out to the first 6–8 weeks following birth, as well as newborn care. Most birth centers provide pre-conception care and well-woman services to nonpregnant clients (American Association of Birth Centers, 2016a).

Typically, birth centers are designed to resemble a home environment and routinely offer some nonmedical interventions during labor and delivery that are not always available in hospital settings. For example, birth centers encourage walking and position changes during active labor, encourage oral fluid and food intake as tolerated, offer round and peanut-shaped birth balls to facilitate comfort and effective positioning, often offer a tub for laboring and birth, and provide options such as nitrous oxide and acupressure for managing pain. After birth, care is provided with the infant skin to skin, and breastfeeding is encouraged. After discharge from the birth center, the birth center nurse or midwife typically makes a home visit at approximately 24 hours and again at 3 days postpartum (varies based on midwifery practice). The initial postpartum home visits are commonly followed by office visits at 10 days to 2 weeks, and 4 to 6 weeks postpartum; follow-up is provided by phone and additional visits as needed (American Association of Birth Centers, 2016b).

In the birth center, care is woman- and family-centered, and families are invited to participate in the experience as desired by the woman. Within the birth center framework, care is provided for healthy, uncomplicated pregnancies and births and for first-line complications. First-line complications such as maternal hemorrhage or initial resuscitation of a compromised infant are managed by midwives and birth center staff, and transfer to a higher level of care is available when needed. Compared with hospitals, birth centers have fewer resources available for emergency situations, such as those requiring cesarean birth or blood transfusion. When a transfer for higher-level care is indicated during labor or postpartum, the woman must be physically transported by ambulance or private car from the birth center to a hospital. The birth center prepares for emergencies by having plans and emergency medications in place for stabilization and transfer to an acute care facility if needed (American Association of Birth Centers, 2016c). The American Association of Birth Centers (AABC) describes the birth center as a "maximized home rather than a mini-hospital" (American Association of Birth Centers, 2016c).

Birth centers can be accredited by the CABC, but accreditation is not mandatory. CABC-accredited birth centers must follow the standards of the

TABLE 2-3 Percentage of Births Attended by Physicians, Certified Nurse Midwives (CNMs)/Certified Midwives (CMs), and Other Midwives by Place of Birth, United States, 2017

Attendant at Birth (%)	All Births (n = 3,855,500)	Hospital (n = 3,793,272)	Out of Hospital[a] (n = 62,228)	Birth Center (n = 19,878)	Home[b] (n = 38,343)	Planned Home[b,c] (n = 28,994)
Physician	89.2	90.6	4.3	2.7	3.7	0.7
CNM/CM	9.1	8.7	34.1	56.6	24.4	29.4
Other midwife[d]	0.8	0.1	41.2	36.7	45.6	50.7
Other	0.8	0.5	20.3	3.9	26.4	19.1

NOTES: Column percentage computed per 100 women in specified group. Not-stated responses (<4% for all variables) were dropped before percentages were computed.

[a]Category includes 3,273 "other," 553 "clinic or doctor's office," and 181 "unknown" location.
[b]Does not include planned home births that were transferred to hospitals.
[c]Excludes data from California, which did not report the planning status of home births.
[d]Includes all non-CNM/CM midwives, including certified professional midwives (CPMs) and licensed and direct entry midwives.
SOURCE: MacDorman and Declercq (2019).

AABC, which require, among other things, that the birth center practice the midwifery model of care; honor the mother's needs and desires throughout labor; and avoid the use of certain interventions, including vacuum extraction and continuous electronic monitoring (American Association of Birth Centers, 2019). All accredited birth centers must also have emergency supplies on hand for woman and newborn, and they must have a specific plan for transfer to a hospital if required.

Home Births

Home births occur at a person's residence and can be either planned or unplanned. Most home births are planned, although about 15 percent are unplanned (MacDorman and Declercq, 2019). A home birth may be attended by a midwife, physician, or other attendant, or by no medical attendant at all, as is preferred by a small number of "freebirthers"[5] or when unplanned. For planned home births only, about 80 percent are attended by midwives, 0.7 percent by physicians, and 19.1 percent by "other."[6] (See Table 2-3.)

Women who plan home births may do so out of a wish to experience physiologic childbirth, a desire for a personalized experience, a desire to avoid unneeded medical interventions, a dislike of the hospital atmosphere, a desire for a sense of control, the lack of a hospital in their community, cultural beliefs and practices, financial constraints, or geographic barriers (Declercq and Stotland, 2017). Like birth center births, planned home births may result in transfer to a hospital for nonemergency or emergency care.

Midwives[7] provide care throughout the prenatal period for families planning a home birth. Home birth clients must remain low-risk throughout the pregnancy and must typically reach 37 weeks' gestation to be eligible for a home birth. During labor, midwives monitor the woman and fetus, providing one-to-one care and continuously assessing for complications. As a best practice, a birth assistant (who may be another midwife or someone who is trained as a birth assistant) is used as a second attendant

---

[5]A "freebirther" is a woman who gives birth without a physician or midwife in attendance (Hickman, 2009).

[6]Of all home births (planned and unplanned), 70 percent are attended by a midwife (including CNMs, CMs, CPMs, and other midwives); 3.7 percent by a physician; and 26.4 percent by "other," which includes family members, emergency medical technicians, and no attendant (MacDorman and Declercq, 2019).

[7]The majority of home births are attended by a midwife, although a small percentage are attended by physicians. For brevity's sake, home birth providers are most often referred to as midwives in this report.

BOX 2-1
Typical Home Birth Supplies and Medications

Whereas hospitals and birth centers are already equipped with supplies and medications that are commonly used during birth, midwives must bring these items with them to a home birth. At the onset of labor, the midwife travels to the client's home with supplies that include the following:

Birth supplies: blood pressure cuff and stethoscope, pediatric stethoscope, thermometer, fetal Doppler, paper or electronic chart forms, infant scale, cord clamps, sterile instruments for cutting the cord and suturing, suctioning equipment (bulb syringe, DeLee suction trap), urinary catheter equipment, amnihook, heating pad, sterile gloves, absorbable underpads, gauze sponges.

Supplies for labor support and pain relief: deep tub; hot/cold compresses; a transcutaneous electrical nerve stimulation (TENS) machine; items such as a sling, yoga ball, and peanut balls for comfort and positioning.

Resuscitation equipment: firm surface for neonatal resuscitation; bag and mask in adult and newborn sizes; a laryngeal mask airway; epinephrine for adult anaphylaxis and/or newborn resuscitation.

Medications: oxygen tank(s); medications for preventing or treating postpartum hemorrhage (Pitocin, methergine, misoprostol); IV equipment and fluids; antibiotics for Group B strep prophylaxis; local injectable anesthetic for suturing; vitamin K and erythromycin eye ointment for the newborn; hepatitis B vaccine and immune globulin for infants born to mothers with hepatitis B.

Some states have laws that restrict midwives' ability to carry or administer certain medications. For example, in Virginia, licensed certified professional midwives are prohibited from carrying any controlled substance, including antihemorrhagic medicines, oxygen, or antibiotics (Virginia Law, 2013).

---

when birth is drawing near.[8] Once the baby is born, the newborn is assessed and stimulation is performed in place as needed. Resuscitation equipment is assembled during labor and located proximal to where the birth is likely to occur, although it can be moved as needed. As one attendant is attending to the newborn, the other is attending to the delivery of the placenta and administering medications as needed (if licensed to do so) to treat a postpartum hemorrhage. In states where midwives are not able to access licensure for carrying these medications, they may utilize herbal medicine and manual skills to stop a postpartum hemorrhage. Box 2-1 provides further detail on typical home birth supplies and medications.

---

[8] State licensure statutes typically require that two attendants be present at every birth because two people are required for neonatal resuscitation. (See, e.g., statutes in Oregon, Washington, and California.)

After birth, attendants assist with breastfeeding; monitor the mother's and newborn's vital signs; inspect and repair the perineum as needed; assess uterine involution and bleeding; ensure that the mother is able to empty her bladder; and conduct a full newborn exam, administering vitamin K and erythromycin eye ointment (if licensed to do so) with the consent of the parents. If at any point the woman or the newborn develops complications, hospital transport is initiated. When assured that the woman and newborn are stable and without complications, the attendants give instructions to the parents, including warning signs that call for paging the midwife, and they depart the client's home within 4–6 hours after the birth. A midwife typically returns to the client's home between 24 and 48 hours postpartum for a full checkup on both mother and newborn, with another home visit on day 3. Often another postpartum visit is conducted at 1–2 weeks, another at 3–4 weeks, and a final visit at 6 weeks postpartum. Prenatal and postpartum visits may occur in the woman's home or in an office setting. Well-newborn care is also usually managed by the midwife for the first 2–6 weeks of life, with consultation or referral to the newborn's pediatric provider as needed or desired. As with most practices surrounding birth, birth and postpartum care are influenced by the licensure of the provider and insurance coverage or source of payment, which are discussed later in this chapter.

Transfer to Hospital Settings

Because health professionals attending birth center and home births do not offer some services during labor (e.g., epidural pain relief, induction or augmentation with medications) and do not have the capacity to provide certain emergency services (e.g., cesarean capability, neonatal intensive care unit), some women need to transfer to a hospital during or after birth. A meta-analysis of studies in the United States and other Western countries found that the rates of transfer for nulliparous women ranged from 23.4 percent to 45.4 percent, and for multiparous women ranged from 5.8 percent to 12.0 percent (Blix et al., 2014). Emergency transfers made up a small percentage of transfers. Although the definition of "emergency" varied across studies, the rates ranged from 0 percent to 5.4 percent (Blix et al., 2014). The authors note that transfers were more common in settings where home birth was regulated and integrated with the health care system, and less common in settings with unregulated midwives. Unfortunately, in the United States, integration and coordination among providers and settings is uncommon, and clear protocols for when and how to transfer patients to risk-appropriate facilities are lacking (Shah, 2015).

Freestanding birth centers are only partially integrated into the U.S. maternity care system. Nine states currently do not license or regulate freestanding birth centers, and variation in regulations and hospital policies across the United States makes it difficult for birth centers in some regions to form collaborative relationships with transfer hospitals and physicians (American Association of Birth Centers, 2016d). Further research is needed to evaluate the impact of integration of maternity systems on outcomes for planned birth center births, although one large U.S. study has shown a positive correlation between midwifery integration across birth settings and improved maternal and neonatal outcomes (Vedam et al., 2018). (See Chapter 6 for further discussion of outcomes.)

Model transfer guidelines for home births have been developed through a multidisciplinary, multistakeholder process (Home Birth Summit, n.d.). (See Chapter 7 for further discussion of these guidelines.)

MATERNAL AND NEWBORN CARE TEAM

Nurses, physicians, and midwives provide the majority of maternal and newborn care across birth settings. Other members of the care team who also provide care include social workers, psychologists and psychiatrists, dietitians, anesthesia professionals, lactation consultants, and physical therapists. The care team also encompasses pregnant individuals and their partners, family, and friends; doulas; community health workers; childbirth educators; breastfeeding peer counselors; and pregnancy fitness educators. Members of the maternal and newborn care team educate, support, and care for women and newborns before and throughout pregnancy, during labor and birth, and after birth. This section provides details about the practice, education, training, and licensing of members of the care team.

Registered Nurses

The majority of nurses working in hospital labor and delivery units are RNs. RNs monitor the woman and baby during labor and birth; assess the woman's progress through the stages of labor; identify potential complications; administer medications; monitor the newborn after birth; help new parents learn about baby care; and communicate with the woman, her family, physicians, midwives, and other members of the care team. The specific ways in which nurses work in different hospitals vary considerably (see Box 2-2). RNs also contribute to maternal care through public health nursing (see Box 2-3), and they may work in birth centers as well.

RNs must have either a diploma in nursing, an associate's degree in nursing, or a bachelor's degree in nursing, and have passed the National Council Licensure Examination (NCLEX-RN) exam. After licensure, an RN may choose to obtain certification in a specialty area of nursing

---

BOX 2-2
Variety of Nursing Work Structures in Hospitals

Such factors as birth volume, philosophy of the leadership team, and physical design of the maternity unit directly influence how nurses are assigned to specific patients and what type of care each nurse provides. In small-volume perinatal services, nurses care for women across the course of their childbirth hospitalization, including the admission assessment, labor, birth, and postpartum/newborn periods. Some small-volume services use perioperative nurses to care for women who have cesarean birth during the intraoperative and post-anesthesia recovery periods. Moderate- to high-volume perinatal services often have designated nurses with specific skill sets and have separate units for antepartum, obstetric triage, intrapartum, postpartum, well-baby, and high-risk baby care. Nurses in high-volume units are less likely to care for women over the course of their entire hospitalization. Hospitals with high birth volumes are more likely to have specialization of nurses, categorizing them as labor and delivery, mother–baby, and special care or neonatal intensive care nursery nurses.

In some hospitals, the physical design is single-room maternity care, where the mother labors, gives birth, and spends the postpartum period in the same room. Single-room physical design does not guarantee continuity of nursing care. Birth volume, leadership team philosophy, and shift scheduling are factors in how maternal–newborn care is provided in the context of a single-room physical design and the priority placed on continuity of care (Association of Women's Health, Obstetric and Neonatal Nurses, 2010, 2018). Labor nurses at times turn the patient care assignment over to a mother–baby nurse after the 2-hour immediate postpartum recovery period. In some hospitals, new mothers are cared for by postpartum nurses and well babies are cared for by nursery nurses, even in models where mother–baby rooming-in has been established. In some hospitals, there is an effort to assign the same nurse each day to the mother–baby couplet. Nurses in many hospitals choose their patient assignments. Therefore, the type of nursing care a woman receives is influenced by her choice of birthing hospital, as each hospital has a unique culture, operations, staffing model, and routine unit flow that determine how nursing care is provided and by which nurses. Education, skill level, personal philosophy, and experience of the nurses are further influences (Association of Women's Health, Obstetric and Neonatal Nurses, 2010, 2018).

---

practice within maternity and newborn care, including low-risk neonatal nurse, maternal newborn nurse, neonatal intensive care nurse, or inpatient obstetric nurse. Certification in one of these specialties requires 2 years of experience as an RN in that specialty, comprising at least 2,000 hours of practice time, and passing the National Certification Corporation exam in the specialty.

BOX 2-3
Public Health Nurses

Public health nurses play an important role in maternity care through delivery of a range of services, including pregnancy screening; family planning services; assistance with Medicaid applications; enrollment in the Supplemental Nutrition Program for Women, Infants, and Children (WIC); patient education; lead screening; breastfeeding support; and social service referrals. These nurses—most of whom are registered nurses—often provide these services through pregnancy and postpartum home visits. One public health nursing program that has demonstrated particular success is the Nurse-Family Partnership (NFP), an evidence-based, nurse home-visiting program that has been shown through randomized controlled trials to improve maternal and child outcomes. The NFP is a program, funded by a variety of public and private sources, that sends nurses into the homes of mostly low-income and unmarried first-time mothers. Nurses visit the mothers about once a month during pregnancy and the first 2 years after they give birth, and they teach positive health behaviors, care of children, and maternal personal development. The NFP has been shown to have positive impacts on maternal and child well-being, including lower rates of pregnancy-induced hypertension and preterm births (Laura and John Arnold Foundation, 2017; Nurse-Family Partnership, 2019).

Advanced Practice Registered Nurses (APRNs)

APRNs have the broadest scope of practice among nurses, although the specific rules regarding their practice vary by specialty and by state. In the labor and delivery setting, APRNs—depending on their specialty—may administer epidurals and other pain medications, diagnose and treat complications during labor, attend births, and monitor and diagnose postpartum complications.

APRNs often, but not always, begin their career as RNs, gain experience, and then pursue further education. APRNs hold either a master of science in nursing (MSN) degree, a doctor of nursing practice (DNP) degree, or a Ph.D. in nursing, and choose one of four specialty tracks on which to focus. APRNs must complete a specific number of hours of training in their specialty, and each specialty has its own clinical requirements and exam (see Table 2-4).

Midwives

Midwives specialize in the management of pregnancy, birth, and newborn care. The United States is unique among nations in that it has three types of midwives with nationally recognized credentials: CNMs, CMs,

TABLE 2-4 Educational and Licensure Requirements for Nurses Providing Maternal and Newborn Care

Requirements	Registered Nurse	Advanced Practice Registered Nurse
Required education	Diploma, ADN, or BSN	MSN, DNP, or Ph.D.
Required training	Training included in educational experience	Depends on specialty track; usually at least 500 hours clinical training
Exams	NCLEX-RN	NCLEX-RN; certification exam(s) depends on specialty

NOTE: ADN = associate's degree in nursing; BSN = bachelor of science in nursing; DNP = doctor of nursing practice; MSN = master of science in nursing.

and CPMs (Cheyney et al., 2015; Vedam et al., 2018). Competencies are aligned across these three credentials and with those of the International Confederation of Midwives (U.S. Midwifery Education, Regulation, and Association Professional Regulation Committee, 2015b). Although distinct, these credentials share some key similarities. For example, all credentialed midwives in the United States are differentiated from "lay," "traditional," or "plain" midwives, who practice without having completed formal educational and national certification requirements (Davis-Floyd and Johnson, 2006; Cheyney et al., 2019). Each of the three types of nationally credentialed midwives must fulfill different education, training, and licensing requirements (Table 2-5), but they share a commitment to the midwifery model of care (Citizens for Midwifery, 2008). Some of the important distinctions among midwives are tied to the "unique cultural and socio-political histories of obstetrics and regional midwifery traditions in the United States" (Cheyney et al., 2015, p. 2). (See also Davis-Floyd, 2018, Chapter 6; and Davis-Floyd and Johnson, 2006, for detailed explications of the complexities of U.S. midwifery.)

Nationally credentialed midwives attend births in all settings, including hospitals, birth centers, and homes. Most CNMs and CMs work in hospitals, although they also work in birthing centers and attend home births. CPMs provide care only in birth centers and at home births, as they have not been granted hospital privileges in most areas (Cheyney et al., 2015). There are approximately 12,000 CNMs, 100 CMs, and 2,500 CPMs in the United States (American College of Nurse-Midwives, 2019; National Association of Certified Professional Midwives, 2014).[9]

---

[9]Some licensed midwives (LMs) are CPMs, but because the credential is not a requirement for licensing in all states, there are a number of LMs who do not hold the CPM credential. Examples of these states are California, Arizona, New Mexico, and Florida.

TABLE 2-5 Educational and Licensure Requirements for Credentialed Midwives

Requirements	Certified Nurse Midwife (CNM)	Certified Midwife (CM)	Certified Professional Midwife (CPM)
Minimum required education	Registered nurse (RN) + master's degree	Master's degree	High school diploma or equivalent; some earn a certificate or an associate's, bachelor's, or master's degree
Required training	Training offered during educational program, primarily in the hospital setting		Training offered during educational program, or through at least 2 years of apprenticeship, primarily in birth centers or home settings
Exams	National Council Licensure Examination (NCLEX-RN) + American Midwifery Certification Board (AMCB) exam	American Midwifery Certification Board (AMCB) exam	North American Registry of Midwives (NARM) exam
Legal status[a]	Legally permitted to practice and prescribe medication in all 50 states, District of Columbia, and U.S. territories	Legally permitted to practice in Delaware, Maine, New Jersey, New York, Rhode Island, Hawaii; prescriptive authority in New York, Rhode Island, Maine	Legally permitted to practice in 33 states[b]

[a]Status is considered legally permitted if licensure, permits, registration, or certification are available at the state level for the given credential (CNM, CM, or CPM).

[b]As of May 2019, CPMs have a path to licensure in Alabama, Alaska, Arizona, Arkansas, California, Colorado, Delaware, Florida, Hawaii, Idaho, Indiana, Kentucky, Louisiana, Maine, Maryland, Michigan, Minnesota, Montana, New Hampshire, New Jersey, New Mexico, Oregon, Rhode Island, South Carolina, South Dakota, Tennessee, Texas, Utah, Vermont, Virginia, Washington, Wisconsin, and Wyoming (National Association of Certified Professional Midwives, 2019).

Certified Nurse Midwives

CNMs are APRNs who are trained in both nursing and midwifery. CNMs provide a range of health and gynecologic services, including preconception care; family planning; and care during pregnancy, childbirth, and the postpartum period (American College of Nurse-Midwives, 2017a). CNMs can assess, diagnose, and treat conditions, conduct examinations, order diagnostic tests, and prescribe medications (American College of Nurse-Midwives, 2011). CNMs are licensed to practice in all 50 states plus the District of Columbia, but their ability to practice independently varies by state. Twenty-seven states allow CNMs full scope of practice including prescriptive authority; other states require supervision by or a collaborative agreement with a physician for some aspects of practice (American College of Nurse-Midwives, 2018). CNMs work in a wide variety of settings, including hospitals and birth centers; 94 percent of CNM-attended births in the United States occur in a hospital (Martin et al., 2019).

Like other APRNs, CNMs must be licensed RNs; obtain an MSN or DNP degree; and pass a specialty exam, which is administered by the American Midwifery Certification Board. There are currently 37 accredited nurse midwifery education programs in the United States, all affiliated with universities (American College of Nurse-Midwives, n.d.c.). CNMs are generally regulated under nursing boards in their respective states.

Certified Midwives

CMs provide all of the same services as CNMs; the primary difference between the two credentials is that CMs are not nurses. Like CNMs, CMs provide the full range of women's health care, including primary care, preconception and prenatal care, and birth and postpartum care. The first accredited CM educational program began in 1996 for those seeking a pathway to midwifery without first obtaining a nursing credential (American College of Nurse-Midwives, 2019).

Aspiring CMs obtain a bachelor's degree in any field and go on to graduate from an accredited midwifery education program. Standards for education and certification in midwifery are identical for CNMs and CMs (American College of Nurse-Midwives, 2019). Only 2 of the 37 nurse midwifery programs are structured to also graduate CMs; in these programs, CNM and CM students sit in the same classrooms, learning the same midwifery skills and body of knowledge. Both CNMs and CMs must pass the American Midwifery Certification Board exam. CMs are licensed to practice in only six states (Delaware, Maine, Hawaii, New Jersey, New York, and Rhode Island) and have prescriptive authority in three (Maine, New York, and Rhode Island) (American College of Nurse-Midwives, 2019).

Certified Professional Midwives

CPMs are independent clinicians who offer care, education, counseling, and support to women and their families throughout pregnancy, birth, and the postpartum period, as well as preconception care and ongoing well-woman care. In states where CPMs are able to access licensure, they typically carry and administer lifesaving medications, order and interpret laboratory and diagnostic tests, and order the use of medical devices. Like all midwives, CPMs are trained to recognize when the condition of a woman or infant requires consulting with or referring to another health care professional (American College of Nurse-Midwives, 2017a). CPMs attend the majority of home births (MacDorman and Declercq, 2016), and they also attend births in freestanding birthing centers.

The credential for CPMs was first offered in 1994 for those seeking a national professional credential for what had formerly been called "lay midwives" (Cheyney, 2010; Davis-Floyd and Johnson, 2006; North American Registry of Midwives, n.d.). Aspiring CPMs must have a high school diploma or the equivalent before beginning their midwifery training, and they can pursue several different paths toward certification and licensure. The North American Registry of Midwives (NARM), the certifying organization for CPMs, uses a competency-based approach to certification that allows applicants to demonstrate and apply knowledge, skills, and experience they have gained through a variety of means. The two primary paths to certification are (1) the portfolio evaluation process (PEP) and (2) graduation from a program accredited by the Midwifery Education Accreditation Council (MEAC), which is recognized as an accrediting body by the U.S. Department of Education (American College of Nurse-Midwives, 2017a). Other, lesser-used paths toward certification include reciprocity for midwives licensed through state-established programs that predate the CPM credential, midwives who are CNMs/CMs, and some internationally educated midwives. A 2015 study found that 48.5 percent of current CPMs utilized the PEP, 36.9 percent graduated from an MEAC-accredited school, 14.5 percent were already licensed by a state as a direct-entry midwife (i.e., a midwife who is not first a nurse) prior to the advent of the CPM credential, and 0.7 percent were already a CNM or CM (Cheyney et al., 2015).

The PEP is a comprehensive evaluation of the skills, knowledge, and competencies of the midwife candidate. It requires, among other requirements, fulfillment of NARM's general education requirements; verification of proficiency in specific skills, knowledge, and abilities; certification in adult cardiopulmonary resuscitation (CPR) and neonatal resuscitation; affidavits from preceptors attesting that the candidate has developed and utilized practice guidelines; an emergency care plan; three professional letters of reference; and completion of a cultural competency course (North American Registry of Midwives, 2019). Alternatively, aspiring midwives may attend MEAC-accredited midwifery education programs, which incorporate NARM competency requirements and the essential competencies of the International Confederation of Midwives (ICM) into their curricula. MEAC-accredited programs may include classroom-based courses, online courses, hybrid classroom/online courses, and/or independent study, and clinical education generally takes place in homes or birth centers. In contrast to the skills examination used by PEP candidates, students who attend MEAC programs have their skills verified by preceptors during the provision of care or using simulations (Cheyney et al., 2015, p. 2).

Regardless of which education route they choose, all CPMs must pass the NARM board examination to be certified, and their education and training must meet NARM standards. NARM requires that the clinical component of a midwife's training be at least 2 years in duration and include a minimum of 55 births. Clinical education must occur under the supervision of a licensed midwife or physician.

In 2013, a coalition of midwifery organizations recommended that starting in 2020, all states newly offering licensure for CPMs require that applicants be educated through MEAC-accredited programs and that CPMs who had already received certification through PEP complete an additional 50 hours of education to obtain a "bridge" certificate (U.S. Midwifery Education, Regulation, and Association Professional Regulation Committee, 2015a).[10]

Physicians

Physicians providing maternal and newborn care evaluate, diagnose, manage, and treat patients; order and evaluate diagnostic tests; prescribe medications; and attend births. After graduating from a 4-year college, all physicians must attend an accredited medical school and receive a doctor of medicine (MD) or a doctor of osteopathy (DO) degree. After 4 years of medical school, MDs and DOs must complete a residency program, which is usually 3 to 7 years, depending on the field of medicine. The first year of residency is commonly called an internship.

---

[10]U.S. MERA (for Midwifery Education, Regulation, and Association) worked to achieve consensus around educational and licensing standards, based on the ICM's global standards for midwifery education and regulation. U.S. MERA published two legislative statements. The first, titled "Statement on the Licensure of Certified Professional Midwives" (U.S. Midwifery Education, Regulation, and Association Professional Regulation Committee, 2015a), codified the coalition's consensus resolution to support legislation in states that do not currently license CPMs. The coalition developed model legislative language stating that by 2020, new applicants for licensure should have a MEAC-accredited education and hold the CPM credential. For those who became CPMs via a nonaccredited pathway prior to 2020, NARM created a Midwifery Bridge Certificate comprising an additional 50 hours of continuing education on topics addressing the ICM essential competencies. The second legislative statement, titled "Principles for Model U.S. Midwifery Legislation and Regulation" (U.S. Midwifery Education, Regulation, and Association Professional Regulation Committee, 2015b), proposed legislative language for the regulation of midwifery practice, including education requirements, standards for practice, and management of complaints. The U.S. MERA leadership team last met in 2016.

Physicians complete a three-step licensing process, consisting of three separate exams, in order to practice medicine. MDs take the United States Medical Licensing Examination (USMLE), while DOs take the Comprehensive Osteopathic Medical Licensing Examination (COMLEX-USA). After residency—and possibly additional training in a subspecialty—doctors may take the relevant board exam(s) to become a board-certified specialist. Education, training, and licensing requirements for physicians are summarized in Table 2-6. Physician specialists that may be involved in maternal and newborn care are as follows:

- *Obstetrician/gynecologists (OB/GYNs)* specialize in women's reproductive health. They may provide preventive care for women, counsel women about reproductive options and prescribe methods of contraception, provide prenatal and postpartum care, attend births, and perform surgeries such as cesarean birth.
- *Maternal-fetal-medicine specialists (MFMSs)*, also called perinatologists, are OB/GYNs who undertake additional years of training to specialize in high-risk pregnancies.
- *Family physicians* often care for an entire family, including pregnant women and babies. The proportion of family physicians who offer maternity care has declined in recent years, and many provide only prenatal and postpartum care, with fewer attending vaginal births and even fewer offering cesarean birth (Rayburn et al., 2014).
- *Pediatricians* specialize in the care of children from birth to young adulthood.
- *Neonatologists* are pediatricians who undertake additional years of training to specialize in the care of premature and critically ill newborns.

TABLE 2-6 Education and Licensure Requirements for Physicians Providing Maternal and Newborn Care

Requirements	All Physicians
Required education	Bachelor's degree, followed by a doctor of medicine (MD) or doctor of osteopathy (DO) degree
Required training	3–4 years residency in the specialty area; additional years of residency for subspecialties
Exams	United States Medical Licensing Examination (USMLE) or Comprehensive Osteopathic Medical Licensing Examination (COMLEX); board certification exam(s) depending on area of specialty and subspecialty

- *Anesthesiologists* provide women with pain relief during labor and birth, such as epidurals, and also provide anesthesia for surgeries, such as cesareans.

Laborists/Obstetric (OB) Hospitalists

Laborists, also referred to as OB hospitalists, are obstetricians, family physicians, or CNMs/CMs who provide care only during OB triage, birth, and the immediate postpartum period (Krolikowski-Ulmer et al., 2018). In the hospital setting, laborists focus solely on pregnant women who present for care and those who are admitted for birth, and they typically do not provide prenatal, postpartum, or gynecological care while in the laborist role. The aims of the laborist model are to provide timely high-quality care, to increase patient safety and reduce litigation by ensuring immediate availability of a provider in the labor and delivery unit, and to support obstetricians in reducing burnout and improving their well-being and professional satisfaction (Olson et al., 2012). The use of laborists may allow other providers to sleep, conduct office visits, or care for other patients, and laborists also can develop advanced skills in handling critical OB emergencies.

Physician Assistants (PAs)

PAs are health care professionals who work closely with physicians to extend and support the physicians' practice. PAs can care for mothers and babies in a number of ways, including conducting well-woman exams, providing prenatal and postpartum care, and assisting with cesarean births. PAs attend an accredited 3-year graduate program and receive a master's degree. The program includes both classroom instruction and clinical rotations in a variety of medical areas of practice. Graduates of a program take the Physician Assistant National Certifying Exam (PANCE), administered by the National Commission on Certification of Physician Assistants (NCCPA), and then seek state licensure (American Academy of Physician Assistants, 2019).

Other Members of the Care Team

While nurses, physicians, and midwives provide the majority of care for women during pregnancy, birth, and the postpartum period, others, such as doulas and community health workers, can also play a critical role in ensuring that the needs of pregnant people and babies are met.

Doulas

The role of doulas is to provide nonclinical support during labor and birth, as well as during the prenatal and postpartum periods. While doulas, nurses, and midwives all provide labor support to the woman, doulas focus on only one laboring woman at a time, providing continuous support without other concurrent responsibilities, such as recordkeeping or monitoring of equipment. Doulas do not perform any clinical tasks, such as giving medication or conducting examinations. In addition to supporting the woman, the doula can also offer emotional support to the woman's partner and family. In the postpartum setting, the doula may assist the new mother with breastfeeding and newborn care, and may also help with light housekeeping and cooking duties at home. Doulas care for women in every birth setting—home, birth center, and hospital. Some women use doula support services in an "extended" model throughout all phases of childbearing—prenatal, labor and birth, and postpartum—while others use them during only one of the phases.

Being a doula does not require formal education or training, although an individual who has experience working in health care may elect to train as a doula. Certification is not required to practice as a doula, though it may be required for reimbursement. Doulas who pursue certification generally must complete a training session of several days and practice their doula skills at a certain number of births.

Community Health Workers

Community health workers provide family-centered support. Usually, they live in the communities they serve and meet individuals in their homes, in clinics, or in community settings (American Public Health Association, 2019). Many community-based perinatal health worker organizations are forming across the country to provide culturally concordant support to childbearing women and families in maternity care deserts and other areas where standard maternity services are sparse and outcomes are poor. These groups, rooted in social, reproductive, and birthing justice frameworks, recognize that women of color face systemic racism, inequities, and other barriers. The groups work to provide trauma-informed, multigenerational support that is tailored to communities and individuals, and focus on respect, empowerment, and choice without judgment. The diverse services of these groups can include mental health, labor, breastfeeding, and parenting support; referral to needed social and community services; and midwifery care. They have various degrees of sustainability and sources of revenue, and some have training programs and are active in shaping policy (National Partnership for Women & Families, 2019).

Education and training requirements for community health workers vary by state and by the type of work they perform. Some states offer certifications for community health workers. For example, certified community health workers in Texas must complete a 160-hour training or have at least 1,000 hours of experience in community health work (Texas Department of State Health Services, 2019).

POLICY AND FINANCING

Although there are multiple options for where to give birth in the United States and a variety of providers of maternity care, the choice of setting and provider is greatly constrained by policies and financing. Federal and state laws and regulations help determine which settings and providers are legally able to provide maternity care, and set rules about Medicaid eligibility. Additionally, federal and state laws and private insurance policies determine what services are covered and which providers will be reimbursed. For example, Medicaid typically looks to Medicare when making coverage decisions, and Medicare does not reimburse certain types of midwives. State regulation of insurance coverage, Medicaid coverage and eligibility, licensing of providers and facilities, and scope of practice for health professionals vary widely by state. These variations may in part explain some of the differences across states between the number of women who give birth in the hospital and those who give birth at home or in a birth center (Yang et al., 2016; MacDorman and Declercq, 2019). For example, in a state where policy and financing facilitate easy access to midwifery care and birth in home or birth center settings, women of many socioeconomic backgrounds may be able to access these options if they choose to do so. By contrast, in a state where policies restrict these choices—for example, by not offering licensure or coverage for settings other than the hospital, or through reduced scope of practice for providers and limited Medicaid options—giving birth at home or in a birth center will likely remain the domain of women who can afford to pay out of pocket.

Financing

Women pay for maternity care in several ways: private insurance (either employer sponsored or individually purchased), Medicaid, self-payment, or Medicare (for some disabled women). The availability and type of coverage greatly influence a woman's choice of care provider and her access to various types of care. States can require that certain minimum benefits be covered by private insurance and Medicaid, and states also can set eligibility rules for Medicaid, which determine when and whether individuals may access different types of maternity care above the federal minimum standards.

Because of federal and state policies, some women are not able to access any form of insurance, leaving them with the entire bill for pregnancy care. For example, the working poor in some states fall into the "coverage gap," in which their income is too high to qualify for Medicaid but too low to receive tax credits for marketplace plans through the Affordable Care Act (ACA) (Garfield et al., 2019). Undocumented immigrants in the United States are not eligible to enroll in Medicaid or to purchase ACA marketplace plans, leaving many without any type of insurance. Undocumented immigrants face additional barriers to care, such as fears about becoming ineligible for lawful permanent residency (Ponce et al., 2018). However, 16 states do permit undocumented women to receive some pregnancy care by extending Children's Health Insurance Program (CHIP) coverage to their unborn child (Artiga and Diaz, 2019).

Costs

Giving birth in the United States is expensive. A national analysis using proprietary data of payments made on behalf of the woman and newborn across the full episode, from pregnancy through postpartum and newborn care, revealed significant expenditures in 2010 (which would be higher as of this writing because of inflation) (Truven Health Analytics, 2013). Payments differed by type of payer and mode of birth. Total payments for privately insured births averaged $18,329 for vaginal and $27,866 for cesarean births. Total payments for Medicaid-insured births averaged $9,131 for vaginal and $13,590 for cesarean births. Payments for privately insured births were about twice as high as those for births covered by Medicaid. When the birth was cesarean, payments were about 50 percent higher than when the birth was vaginal. For privately insured individuals, these payments included substantial average out-of-pocket costs for both vaginal ($2,244) and cesarean ($2,669) births, whereas such costs were negligible for individuals with Medicaid coverage. A major finding from this analysis is that about 4 of 5 dollars paid on behalf of the woman and newborn across the full episode of care went to intrapartum care, while only 1 in 5 dollars went to prenatal and postpartum/newborn care. As these figures indicate, the amount actually paid to the provider and the facility may differ depending on whether it is paid for by private insurance, Medicaid, or self-pay.

Actual expenditures for maternity care depend on the type of provider, the specific services used, and the birth setting. Because most of the births in the United States occur in a hospital, the numbers discussed above reflect primarily the cost of delivery in a hospital. However, those costs can vary significantly from hospital to hospital. For example, the rate of cesarean birth will impact average costs, and these rates can vary dramatically among hospitals (Main et al., 2011).

Birth center and home birth costs are typically lower in price for vaginal births than hospital vaginal births. An Urban Institute study comparing birth center births with hospital births found a savings (in 2008 constant dollars) of $1,163 per birth for Medicaid births (Howell et al., 2014). Another study in Washington state found the impact of the cost savings from the practice of licensed midwifery on the cost of deliveries to all payers to be significant; the study found that there would be an additional $2,713,072 in costs if births that took place out of the hospital or in the hospital with a midwife attendant were moved into the hospital setting with a non-midwife attendant (Health Management Associates, 2007).

Payers

Private insurance, which includes both insurance purchased by individuals directly from an insurer or on the marketplace, as well as employer-sponsored insurance, financed about half (49.6%) of all births in the United States in 2018, with Medicaid close behind at 42.3 percent of all births (Martin et al., 2019) About 4 percent of births were self-paid, and another 4 percent were paid for by other means. Medicare plays a very limited role in financing maternity care, primarily for beneficiaries who are disabled. Coverage by the various payers is detailed below. Box 2-4 summarizes coverage for doulas and other nonclinical support.

Private Insurance   Under the ACA, nearly every insurance plan is required to cover maternity care in general (Cuellar et al., 2012). According to the AABC, most major private health insurers will cover care and delivery at birth centers in some, but not all, states. A national survey indicated that Aetna/US Healthcare, Blue Cross/Blue Shield, TRICARE, and Humana are among those that cover birth center care (American Association of Birth Centers, 2016e). Fewer private insurers cover home births; for example, Aetna (2019) does not cover home births because it "considers planned deliveries at home and associated services not medically appropriate." Aetna notes, however, that it will consider coverage when mandated by state law. A few states, including New Hampshire, New York, New Mexico, and Vermont, do require private insurers to cover home births (Rathke, 2011). However, even in states where insurers must cover home births, insurance companies may have certain requirements for coverage, which can sometimes result in denial of reimbursement. For example, an insurance company might deny coverage for a midwife who does not carry malpractice insurance (which many do not) (Fisch, 2012; The Editorial Board, 2014). In addition, if home and birth center providers are considered out of network, the process of getting reimbursement can be

---

BOX 2-4
Coverage for Doulas and Other Nonclinical Support

As of this writing, few insurance plans cover the costs of doula or other nonclinical support services. Initially, use of doulas was concentrated among interested families with the ability to pay out of pocket. However, there is a growing trend in the rise of programs to provide low-income women of color with community-based, culturally concordant support services, with various types of financing. Many states are now considering or implementing legislation to create such programs as a way to address disparities in maternal health outcomes (Association of State and Territorial Health Officials, 2018).

A primary way of covering the costs of nonclinical support is through Medicaid reimbursement. In 2013, a Centers for Medicare & Medicaid Services (CMS) Expert Panel on Improving Maternal and Infant Health Outcomes in Medicaid/CHIP recommended that doula support during labor be covered (Centers for Medicare & Medicaid Services, 2013). In the years since, only a few states have passed legislation to obtain Medicaid reimbursement for doulas, and the reimbursement rates can be low (Quinn, 2018). Some organizations have negotiated Medicaid reimbursement for nonclinical support directly from managed care organizations (MCOs). For example, Mamatoto Village in Washington, DC, has secured reimbursement from four MCOs for the services of community health workers who support women of color through pregnancy and birth (Commonwealth Fund, 2018).

However, getting reimbursement from Medicaid for nonclinical services entails challenges even in the states that have passed legislation to do so. For example, the New York pilot project requires doulas to be enrolled as providers with the state Medicaid program, which in turn requires completion of a doula training course, as well as of a specific number of hours of education and training. These requirements can be burdensome for doulas who are part of the lower-income communities of color that the pilot project is designed to help (New York State, 2019).

---

onerous, and payment levels may be set at rates that limit the providers' ability to provide services to certain enrollees.

Medicaid   Medicaid is a joint federal and state program, and therefore its policies are determined at both the federal and state levels. Federal and state laws dictate who is eligible for Medicaid, the care that must be covered, and what facilities or providers can be reimbursed. The federal government mandates certain groups that must be eligible for Medicaid, including pregnant women whose income level is at or below 133 percent of the federal poverty level (FPL) (Kaiser Family Foundation, 2017). Further, federal Medicare policy related to covered providers typically drives Medicaid policy; Medicare currently covers nurse midwives but not CPMs. States set additional rules about who is eligible for Medicaid; for example, a state may extend eligibility to women with higher-income levels than the federal minimum (Kaiser Family Foundation, 2017). Undocumented women are not eligible for Medicaid under federal law, although some states find other avenues to pay for the care of these women (Artiga and Diaz, 2019).

There are different eligibility pathways to Medicaid for pregnant women:

- *Pregnancy-only eligibility:* Medicaid coverage available prior to the ACA for pregnant women through 60 days postpartum; all states required to cover pregnant women with incomes up to at least 133 percent of the FPL.
- *Traditional Medicaid:* Medicaid coverage available prior to the ACA based on an individual having income below a state's threshold, as well as being in one of the program's eligibility categories: pregnant woman, parent of children 18 and younger, disabled, or over age 65.
- *ACA Medicaid expansion:* The ACA allowed states to eliminate categorical requirements and extend Medicaid to most women and men with family incomes at or below 138 percent of the FPL. States that have adopted this expansion must cover all recommended preventive services without cost sharing for beneficiaries in this pathway (Kaiser Family Foundation, 2017, p. 2).

In addition, some states have implemented presumptive eligibility, in which pregnant women may receive immediate care while their eligibility for Medicaid is being determined (Kaiser Family Foundation, 2017).

Coverage for prenatal services (e.g., ultrasounds, genetic testing) and labor and birth services (e.g., induction, epidurals, elective cesareans) depend on a woman's eligibility status and state of residence, and it can be difficult for women to determine ahead of time which services will be covered (Haney, 2017). For women with incomes at or below 133 percent of the FPL, the federal government requires that the state Medicaid plan provide, at a minimum (Gurny et al., 1995), the following:

- "Those services that are necessary for the health of the pregnant woman and fetus, or that have become necessary as a result of the woman having been pregnant. These include, but are not limited to, prenatal care, delivery, postpartum care, and family planning services."
- "Services for other conditions that might complicate the pregnancy [including] those for diagnoses, illnesses, or medical conditions which might threaten the carrying of the fetus to full term or the safe delivery of the fetus."

As of 2019, 36 states and the District of Columbia had expanded Medicaid under the ACA (Kaiser Family Foundation, 2019a), making low-income women eligible for coverage before, during, and after the period of pregnancy, labor and birth, and the conventional 2-month postpartum period. Several other states have passed Medicaid expansion ballot initiatives, which have not been implemented.

Section 2301 of the ACA requires state Medicaid programs to cover the costs of services at freestanding birth centers, to the extent that the state licenses or otherwise recognizes these providers and facilities under state law (Centers for Medicare & Medicaid Services, 2011). However, this provision has been implemented inconsistently and inadequately by states, meaning that birth centers are not covered in every state in which they are licensed (Bauer et al., n.d.). In a 2017 survey, 32 states plus the District of Columbia reported that they covered births at birth centers, and 11 states reported that they did not (the remaining states did not respond) (Kaiser Family Foundation, 2019c). Because Medicaid is administered by the state, coverage and reimbursement of birth center services face other barriers. Medicaid MCOs, which administer Medicaid in 38 states plus the District of Columbia (Kaiser Family Foundation, 2019b), can limit which providers are in their networks, negotiate very low rates such that only hospitals can afford to take Medicaid patients, and make it difficult for providers to get paid through requirements such as prior authorization. Coverage of birth center services may be contingent on meeting certain state requirements, for example, accreditation of the birth center or certain limits on liability insurance. If these requirements are not met, Medicaid may not cover the costs of the birth.

Home birth expenses are less likely to be covered by Medicaid either in policy or in practice. Many states will cover home birth only if certain requirements are met; for example, the midwife must have malpractice insurance. A 2018 survey found that 21 states allowed Medicaid coverage for home births, out of 41 states that responded (Kaiser Family Foundation, 2017). There is also great variation in the extent to which Medicaid covers certain providers. Currently, all states reimburse for CNM and CM services, some at the level of a physician providing the same service and some at a lower level. Whether states reimburse CPMs for services is determined on a state-by-state basis (Kaiser Family Foundation, 2017).

Medicare Medicare pays for relatively few births compared with private insurance and Medicaid. However, Medicare coverage rules have a large impact on coverage and payment in other plans, in that most private plans and Medicaid follow Medicare's lead on which types of providers are covered and on reimbursement amounts for providers and services. This is relevant to maternity coverage in two areas. First, Medicare does not recognize CPMs as eligible providers at the federal level. By extension, many private insurers and Medicaid state plans do not cover CPM services. Second, federal law dictates that Medicare pay the same rate for the same services provided by CNMs and physicians. Previously, CNMs were reimbursed at 65 percent of the physician level; advocacy from the American College of Nurse-Midwives (ACNM), ACOG, and others resulted in equitable reimbursement as part of the ACA (American College of Nurse-Midwives, 2009). This equitable reimbursement of CNMs and physicians is expected to trickle down into the reimbursement policies from other insurance plans, including Medicaid (American College of Nurse-Midwives, n.d.b.).

Self-Financing Only about 4 percent of all births are self-paid, although women who use birth centers or home birth are more likely to self-pay. More than two-thirds (67.9%) of planned home births and almost one-third (32.2%) of birth center births were self-paid in 2017, while only 3.4 percent of women self-paid for hospital birth (MacDorman and Declercq, 2019).

Licensing and Scope of Practice

States are responsible for licensing health care professionals and for dictating where they can practice, what services they can provide, and whether they are required to be supervised. Physicians and nurses are licensed and recognized in all states, although scope-of-practice rules vary for APRNs. For example, 22 states allow full-practice nurse practitioners (NPs), meaning that NPs can prescribe medication, diagnose patients, and provide treatment without the presence of a physician. Seventeen states allow reduced-practice NPs; in these states, NPs need a physician's authority to prescribe medication. Twelve states restrict the autonomy of NPs and require a physician's oversight for all practice (American Association of Nurse Practitioners, 2019). Still other states stipulate the type of medication that NPs can prescribe. Arkansas, Georgia, Louisiana, Missouri, Oklahoma, South Carolina, Texas, and West Virginia, for instance, do not allow NPs to prescribe any Schedule II medications (American Medical Association, 2017).

Midwife licensing and scope-of-practice rules vary by state and type of midwife. Currently, CNMs are licensed in all 50 states, CPMs are licensed in 33 states, and CMs are licensed in only 6 states. Twenty-seven states and the District of Columbia allow CNMs to practice independently, 19 require a collaborative agreement with a physician, and the remaining 4 allow CNMs to practice independently but without the ability to prescribe medications (American College of Nurse-Midwives, 2015). States can also place specific limits on the settings in which providers can practice. In Nebraska, for example, it is illegal for CNMs to attend home births (Nebraska Legislature, 2007).

States also license and regulate facilities such as hospitals and free-standing birth centers. Some states have birth center regulations, such as a requirement for a medical director who is a physician, which makes it difficult for new birth centers to obtain recognition and licensure if no physician is willing or able to serve in this role. Steps taken to meet other requirements, such as a written agreement with the area hospital regarding transfers, can easily be lost with administrative changes within hospitals, causing existing birth centers to close. One state—North Dakota—does not permit freestanding birth centers to operate at all (Alliman and Phillippi, 2016).

CONCLUSION

Pregnant people who give birth in the United States can have vastly different experiences depending on the setting in which they give birth, the providers who participate in their care, how the birth is financed, and the state in which they give birth. Hospitals, home births, and birth centers offer different resources, services, and care options. For example, hospitals offer more intensive interventions, such as induction and augmentation of labor, epidural pain relief, and cesarean birth, whereas birth centers and home births do not offer similar interventions and instead put more emphasis on supporting physiologic birth. Even among different hospitals, the resources, providers, services, and outcomes can vary widely, depending on such factors as the level of care, geographic location, staffing, and culture. In some circumstances, individuals may need to be transferred from home or a birth center to a hospital, and such transfers are more complicated and difficult in areas where midwives and out-of-hospital birth options are not well integrated into the health care system.

A number of different clinicians participate in birth care, including physicians, nurses, and midwives, in addition to other members of the health care team, such as doulas. In the United States, all credentialed providers must meet specific education and training requirements and must pass standardized exams in order to be licensed by the state.

While the vast majority of women give birth in a hospital, the percentage of women choosing to give birth at home or in a freestanding birth center has been rising steadily; however, the rate still represents a small proportion of overall births, and the increase has been primarily among certain groups of women. In 2017, 0.99 percent of all births took place in the home and 0.52 percent in a freestanding birth center (MacDorman and Declercq, 2019). These rates vary substantially by state and region of the country, and women who plan to give birth at home or in a birth center are more likely to be White, more highly educated, older, and able to pay for the birth out of pocket.

State financing and policy choices have a large impact on women's access to different birth options. For example, women who are covered through Medicaid may not be covered for births at home or in a birth center, depending on the state in which they live. Other state policies may restrict the types of providers who are licensed, the types of birth settings that are legal, and the scope of practice for different providers.

In addition to these factors, pregnant people's birth experiences may be shaped by social determinants and medical risk profile. Social determinants include such factors as racism, geographic location, and socioeconomic conditions; these factors can substantially impact the choices they have, their access to care, and the outcomes of their birth experience. A pregnant individual's experience and outcomes are also impacted by medical risk profile, such as whether complicating health conditions are present, whether the individual is carrying twins, and the position and health of the fetus. These factors can restrict choice of setting and provider because of the possibility that quick access to medical expertise or knowledge of the condition and its management along with interventions may be necessary. Social determinants and medical risk profile, and how they affect choices and outcomes, are discussed in the subsequent chapters.

3

Epidemiology of Clinical Risks
in Pregnancy and Childbirth

isk is defined as "the chance of danger, loss, injury or other adverse consequence." Generally, risk is thought of as the potential for or probability of harm. When health care providers use the term "high-risk pregnancy," therefore, they are typically describing a situation in which the pregnant woman, fetus, or both have an increased likelihood or odds of a pregnancy complication, adverse event, or poor outcomes occurring during or after the pregnancy or birth as compared with an uncomplicated or "low-risk" pregnancy. It is important to note that an exact definition of a "high-risk pregnancy" is not available, because the term lacks conceptual precision in maternity care. Pregnancy is never without some risk; however, most studies use the absence of identified risk factors for poor outcomes as the comparator. Also worth noting is that risk in pregnancy and risk in labor are separate concepts. A person can have pregnancy risk factors such as obesity or hypertension but still have an uncomplicated labor and birth, and vice versa. Finally, all risk factors are not equally significant. Age, for example, is an independent risk factor but confers different risks from those of preeclampsia (both discussed in the text below). Nonetheless, both are similarly labeled as representing "high-risk pregnancies."

The increased likelihood of an adverse event conferred by risk may be attributable to structural or environmental exposures; inherited or congenital conditions; chronic or acquired health problems, such as diabetes or high blood pressure; infections; complications from a previous pregnancy; risk behaviors; or other issues that might unexpectedly arise during the course of pregnancy. Moreover, these risk factors may interact and intersect. For example, maternal age is associated with diabetes and hypertension, as well as poor outcomes such as stillbirth independently. In short, risk during pregnancy and labor can arise from many sources, both clinical and societal.

In epidemiological terms, risk takes into account not only the probability of harm but also the impact or consequence of the adverse event. In the setting of pregnancy, this becomes relevant because catastrophic losses—those resulting in the death of a pregnant woman or newborn—are infrequent events. However, the severity of these outcomes, the fear of litigation and liability on the part of providers, and the lifelong implications of loss for families have centered the practice of "high-risk" obstetrics on the prevention and mitigation of these and other types of rare but severe events.

Fortunately, the majority of pregnancies that occur in the United States are not high-risk pregnancies. The rates of diabetes, hypertension, obesity, and advanced maternal age among women of reproductive age, however, are on the rise. And while these pregnancies may not ultimately end in adverse events, they warrant additional surveillance and monitoring for disease progression and fetal compromise in women with medical, social, or obstetrical histories that confer increased risk of an adverse pregnancy outcome.

In this context, appropriate risk assessment by qualified providers to match pregnant people with the most appropriate setting and provider for their care during pregnancy and childbirth is critical. This includes consideration of the risks inherent in different settings, including iatrogenic injuries in hospitals, as well as the risk of potentially avoidable interventions. Cesarean rates in particular are known to vary widely and arbitrarily among hospitals, suggesting that hospital choice may be among the biggest independent risk factors for undergoing major surgery. The immediate risks of cesareans include three-fold higher odds of surgical complications, such as infection and hemorrhage, as well as risks in future pregnancies caused by uterine scarring, including uterine rupture and placenta accreta. In addition, as more women desire and choose birth settings other than hospitals, understanding, screening, and monitoring of the medical, obstetrical, and psychosocial risk factors that affect the care needs of women are increasingly important. At the same time, unforeseen emergencies related to either the birth process or an unrecognized condition may require immediate skilled intervention on behalf of the pregnant woman, fetus, or newborn, including cesarean birth or neonatal resuscitation. After birth, for example, the newborn may encounter difficulties adapting to the neonatal environment, suffer consequences of blood flow or oxygen deprivation during the birth process, or experience a problem based on a congenital anomaly. In light of such events, the ability to access higher-level care without delay is critical for the safety of the woman, fetus, and newborn. Moreover, because risk is not static and can change rapidly during pregnancy and the intrapartum period, risk assessment must be continuous. Ensuring that women are effectively matched to risk-appropriate care contributes to quality and safety throughout the maternity care system.

In this chapter, we consider medical and obstetrical factors that can increase a woman's risk of an adverse pregnancy outcome, including both maternal and fetal characteristics, and the ways in which those risk factors affect the decision making of pregnant people and their providers. Common clinical risk factors in pregnancy and childbirth and their clinical implications are described in Table 3-1 and discussed in detail in the following sections. Although this chapter focuses on individual risk factors, it is important to note that many of these factors are the result of structural conditions and societal trends. Demographic trends, such as the increasing age at first pregnancy and increased use of fertility treatments, can contribute to higher pregnancy risk profiles. The social determinants of health (discussed in greater detail in Chapters 1 and 4) also contribute to such preexisting health conditions as obesity, type 2 diabetes, and hypertension among women of reproductive age. These and other system-level risk factors are discussed in the following chapter.

MEDICAL RISK FACTORS

Medical risk factors—for example, such chronic conditions as diabetes and hypertension—are an important consideration in risk assessment for maternity care. Women with preexisting chronic conditions (such as hypertension or obesity) or conditions that develop during pregnancy (such as gestational diabetes) require more intensive care relative to women without these conditions. Demographic shifts, such as people having children later in life, and a number of growing public health challenges, such as increased opioid use, have changed the risk profile of childbearing women on a population level, increasing the proportion of people entering pregnancy with chronic conditions, including substance abuse.[1] This section examines some of the medical risk factors that are present during pregnancy.

Hypertensive Diseases

Hypertension during pregnancy can take several forms. Women may enter pregnancy with hypertension (chronic hypertension) or develop it during pregnancy (gestational hypertension). In addition, pregnant women can develop preeclampsia or eclampsia, conditions in which women develop high blood pressure and signs of damage to another organ system, most

---

[1]The number of opioid-related births in hospitals has tripled since 2005 (Admon et al., 2019).

TABLE 3-1 Clinical Risk Factors in Pregnancy and Childbirth and
Clinical Implications

	Causal Factors
Medical Risk Factors	
Preexisting Diabetes (type 1 or type 2)	Type 1: • Hypothesized to be caused by genetic or environmental factors (National Institute of Diabetes and Digestive and Kidney Diseases, 2017) Type 2: • Obesity and overweight • Physically inactive • Older age • High blood pressure • History of gestational diabetes • History of polycystic ovary syndrome (PCOS) (National Institute of Diabetes and Digestive and Kidney Diseases, 2016)
Gestational Diabetes	• Prepregnancy overweight and obesity • Family history of diabetes
Preexisting Hypertension	• Diet • Physical inactivity • Obesity • Tobacco use • Type 2 diabetes • Family history of hypertension

Maternal and Neonatal Outcomes	Clinical Implications
Diabetes that is not well controlled during pregnancy can increase the risk of: • birth defects • macrosomia • neonatal hypoglycemia • preeclampsia • cesarean birth • miscarriage and stillbirth (Centers for Disease Control and Prevention, 2018)	• Women who enter pregnancy with diabetes are recommended to self-monitor blood glucose to achieve glycemic control and achieve an A1C level of less than 6 percent. • Insulin is the preferred agent for management of preexisting diabetes during pregnancy as it does not cross the placenta to a measurable extent, while oral agents such as metformin and glyburide do (American Diabetes Association, 2019).

Increased neonatal risk of:
• macrosomia
• hypoglycemia
• preterm delivery
• instrumental delivery
• type 2 diabetes and overweight/ obesity later in life
• stillbirth and miscarriage
Increased maternal risk of:
• preeclampsia
• cesarean birth
• developing type 2 diabetes postpregnancy
	• Women who develop gestational diabetes mellitus during pregnancy are recommended to:
	  o self-monitor blood glucose to achieve glycemic control, and
	  o make lifestyle changes to control blood glucose.
	• Insulin is the preferred first-line treatment for gestational diabetes mellitus as it does not cross the placenta to a measurable extent. Metformin and glyburide should not be used as first-line agents (American Diabetes Association, 2019).

Increased risk of preeclampsia and its negative sequelae	Pregnant women with chronic hypertension may require additional monitoring prior to delivery. • Depending on other risk and lifestyle factors, women with chronic hypertension may be prescribed low-dose aspirin for preeclampsia prophylaxis. • Magnesium sulfate should be administered to prevent and treat seizures with gestational hypertension, preeclampsia with severe features, or eclampsia (American College of Obstetricians and Gynecologists, 2018c).

continued

TABLE 3-1 Continued

	Causal Factors
Hypertensive Diseases of Pregnancy (gestational hypertension, preeclampsia, and eclampsia)	• History of preeclampsia or eclampsia • Previous adverse pregnancy outcomes • Maternal comorbidities (including preexisting hypertension, gestational diabetes, type 1 or type 2 diabetes, and renal disease, among others) • Primiparity • Multifetal gestation (U.S. Preventive Services Task Force, 2017)

Obstetrical Risk Factors

Breech Presentation	• Preterm labor • Abnormally shaped uterus, fibroids, or too much amniotic fluid • Multifetal gestation • Placenta previa
Multiple Gestation	• Use of fertility drugs to induce ovulation • In vitro fertilization • Older maternal age
Previous Caesarean Birth	• Cesarean birth can be medically indicated or elective

Maternal and Neonatal Outcomes	Clinical Implications
• Induction of labor • Seizures • Stroke • Kidney failure • Hepatic rupture • Heart failure • Death	• For women with gestational hypertension or preeclampsia without severe features at 37 weeks gestation or more, delivery upon diagnosis, rather than expectant management, is recommended by the American College of Obstetricians and Gynecologists (ACOG). • Magnesium sulfate should be administered to prevent and treat seizures with gestational hypertension, preeclampsia with severe features, or eclampsia. • Delivery is recommended at 37 weeks of gestation for women with gestational hypertension or mild preeclampsia and no severe features, and at 34 weeks for women with severe preeclampsia (Roberts et al., 2013). Women with severe preeclampsia at less than 34 weeks of gestation with stable maternal and fetal conditions are recommended to "continue pregnancy...only at facilities with adequate maternal and neonatal intensive care resources" (Roberts et al., 2013).
• Increased risk of perinatal and neonatal mortality and neonatal morbidity (including birth trauma and hypoxic ischemic encephalopathy) compared with planned cesarean birth with breech presentation (Berhan and Haileamlak, 2015; Hannah et al., 2000)	• The decision regarding the mode of delivery should consider patient wishes and provider experience with breech birth. • Women with term singleton breech presentations should be offered external cephalic version (ECV), a procedure to rotate the fetus into vertex position. The procedure should be performed in facilities with capabilities for caesarean births. • Planned vaginal delivery of a term singleton breech fetus may be reasonable under hospital-specific protocol guidelines for eligibility and labor management. • If a vaginal breech delivery is planned, a detailed informed consent should be documented—including risks that perinatal or neonatal mortality or short-term serious neonatal morbidity may be higher than if a cesarean delivery is planned (American College of Obstetricians and Gynecologists, 2018d).
• Preterm birth • Low birthweight • Cerebral palsy	Newborns need to be evaluated for a variety of potential adverse consequences based on the details of the twinning process, pregnancy and birth events.
• Vaginal birth after a previous cesarean birth can increase risk of uterine rupture; multiple cesarean births increase risk of maternal morbidities	Newborns may require monitoring based on the details of the specific birth circumstance.

commonly the liver or kidneys.[2] In general, chronic and gestational hypertension without severe features can be managed pharmaceutically during pregnancy, while the only known treatment for preeclampsia is giving birth.[3]

Hypertensive disorders affect 10 percent of all pregnant women in the United States (Leeman et al., 2016) and were the cause of 6.8 percent of maternal deaths between 2011 and 2015 (Centers for Disease Control and Prevention, 2019a). About 7.7 percent of reproductive-age women in the United States have chronic hypertension (Bateman et al., 2012), which affects 2 percent of all hospital births, while gestational hypertension, preeclampsia, and eclampsia affect 9 percent of hospital births and chronic hypertension 2 percent (Centers for Disease Control and Prevention, 2019c). The prevalence of hypertensive disorders of pregnancy, including preeclampsia, has increased substantially in recent decades, from 528.9 per 10,000 deliveries in 1993 to 912.4 per 10,000 deliveries in 2014 (Centers for Disease Control and Prevention, 2019c). Both chronic and gestational hypertension can lead to such complications as preeclampsia and eclampsia, which can be life-threatening.

Preeclampsia occurs in 5 to 8 percent of all pregnant women (National Institutes of Health, 2019). All pregnant women are at risk of preeclampsia, but some women are at higher risk (refer to Table 3-1). Black women, women of lower socioeconomic status, women of advanced maternal age, and women with obesity are at greater risk of preeclampsia (U.S. Preventive Services Task Force, 2017). Although Black and White women experience preeclampsia at similar rates, Black women die of preeclampsia-related causes at three times the rate of non-Hispanic White women, which may be attributable to inequities in access to prenatal care (U.S. Preventive Services Task Force, 2017), as well as to unequal treatment within the health care system and structural racism (discussed in greater detail in the section "Race, Racism, and Risk" in Chapter 4).

Maternal Age

A woman's age when she enters pregnancy can contribute to her risk profile in birth. Advanced maternal age, defined as pregnancy at

---

[2]In severe cases, preeclampsia can damage the mother's organs and restrict oxygen and blood flow to the fetus. If eclampsia develops, women may experience seizure or stroke (National Institutes of Health, 2019). Women with preeclampsia may need close monitoring, specialized drugs, or treatments to prevent further complications or support fetal maturity (American College of Obstetricians and Gynecologists, 2018e).

[3]In cases of severe, acute-onset hypertension in pregnancy or the postpartum period, immediate treatment to reduce the risk of maternal stroke is needed (American College of Obstetricians and Gynecologists, 2017a). Moreover, since preeclampsia usually resolves after delivery, induction of labor may be medically indicated. (Refer to Table 3-1.)

age 35 and above, is associated with greater risk of maternal mortality, preeclampsia, poor fetal growth, fetal distress, and stillbirth compared with mothers ages 25–29 (Society for Maternal and Fetal Medicine, 2014; Cavazos-Rehg et al., 2015). Likewise, teenage pregnancy is associated with a greater likelihood of endometritis, postpartum hemorrhage (ages 15–19), and mild preeclampsia and an overall likelihood of having any complication during labor and delivery for those ages 11–14 (Cavazos-Rehg et al., 2015). Pregnancy both during the teenage years and later in reproductive life is associated with higher rates of preterm birth compared with pregnancy among women in their 20s (Ferré et al., 2016). The elevated risk of preeclampsia among women with advanced and early maternal age and the higher rate of maternal mortality among women ages 35 and above frequently necessitate more intensive care during pregnancy and childbirth. Nationwide, about 5 percent of births occurred to mothers less than 20 years old in 2017, while almost 18 percent occurred to mothers ages 35 and older.

In the United States, an increasing number of births occur to women ages 35 and older. Women in this age group account for 9.1 percent of all first births in the United States, and rates of first births to these women increased by 23 percent between 2000 and 2014 (Mathews and Hamilton, 2016). Asian, Hispanic, and Native Hawaiian and Other Pacific Islander women have the highest birth rates at ages 35 and older compared with American Indian/Alaska Native, Black, and White women (Martin et al., 2018a).

Rates of first birth in the teenage years (ages 15–19) decreased by 42 percent between 2000 and 2014 (Mathews and Hamilton, 2016). Yet while teenage pregnancy rates have declined for almost all racial groups, the rates among American Indian/Alaska Native, Latinx, and non-Hispanic Black youth are substantially higher than those among their White peers (Centers for Disease Control and Prevention, 2019c).[4] Teen pregnancy is highest in rural counties, followed by medium and small urban counties, and the rate is lowest for those residing in large urban counties (Hamilton et al., 2016).

Weight Status

Rates of overweight (body mass index [BMI] between 25.0 and 29.9) and obesity (BMI of 30.0 or higher) in the United States have been in-

---

[4]For example, the birth rate among American Indian and Alaska Native youth ages 15–19 was 32.9 per 1,000, compared with 13.2 per 1,000 births among White youth (Centers for Disease Control and Prevention, 2019c).

creasing for several decades (Hales et al., 2017).[5] Entering pregnancy with overweight or obesity may necessitate more intensive care during pregnancy and birth.[6] Prepregnancy overweight or obesity increases the likelihood of developing gestational diabetes or a hypertensive disorder of pregnancy compared with women who enter pregnancy at a lower BMI (Institute of Medicine and National Research Council, 2009; Kim et al., 2010). These antepartum complications increase the risk of indicated preterm and cesarean birth, but women with higher prepregnancy BMI are also at greater risk of miscarriage, stillbirth, shoulder dystocia, and spontaneous preterm birth compared with normal-weight women (Declercq, et al., 2016; Catalano and Shankar, 2017; Schummers et al., 2015). The relationship between prematurity and obesity is not well understood, although maternal inflammation is hypothesized to play a role (Catalano and Shankar, 2017).

Obesity affects more than one-third of U.S. women aged 20–39 (Hales et al., 2017). Black and American Indian/Alaska Native women experience obesity and overweight at higher rates (66.7% and 73.6%, respectively) compared with non-Hispanic White and Asian women. In addition, the prevalence of obesity is estimated to be higher among women of lower socioeconomic status and women in rural areas (McLaren, 2007; Lundeen et al., 2018). For example, rates of prepregnancy obesity among non-Hispanic White, college-educated, and married women are half those of non-Hispanic Black, unmarried women with less than a high school degree (14% and 28%, respectively) (Aizer and Currie, 2014). Rates of prepregnancy obesity in the United States are highest among women of Samoan, American Indian/Alaska Native, Black, and Native Hawaiian ancestry (Singh and Dibari, 2019).

In addition to its clinical implications, having overweight and obesity may make women vulnerable to experiencing weight stigma—the societal devaluation of people with overweight or obesity—in daily life and in the health care system (Andreyeva et al., 2008; Phelan et al., 2015; Pont et al., 2017). In health care, weight stigma can manifest in negative provider attitudes or ambivalence toward patients with obesity (Phelan et al., 2015; Puhl

---

[5] Obesity is further broken down into three categories: class 1 obesity (BMI between 30.0 and 34.9); class 2 (BMI between 35.0 and 39.9); and class 3, or extreme obesity (BMI of 40.0 and above). Each class of obesity is associated with a higher risk of type 2 diabetes, hypertension, and cardiovascular disease (National Heart, Lung, and Blood Institute, n.d.).

[6] Like obesity and overweight, entering pregnancy with underweight can contribute to adverse pregnancy and birth outcomes, although it affects far fewer women. Entering pregnancy underweight—at a BMI of 18.5 or lower—increases the risk of preterm birth and low birthweight compared with normal-weight women (Han et al., 2011). About 4 percent of women enter pregnancy with underweight (Deputy et al., 2018). Underweight women are recommended to gain more weight during pregnancy to support fetal growth (Institute of Medicine and National Research Council, 2009).

and Latner, 2008; Puhl and Brownell, 2001), and studies from Australia and the United Kingdom document weight bias among maternity care providers (Mulherin et al., 2013; Furber and McGowan, 2011). For example, in an Australian study of 627 women, women with higher prepregnancy BMI reported poorer perceived quality of treatment during pregnancy and after birth relative to normal-weight women (Mulherin et al., 2013).

Diabetes

Nationwide, about 1 percent of women enter pregnancy with pre-existing diabetes[7] (Centers for Disease Control and Prevention, 2018), and between 6 and 9 percent of women develop gestational diabetes (glucose intolerance that develops during pregnancy) over the course of their pregnancy (American College of Obstetricians and Gynecologists, 2018c; DeSisto et al., 2014). While type 1 diabetes is hypothesized to be caused by genetic or environmental factors, type 2 diabetes is associated with obesity and overweight, physical inactivity, older age, high blood pressure, family history of diabetes, and history of polycystic ovarian syndrome (National Institute of Diabetes and Digestive and Kidney Diseases, 2016, 2017). Similarly, gestational diabetes is associated with overweight and obesity and previous pregnancies complicated by gestational diabetes.

Rates of prepregnancy diabetes are highest among American Indian/Alaska Native (2.1%) and Native Hawaiian and Pacific Islander (1.8%) women, followed by African American and Hispanic (1.2% and 1.0%, respectively), Asian (0.9%), and White (0.7%) women. Rates of gestational diabetes are higher among older women compared with younger women; women with obesity and overweight compared with normal-weight women; and Asian, American Indian/Alaska Native, Native Hawaiian/Pacific Islander, and Hispanic women compared with non-Hispanic White women.

Diabetes during pregnancy that is not well controlled is associated with a greater risk of several adverse maternal and neonatal outcomes, including the risk to both birthing women and infants of developing type 2 diabetes later in life (Centers for Disease Control and Prevention, 2018; American College of Obstetricians and Gynecologists, 2018c). Specifically, gestational diabetes increases the risks for preeclampsia, cesarean birth, fetal macrosomia (fetal weight of 9 or more pounds, which can make delivery difficult), neonatal hypoglycemia (low blood sugar immediately after birth), and birth trauma (American College of Obstetricians and Gynecologists, 2018c). Women with pregnancies complicated by diabetes may require additional resources for safe care of the women and their neonates. For

---

[7]This includes type 1 and type 2 diabetes.

example, the American College of Obstetricians and Gynecologists (ACOG) recommends increased monitoring for women with gestational diabetes (2018d), and macrosomia may necessitate cesarean birth.

Substance Use

Substance use during pregnancy is associated with several adverse outcomes, such as premature birth, low birthweight, neonatal abstinence disorder,[8] fetal alcohol syndrome and fetal alcohol spectrum disorder, miscarriage, stillbirth, and placental abruption (Centers for Disease Control and Prevention, 2019d; Popova et al., 2017; Forray and Foster, 2016; National Institute on Drug Abuse, 2018). Nicotine is the most commonly used substance in pregnancy, followed by alcohol and marijuana (Forray, 2016).[9] Moreover, opioid use and opioid use disorder (OUD) have increased among pregnant women in recent years. It has been estimated that the number of women with OUD at the time of labor and birth quadrupled between 1999 and 2014, with geographic variation: the lowest rates of OUD were found in Washington, DC (0.7 cases per 1,000 hospital births) and the highest in Vermont (48.6 cases per 1,000 hospital births) (Haight et al., 2018). Opioid use is most common among older pregnant women (over the age of 30) and those who are covered by Medicaid. Moreover, non-Hispanic White women have the highest rate of opioid use, followed by Hispanic and non-Hispanic Black women and those who identify as all other races.

In addition to its deleterious effects, substance use is of particular concern in maternity care because of its frequent co-occurrence with other risk factors. Substance use is often comorbid with other psychiatric illnesses (Swendsen et al., 2010; Forray, 2016). In addition, pregnant women with substance use disorders are more likely to be exposed to other risk factors, such as inadequate prenatal care, chronic medical problems, poor nutrition, and intimate partner violence (Forray, 2016).

Depression

Depression is a common but serious mood disorder that affects 10.1 percent of reproductive-age women in the United States (Brody et

---

[8] Infants who are exposed to opioids during their mother's pregnancy are commonly born with neonatal abstinence syndrome (NAS). In addition to the withdrawal symptoms they experience shortly after birth, children with NAS have disturbances in their gastrointestinal system, autonomic nervous system, and central nervous system (American College of Obstetricians and Gynecologists, 2017b).

[9] The evidence regarding low-to-moderate use of alcohol during pregnancy is mixed, showing either inconclusive results or no increased risk for adverse pregnancy outcomes (Forray, 2016). Therefore, heavy alcohol use is of greatest concern in risk assessment of pregnant women.

al., 2018). Perinatal depression has been associated with increased risk of several adverse maternal and neonatal outcomes, including preeclampsia, gestational diabetes (Kozhimannil et al., 2009), hypertension (Kurki et al., 2000), preterm birth, and low birthweight (Grote et al., 2010). Depression is estimated to affect 12 percent of women during pregnancy (Bennett et al., 2004). Prenatal depression is more common among Black, Hispanic, and non-Hispanic White reproductive-age women compared with Asian women in the United States (Brody et al., 2018).

Women may enter pregnancy with depression or develop depression over the course of pregnancy and the postpartum period. Risk factors for developing depression during pregnancy include a history of depression and discontinuation of antidepressant medications during pregnancy (Becker et al., 2016). In addition, hormone changes during pregnancy are thought to increase vulnerability to the onset or return of depression (Bennett et al., 2004). Moreover, depressive symptoms during pregnancy are a strong predictor of postpartum depression, which affects 10 to 15 percent of people who give birth (Ko et al., 2017; Becker et al., 2016; Pearlstein et al., 2015; Halbreich and Karkun, 2006).

OBSTETRIC RISK FACTORS

As with the medical risk factors discussed above, women enter pregnancy with obstetric histories and characteristics that can confer risk. Like medical risk factors, these obstetric factors require careful consideration during the risk-assessment process. In this section, we discuss two obstetric risk factors that need to be considered when determining appropriate birth settings for pregnant women: breech presentation and previous cesarean birth.

Breech Presentation

Breech presentation refers to situations in which the fetus presents as bottom- or feet-first rather than head-first. Breech presentation occurs in 3–4 percent of term pregnancies (Royal College of Obstetricians and Gynaecologists, 2017) and is more common among nulliparous women (Fruscalzo et al., 2014). In cases of breech presentation with a single fetus, women may be offered a procedure to reposition the fetus (called external cephalic version, or ECV). If the fetus cannot be repositioned, options for birth include planned vaginal breech birth or planned cesarean birth. Planned vaginal birth with breech presentation carries higher risk of perinatal mortality than planned cesarean birth, as well as the possibility that emergency cesarean birth will be needed (Royal College of Obstetricians and Gynaecologists, 2017). However, cesarean birth carries greater risk of maternal morbidity (discussed in the following section).

Previous Cesarean Birth

Over the past five decades, the rate of cesarean birth among U.S. women has increased from 5 percent to 32 percent. This increase has been attributed to changes in medical technology (e.g., the advent of electronic fetal monitoring), decreases in operative vaginal births and attempted breech births, and the assumption that having a prior cesarean birth would disqualify a woman from having a vaginal birth (known as a vaginal birth after cesarean, or VBAC) in the future (American College of Obstetricians and Gynecologists, 2019e).

Having a prior cesarean birth, whether elective or planned, influences a woman's risk status in any additional pregnancies. In the case of previous cesarean birth, a woman may be faced with two options in a future pregnancy: to attempt a vaginal birth or to have another cesarean birth. Both carry risks and benefits for the woman and fetus. Benefits of VBAC include avoidance of major abdominal surgery, lower rates of morbidity (such as hemorrhage, thromboembolism, and infection), and a shorter recovery period compared with women who have an elective repeat cesarean delivery (American College of Obstetricians and Gynecologists, 2019a; National Institutes of Health Consensus Development Conference Panel, 2010). In addition, women who have one successful VBAC are more likely to be able to have a vaginal birth in the future.

Both planned labor after cesarean and repeat cesarean delivery are associated with increased risks. Planned labor after a cesarean birth is associated with greater risk of maternal infection, surgical injury, and uterine rupture (American College of Obstetricians and Gynecologists, 2019e). However, most maternal morbidity related to labor occurs when surgical birth becomes necessary, rather than when vaginal birth is successful (American College of Obstetricians and Gynecologists, 2019e). Women with multiple surgical births are at greater risk for complications associated with repeat abdominal surgeries (such as bowel and bladder injuries) and for issues of placental position and growth[10] in subsequent pregnancies (National Institutes of Health Consensus Development Conference Panel, 2010). In addition, laboring after prior cesarean birth carries some risks for the fetus. Rates of perinatal mortality and hypoxic ischemic encephalopathy associated with labor after prior cesarean birth are higher than those for repeat cesarean birth without labor (National Institutes of Health Consensus Development Conference Panel, 2010).

Given the available evidence on risk and benefit, the *Eunice Kennedy Shriver* National Institute of Child Health and Human Development (NICHD) and ACOG recommend that VBAC birth be offered to women

---

[10]For example, placenta previa, placenta accreta, increta, and percreta.

who meet certain conditions (primarily, one previous cesarean birth with a low-transverse incision, which carries the lowest risk of uterine rupture). However, other risk factors, such as maternal age, weight status, chronic health conditions, and obstetrical history must also be considered (Wu et al., 2019; American College of Obstetricians and Gynecologists, 2019e). In general, ACOG recommends that planned labor after previous cesarean delivery be attempted at facilities capable of performing emergency deliveries (American College of Obstetricians and Gynecologists, 2019e). Moreover, NICHD calls for the use of a shared decision-making process between women and their providers when planned labor and elective repeat cesarean birth are medically equivalent options (National Institutes of Health Consensus Development Conference Panel, 2010).

MEDICAL AND OBSTETRIC RISK FACTORS BY BIRTH SETTING IN THE UNITED STATES

In general, planned home and birth center births are much less likely to be affected by complications than are hospital births because of the risk selection process conducted by providers in those settings. Women with complicated pregnancies, whether due to medical risk factors or previous obstetric outcomes, are more likely to give birth in a hospital. This distribution of risk is reflected in the birth certificate data on risk factor by place of birth (see Table 3-2). Women with planned home and birth center births in 2017 were much less likely to have medical risk factors, such as prepregnancy or gestational diabetes, hypertensive disorders, or obesity, than women who gave birth in hospitals (refer to Table 3-2). Births to adolescents also occurred at a greater rate in hospitals, while a greater proportion of planned home and birth center births than hospital births were to mothers ages 35 and older (23.6 and 18.1%, respectively, compared with 17.5%). However, VBAC occurred more frequently in home and birth center settings (2.0% of hospital births versus 3.4% of out-of-hospital births). This difference was driven by both planned and unplanned home births, of which VBACs made up about 4 percent (refer to Table 3-2).

In light of the various medical, obstetrical, and social risk factors that can affect a woman and fetus during birth, the risk selection process employed by maternity care providers is critical for promoting patient safety. An analysis of birth certificate data by Grünebaum and colleagues (2015a) found that more than 30 percent of midwife-attended planned home births that occurred between 2010 and 2012 were to women that had at least one perinatal risk factor (breech presentation, prior cesarean birth, more than 41 weeks gestation, or twin gestation). Risk assessment and selection is an important process that requires monitoring and evaluation to support patient safety and promote favorable outcomes at the systems level.

TABLE 3-2 Percentage of Births with Selected Risk Factors by Place of Birth, United States, 2017

	All Births (n = 3,855,500)	Hospital (n = 3,793,272)	Out of Hospital (n = 62,228)	Birth Center (n = 19,878)	Home (n = 38,343)	Planned Home (n = 28,994)
Age of mother (years)						
<20	5.1	5.2	1.4	0.9	1.4	0.7
20–34	77.3	77.3	77.1	81.0	74.9	75.8
35+	17.6	17.5	21.5	18.1	23.6	23.5
Live birth order						
First live birth	37.9	38.2	23.3	33.4	18.5	17.7
Second or third live birth	49.3	49.3	49.5	49.7	49.4	47.3
Fourth or higher-order birth	12.8	12.6	27.2	17.0	32.1	34.9
Preterm birth	11.6	11.8	4.5	1.5	5.2	2.1
Low birthweight	8.3	8.4	3.6	0.9	4.2	1.3
Multiple birth	3.4	3.5	0.7	0.2	1.0	0.7
Diabetes[a]	7.3	7.4	1.6	1.7	1.5	1.1
Hypertensive disorders[b]	8.5	8.7	0.8	0.4	1.0	0.5
Prepregnancy body mass index						
Underweight (<18.5)	3.4	3.4	4.3	3.9	4.4	4.2
Normal weight (20.0–24.9)	43.3	43.1	59.5	61.1	59.4	60.4
Overweight (25.0–29.9)	26.2	26.3	22.4	22.0	22.3	22.2
Obesity (30+)	27.1	27.3	13.9	13.0	13.9	13.2
Smoked during pregnancy	6.9	7.0	3.0	1.1	3.3	0.9
Vaginal birth after cesarean section	2.0	2.0	3.4	1.7	4.1	4.2

NOTES: Column percentage computed per 100 women in specified group. Not-stated responses (<4% for all variables) were dropped before percentages were computed.

[a]Includes prepregnancy and gestational diabetes.
[b]Includes prepregnancy hypertension, gestational hypertension, and eclampsia.
SOURCE: Based on birth certificate data.

Despite the fact that hospitals are at present the safest place for women in some high-risk situations to obtain desired care options for vaginal birth (Bovbjerg et al., 2017), many women cannot find hospitals and physicians offering such care, such as VBACs, which may in part explain the higher percentage of women having VBACs in home and birth center settings. Other maternity care services that are often not available in hospital settings include external cephalic version, vaginal breech birth, and planned vaginal twin birth. Further, some women face challenges in finding hospitals that support intermittent auscultation, nonpharmacologic measures for labor comfort and progress, freedom to drink fluids and eat solids, freedom of movement in labor, and freedom of choice of birth positions, as well as the related essential care option of the choice between midwifery- or medical-led care (Bovbjerg et al., 2017).

CHOICE, RISK, AND DECISION MAKING

In the face of a maternal health crisis in the United States, including maternal mortality and severe maternal morbidity, the nation needs to take seriously the reality that birth, a natural process that in a majority of cases occurs without complication, also can result in devastating outcomes for women, their infants, and their families. Importantly, disparities in these outcomes disproportionately affect the most vulnerable populations. Women, however, may conceive of risk differently; may understand risk differently or tolerate risk differently; or may simply have competing values (e.g., control, respect, faith) that they prioritize over and above medical risks.

Given the prevalence of medical and obstetric risks in the U.S. population, risk assessment and risk selection in birth settings are critical to decision making and choice among birth settings. It is clear that some women desire birth setting options other than hospitals, as evidenced by the increased number of women choosing home and birth center births in recent years (MacDorman and Declercq, 2019). Moreover, among participants in the population-based Listening to Mothers in California Survey who had given birth in hospitals in 2016, a majority expressed an interest in midwifery care and doula support, 40 percent in birth center care, and 22 percent in home birth. Box 3-1 further details the literature regarding pregnant people's preferences for birth settings and birth experiences and the cultural, social, and religious factors that influence these preferences.

It is broadly accepted that women with decisional capacity have the right to make informed decisions about their care, including crucial, highly determinative, and interrelated decisions about choice of care provider and choice of place of birth (American College of Nurse-Midwives, 2016; American College of Obstetricians and Gynecologists, 2016a). Informed choice, however, requires a set of real options, accurate information about

BOX 3-1
Preferences in Birth Setting

Pregnant people's values and preferences, in concert with unique cultural, social, and religious factors, influence how much (or what type of) risk a woman is willing to tolerate during birth and her choice of birth setting. Culture can influence what a woman views as "normal" during pregnancy and childbirth, her preferences for her birth experience, and the roles she and her family members are expected to play in the intrapartum period. Among many Native American cultures, for example, pregnancy and childbirth are viewed as normal events that should occur within the context of family and community (Ogburn et al., 2012; Kornelsen et al., 2010). Women are traditionally attended to by their female relatives and tribal midwives (Ogburn et al., 2012; Kornelsen et al., 2010), and birth is viewed as a celebratory event for the entire community. In addition, in indigenous models of health, connection to ancestral lands is considered an important aspect of well-being (Notah Begay III Foundation, 2015). That connection has implications for an individual's physical, spiritual, and emotional health, and its disruption can diminish an individual's well-being (Notah Begay III Foundation, 2015). Thus among many indigenous cultures, giving birth on ancestral lands is important for supporting the well-being of the woman and newborn, as well as maintaining their connection to family and identity, and can outweigh the risks of having less access to specialty care (Chamberlain and Barclay, 2000). In one qualitative study of women from the Heiltsuk community of Bella Bella, British Columbia, for example, postpartum women described the significance of giving birth in their home communities, for reasons ranging from greater levels of support from their family and community to the cultural significance of birthing on traditional lands (Kornelsen et al., 2010).

In addition, a number of qualitative studies have sought to understand women's preferences for their childbirth experience. For instance, the Good Birth Project, a qualitative study of 101 birthing women conducted in 2006, found that women valued five things in childbirth: agency, personal security, connectedness, respect, and knowledge (Lyerly, 2013). Other work on women's preferences during childbirth have highlighted similar sentiments, especially women's valuing of security and safety.

Of course, women perceive and understand safety in a variety of ways. In a study of 17 women of childbearing age, some women interpreted safety as conferred by the competency of the provider, while others perceived it as deriving from providers who listened to their feelings and concerns during the birth experience (Lyndon et al., 2018). In a similar study of 13 childbearing women, some women reported choosing to deliver at home because they felt safest in an environment without medical interventions, they knew their provider well, and they knew medical care (via transfer to a hospital) was available if necessary (Lothian, 2013). For those women who chose a hospital birth, safety was perceived in the structured environment of a hospital with technology available and the belief that a hospital birth would minimize risks (Lyerly, 2013). Miller and Shriver (2012), in a qualitative study of 135 women, similarly found that women who chose hospital births did so since they perceived birthing in a hospital to be the safest choice because of its ability to minimize risks to the woman and the child (Miller and Shriver, 2012). And Sperlich and colleagues (2017), in a study of a convenience sample of 634 women, found that only 12.6 percent of nulliparous women felt safe giving birth outside a hospital, either at a birthing center or at home.

Women may also choose a birth setting based on their preference for the philosophy of care offered in that setting. For instance, in a survey of 160 women who had a home birth, desire for an intervention-free birth was the one of the most cited reasons for choosing that setting (Boucher et al., 2009). For these women, the value of an intervention-free birth outweighed the risk associated with giving birth away from medical resources. Surveys indicate that there is a growing, but still minority, interest in out-of-hospital birth options among some women (Sakala et al., 2018). Among women who gave birth in California hospitals in 2016, the Listening to Mothers in California Survey of 2,539 women found that 11 percent "would definitely want" a birth center birth, and 29 percent "would consider" such a birth should they give birth in the future. Six percent of survey respondents reported that they "would definitely want" a home birth, and 15 percent "would consider" such a birth should they give birth in the future. Among race/ethnicity groups, Black women expressed the strongest interest in these settings, and women with Medi-Cal coverage expressed greater interest than women with private insurance (Sakala et al., 2018).

In the second national Listening to Mothers Survey, differences were seen between first-time and experienced mothers, suggesting a growth in confidence and decrease in fear with experience (see below; Declercq et al., 2006). Looking at responses of women who had had vaginal births, the table below illustrates these contrasts. Although the survey was limited to women with hospital births, these results suggest that experienced mothers may be more open to birth center and home births than first-time mothers.

	First-Time Mothers (%)	Experienced Mothers (%)
Took childbirth class this pregnancy	55	10
Felt confident as approached labor	72	85
Had epidural	81	67
Used no pain medications during labor	8	22
Felt frightened when giving birth	40	25
Felt overwhelmed when giving birth	56	35
Agreed that birth should not be interfered with unless medically necessary	41	55

Taken together, these studies illustrate the ways in which individual values, preferences, and experiences influence perceptions of risk in birth and birth setting. Although perceptions and desires vary across women and settings, the studies reviewed here demonstrate that women desire to feel comfortable, safe, and respected during the birth experience, regardless of setting. What feels comfortable, safe, and respectful varies from woman to woman. In short, patient-centeredness[a] is not necessarily determined by place of birth or birth attendant.

[a]Patient-centered health care is "a method of care that relies upon effective communication, empathy, and a feeling of partnership between doctor and patient to improve patient care outcomes and satisfaction, to lessen patient symptoms, and to reduce unnecessary costs" (Rickert, 2012).

the risks and benefits of those options, appropriate and ongoing medical/ obstetrical risk assessment, respect for women's informed decisions, and recognition that those choices may change over the course of care. Indeed, true choice requires both that obstetricians inform patients of the availability of alternative care settings and midwifery providers, and that midwives inform patients about the limits of their scope of practice and when medical and/or hospital-based care would be more appropriate.

The discussion in this section considers the concept of risk—how it is assessed (by physicians and midwives versus by pregnant women) and how that risk assessment can and should factor into a provider's recommendation for a given birth setting. We consider how the skills of shared decision making might facilitate provider–patient communication regarding risks, benefits, and alternatives, as well as elicit values and help women negotiate competing priorities to make the choice that best aligns with their risk profile and values. Recognizing that not all women are candidates for birth center and home birth based on medical and obstetric risks and that women in hospital settings may decline some interventions, providers will inevitably find themselves in a position in which a patient declines or refuses medically recommended care. Therefore, we discuss the provider's professional and ethical obligation to ensure that a refusal is an informed one and consider best options for respecting patient autonomy while supporting patient safety.

In all of these areas, of course, there is the risk of decisions being made because of unacknowledged normative assumptions. Using end-of-life decision making as an analogy, for example, a normative assumption might be that life must be preserved at all costs, which could lead to choosing medical interventions at the end of life, regardless of their impact on quality of life. A competing normative assumption might be that quality of life is the most important thing, which could lead to foregoing lifesaving interventions (e.g., chemotherapy) that have uncomfortable side effects. These types of normative assumptions might be the basis for decisions made by policy makers, payers, administrators, or providers, but they might not align with a particular person's or family's values and preferences. In the case of maternity care, for example, a provider might advise a nulliparous woman with a breech fetus to schedule a cesarean in order to minimize risks to the baby, but the woman might prefer to attempt a vaginal birth because of concerns about operative risks and recovery. Thus, it is important to be aware of how normative assumptions may influence decision making, and to be cognizant of when and how different assumptions are in conflict.

When one considers normative assumptions through the lens of population and public health, tensions often emerge between individual rights or preferences and population-based efforts that seek to maximize health and safety. At the bedside, maternity care providers can prioritize patients' individual preferences in light of their individual risk profile. At the population level, policy makers are tasked with developing strategies for minimizing pregnancy-related morbidity and mortality for women and infants. As a result, they may operate under the normative assumption that their role is to drive down perinatal mortality at all cost without recognizing that doing so may cause maternal mortality or morbidity or other neonatal morbidity to rise, or that many potentially avoidable cesareans may lead to life-threatening conditions in future pregnancies. This is particularly the case in settings, such as the United States, where interventions for "safe maternity" are tertiary in nature, relying on obstetric intervention and surgical "rescue" rather than preventive and safety net strategies designed to ensure that all women have an equitable prospect of entering pregnancy in good physical and mental health and with adequate support. This trade-off is not intended to pit women and their babies against one another, as their interests are, in fact, almost always aligned. However, it does raise important considerations for policy makers regarding the normative assumption that "perfect" is possible or that all risk of adverse perinatal outcomes can ever be perfectly known and mitigated. Two normative questions thus arise: What risk of maternal morbidity and mortality is U.S. society willing to accept in efforts to reduce perinatal mortality and morbidity? Conversely, what risk of perinatal morbidity and mortality is U.S. society willing to accept to prevent maternal mortality and reduce morbidity? The answers to these questions are fraught with practical, political, and ideological implications (Cahill, 2001). However, they are central to any discussion of birth setting, and the collective decisions made with regard to these questions communicate, implicitly and explicitly, the nation's norms, values, and biases.

Risk Assessment, Informed Choice, and Shared Decision Making

In the late 1990s, Charles and colleagues (1997) developed the framework of shared decision making (SDM), defining it as the bidirectional flow of information between patient and provider resulting in deliberation and negotiation between the two parties, after which patient and provider jointly decide on a treatment strategy. SDM is distinguished from informed decision making, which involves a one-way communication (provider to patient) of medical information, with patients being left to deliberate and decide on their own. Informed decision making is considered more of a "menu of options" approach, in contrast to the more deliberative and negotiated partnership conceptualized in SDM (Charles et al., 1999). SDM has since been designated the optimal model for treatment decision making to promote patient-centered care, particularly when the treatment decision is preference-sensitive (Institute of Medicine, 2013).

Preference-sensitive decision making has been defined as "medical care for which the clinical evidence does not clearly support one treatment option such that the appropriate course of treatment depends on the values of the patient or the preferences of the patient...regarding the benefits, harms and scientific evidence for each treatment option" (Centers for Medicare & Medicaid Services, 2016). Preference-sensitive care does not mean simply that patients may have preferences about their care, as this can be assumed for almost every treatment decision, but rather that patients' preferences, values, and goals determine which of a number of equally medically indicated treatment alternatives is most suitable and effective for each patient.

Reproductive health in general, and obstetrical care in particular, is replete with preference-sensitive decision making because there is often insufficient or poor-quality evidence to inform treatment decision making, given that it is often infeasible and/or unethical to perform randomized trials of interventions manipulating birth experiences. (See Chapter 5 for further discussion of the strengths and limitations of methodologies used in birth settings research.) Furthermore, pregnant women have historically been excluded from research studies and discoveries, leaving practitioners with little information to guide prescribing practices and clinical management (McCormack and Best, 2014). Accordingly, there is frequently a degree of uncertainty surrounding obstetrical management decision making. However, practitioners may not be skilled or well practiced in navigating or disclosing this uncertainty, and may be biased in their assessments of risks and benefits associated with medical therapies.

Thus, for a maternity care provider, determining the optimal approach to counseling first requires determining whether the *medical* and *obstetric* risk and benefit assessment for a patient results in a clear recommendation for hospital, birth center, or home birth. If risks are comparable in all settings, the "right choice" of birth setting depends entirely on what is "right" for that woman. Similarly, if risks are not equivalent across settings, the pregnant woman must weigh this trade-off. She must assess, through the lens of her personal values, preferences, and lived experiences, the probability and severity of potential adverse outcomes, and make the choice she deems safest for her and her child. The same criteria apply within hospital settings when women need to make informed choices about interventions.

In the absence of a medical recommendation for in-hospital care and/or a provider of high-risk maternity care, decision making with respect to birth setting and maternity care provider requires explicitly eliciting a woman's values, preferences, fears, and concerns regarding her hoped-for birth experience (e.g., family involvement, support persons, pain management, mobility). This includes presenting a full array of options together with an unbiased explanation of the maternal and neonatal risks—both absolute and relative—and benefits associated with each option. These options need to be presented in appropriate language, which considers not only a language other than English if needed, but also health literacy, such as vocabulary, culturally appropriate terminology, and terminology consistent with levels of education and familiarity with the physiology of pregnancy and birth (National Academies of Sciences, Engineering, and Medicine, 2018).

Risk Assessment and Informed Refusal

As pregnancy progresses, assessments need to be ongoing for maternal or fetal risk factors that would place a woman at increased risk of requiring medical therapies and interventions accessible to her or her newborn only in the inpatient setting, and perhaps only at a higher level of hospital care. These risk factors include her medical history (e.g., cardiovascular disease, autoimmune disorders, chronic renal disease), obstetric history (e.g., prior cesarean, shortened cervix), and psychosocial background (e.g., substance use disorder, current or prior trauma, intimate partner violence, homelessness). For example, professionally and ethically speaking, "to provide safe care, midwives need to be able to tell parents that they can no longer participate in their birth because of changes in risk status" (Jankowski and Burcher, 2015). Out-of-hospital providers are encouraged to practice "preventive ethics" by making the parameters of their care explicit at their first visit with the pregnant woman, as well as being transparent about liability coverage and the potential for redress (McCullough and Chervenak, 1994). Similarly, it is incumbent upon in-hospital maternity care providers to be transparent and forthcoming about the harms associated with hospital-based care—specifically, the use of interventions to induce or augment labor, which can introduce their own side effects and risks for maternal morbidity.

Women who "risk out" of or are deemed poor candidates for home or birth center care still have the right to refuse recommended care, and may do so for any number of reasons, including inability to access the type of care they desire, such as VBAC, in a hospital setting. Informed refusal also takes place within hospitals with regard to specific interventions or types of care (Declercq et al., 2007). Maternity care providers have a responsibility to ensure that these are informed refusals, offering resources and information to support informed choice and mitigate bias and misinformation where possible. Nevertheless, "pregnancy is not an exception to the principle that a decisionally capable patient has the right to refuse treatment, even treatment needed to maintain life. Therefore, a decisionally capable pregnant woman's decision to refuse recommended medical or surgical interventions should be respected" (American College of Obstetricians and Gynecologists, 2016a, p. 1). Indeed, a woman's informed refusal provides the challenge and opportunity for in-hospital and birth center and home birth providers to work collaboratively in a fully integrated system to try to work with the woman to facilitate a safe set of alternatives in support of her well-being.

In the face of such refusal to accept a recommendation for a hospital birth, home birth and birth center providers may find themselves in a quandary, wondering whether they do more good or harm by not providing the woman with care that is outside of their scope of practice. Fears of patient coercion and abandonment may lead these providers to accept patients despite or precisely because of the increased risk, particularly when a woman has either refused or been denied in-hospital vaginal birth for a given indication, such as planned VBAC, vaginal twin birth, and vaginal breech birth.

In their review of a case of home birth with anticipated congenital anomalies, Jankowski and Burcher (2015, p. 31) provide the following guidance for out-of-hospital maternity providers: "Careproviders are obligated to define the boundaries of practice for patients, but careproviders cannot be compelled by patients' assertion of their positive right for care that is beyond the careproviders' skill set. To do so, in violation of professional standards, out of a fear that patients will fare even worse if their requests are refused, is a misapplication of the principle of beneficence." The authors remind care providers that speculative fears "do not outweigh a careprovider's professional obligation to recognize her own limitations and act accordingly" (p. 32), reasoning that "if a patient's autonomy could override physicians' and midwives' responsibility to remain within their respective scopes of practice, then a patient's request to her obstetrician to provide a home cesarean section has no grounds for denial" (p. 34). They stress that "careproviders cannot be held hostage by parents' poor choices" (p. 33), concluding that in doing so, a birth center or home birth careprovider "threatens birth options for other women by opening herself, and her profession, up to criticism" and jeopardizing her own "professional status and the perception of her profession in the broader healthcare community" (p. 34). Similar cautions apply in the realm of hospital care, wherein a woman's refusal of interventions must be respected, yet providing care beyond one's scope of practice or skillset places patients and the profession at large at risk.

Risk Communication

Communicating risk in a way that is appropriate for a variety of literacy levels and in culturally and linguistically concordant ways is quite difficult. The literature on health literacy has demonstrated multiple barriers to appropriate risk communication (see, e.g., National Academies of Sciences, Engineering, and Medicine, 2015). Written materials on risk are constrained by requirements for informed consent documents to be written at vocabulary and complexity levels far beyond the average reading level of the U.S. population. In addition to vocabulary, literacy, and numeracy barriers, cultural background and lived experiences can shape how messages are heard (Nielsen-Bohlman et al., 2018). In Spanish, for example, the word "risk" translates directly as "riesgo," but pregnant women in one study said that "peligro"—literally "danger"—better communicated what was meant by risk (Alcalay et al., 1993).

In addition, the limited time that some types of maternity care providers can spend with patients can impede implementation of the shared decision-making model discussed earlier (Luntz, 2007). The midwifery model of care, which as noted can be applied in all birth settings and implemented by all types of clinicians, including physicians, provides the time necessary for shared decision making. Nurse practitioners and labor and delivery nurses also have more time for communication and shared decision making, although this can depend on their patient load and clinic or hospital policies.

Decision aids have been found to be useful and effective adjuncts to provider counseling to help health care consumers access and understand treatment options and their risks and benefits (Stacey et al., 2017). These tools not only present information in support of informed choice, but also can include clarification of values to facilitate deliberation and negation of competing priorities. Evidence suggests that decision support tools can help increase patient knowledge and activation and facilitate shared decision making, and in some cases have been shown to result in patients opting for less interventional and costly treatment options (Alston et al., 2014). Calculators and assessment tools can even be embedded in these decision aids to help tailor decision making to personal medical or obstetric risk factors. Were decision aids available to assist in the related choices of maternity care provider and birth setting at the onset of or even prior to pregnancy, women might enter care more activated, engaged, and knowledgeable about these choices (O'Connor et al., 1999; O'Connor, 2001; Stacey et al., 2017). Practical options include making such decision aids available on the intranets of health plans and employers and on respected websites that support childbearing women.

Social media also can be used for clear communication before and during pregnancy, as well as the postpartum period (Scheufele, 1999; Scheufele and Tewksbury, 2006). Women with access to the Internet and the literacy level and language background to utilize that access can find multiple ways to learn about choices for prenatal and intrapartum care and the risks around those choices. Many women with fewer resources have limited access to the Internet, including linguistic and educational barriers to full understanding of Internet materials, but access is rapidly increasing (Kontos et al., 2014; Kim and Xie, 2017). One report notes that in 2018, 68 percent of Americans used Facebook, and nearly three-quarters accessed YouTube (Smith and Anderson, 2018).

It is also important to note that the potential of social media to facilitate communication about risks and choices in pregnancy and childbirth is complicated by the fact that not all media sources are objective and reliable (Southwell et al., 2018). Some are driven by special interests, and some by individuals or groups with perspectives that are not supported by science and best practices. It remains for respected institutions in government (e.g., the Centers for Disease Control and Prevention, state and local health departments) and the private sector to provide sources that are linguistically, educationally, financially, and culturally accessible (Scrimshaw, 2019).

CONCLUSION

In summary, risk is the potential or probability of harm occurring. In the context of maternity care, clinicians conceive of risk as the potential for pregnancy complications, adverse events, or poor outcomes occurring during pregnancy or after delivery. Risk in this context is influenced by a host of medical and obstetrical factors, as well as systems-level determinants (discussed in the next chapter). Some population groups, particularly women from historically marginalized communities, face a disproportionate burden of pregnancy-related risk, indicating greater care needs that are appropriately provided only in certain birth settings. Although the likelihood of catastrophic losses, such as the death of a pregnant woman or newborn, is low, many pregnancies in the United States warrant additional surveillance and monitoring, and, often, access to medical resources. In addition, members of the maternity care team have a responsibility to inform women accurately and transparently about the risks and benefits of their options, and do so in a way that is culturally concordant, easily understandable, and respectful.

Risk assessment is the process of identifying and assessing sources of risk. In maternity care, the risk-assessment process can be used to match women with the settings and resources they need, focusing more resources on those who need them most and avoiding overuse of technology and intervention for those who do not need them (Institute of Medicine, 2013). In short, the risk assessment process can be used to indicate which settings are most appropriate for a pregnant woman's care during pregnancy and childbirth. Greater understanding of essential resources for each of the various birth settings, predictors of neonatal complications to guide decisions about level of neonatal care, predictors of maternal complications to guide decisions about level of maternal care, and predictors that should prompt maternal transport between birth settings is needed to inform continuous risk assessment and to guide decisions about which level of care a woman should receive (Institute of Medicine and National Research Council, 2013). Appropriate risk communication is also essential.

Such consideration and assessment to match women appropriately to the setting and care they need and desire, when carried out continuously and effectively, results in risk stratification across birth settings. That is, lower-risk women predominate in home and birth center settings, while higher-risk women are generally treated in hospital settings. However, in reality, women's options will be limited by the availability of different types of birth settings and maternity care providers within or near their community, including hospital resources and within-hospital options. Availability is particularly challenging in rural areas and in some inner cities. Also, a woman's choices are further limited by health insurance and Medicaid restrictions; economic circumstances; access to transportation; and cultural and linguistic factors, such as language barriers with providers and her perception of how she will be received and treated. In short, many nonclinical factors, such as where a woman lives, her opportunities for employment and education, her exposure to discrimination and stress, and her access to services, can influence the level of clinical risk she carries into pregnancy and childbirth. These social and environmental factors impact not only her health, but also the health and well-being of her child, both in the immediate postpartum period and for years to come. These system-level influences on access to and choice in birth settings are the focus of the next chapter.

4

Systemic Influences on Outcomes in Pregnancy and Childbirth

The individual-level risks discussed in the previous chapter are just one source of risk during pregnancy and childbirth. As shown in the committee's conceptual model (refer to Figure 1-7 in Chapter 1), systems-level factors can contribute to existing risk factors or create new ones, shaping quality, access, choice, and outcomes in birth settings. These factors include structural inequalities and biases, the social determinants of health, and financing and policy decisions in the health system. In this chapter, we explore these systems-level influences that confer risk during pregnancy and childbirth. First, we discuss the current landscape of inequity in maternal and neonatal outcomes and consider a birthing justice framework for understanding and ameliorating these disparities. Next, we explore the outermost circle of the model, the structural inequities and biases that contribute to disparities in outcomes along racial/ethnic, socioeconomic, and linguistic lines. We then move inward on the model to a discussion of the social determinants of health, which provides a framework for understanding the impact of upstream factors on individual health and risk. Finally, we consider the innermost circle and the role of policy and financing in the health system in patterning women's access to care and risk in pregnancy and childbirth. Our analyses lead to a series of conclusions, which are presented in the final section of the chapter.

INEQUITIES IN MATERNAL AND NEWBORN OUTCOMES

The United States has considerable and persistent racial/ethnic inequities in maternal and newborn outcomes (see Table 4-1; see also, e.g.,

Howell, 2018; Martin et al., 2018a). Across a number of risk and protective factors (e.g., maternal education, early initiation of prenatal care), Black, Hispanic, and American Indian/Alaska Native (AIAN) women fare worse than their non-Hispanic White and Asian counterparts (see Table 4-1). For example, 77.3 percent of White women and 81.1 percent of Asian women entered prenatal care in the first trimester, compared with 72.3 percent of Hispanic women, 66.6 percent of Black women, and 63.4 percent of AIAN women. Asian and White women are also more likely to have private insurance to cover their birth than are Black, Hispanic, and AIAN women. These disparities in protective factors are reflected in disparities in outcomes. Rates of preterm birth and low birthweight are higher among Black, AIAN, and Hispanic women than White women.[1] In the case of low birthweight, Black women are more than twice as likely to have a low-birthweight infant as White women (refer to Table 4-1). Most strikingly, rates of pregnancy-related mortality and infant mortality are substantially higher among Black women compared with White women. The disparity in the White–Black infant mortality rate has persisted for decades (David and Collins, 1997; Collins et al., 2002).

Breaking down these broad racial/ethnic categories into ethnic subgroups reveals further disparities. Among Hispanic women, Puerto Rican, Mexican, Central and South American, and Cuban women all have different levels of risk and protective factors. For example, 82.2 percent of Cuban women initiated prenatal care in the first trimester—a greater proportion than White and Asian women—while only 67.7 percent of Central and South American women did so. Similarly, the infant mortality rate among births to Cuban women is 4.0 in 1,000, compared with 6.5 in 1,000 for Puerto Rican women.

There are many factors that may contribute to these racial/ethnic disparities in maternal and infant health outcomes. One factor that we consider here is the concept of "weathering." Researchers have proposed that exposure to experiences of discrimination across the lifespan has the effect of "weathering" women of color, increasing their allostatic load,[2] and, ultimately, physiologically compromising their health and pregnancies (Geronimus et al., 2006; Holzman et al., 2009; Lu and Halfon, 2003). In light of these realities, a thoughtful discussion of risk and birth settings must be placed in the context of historical and present-day inequities that may contribute to risk and impede equitable access to birth settings for

---

[1] Asian women have higher rates of low birthweight but lower rates of preterm birth compared with White women.

[2] Allostatic load refers to the "dysregulation of the stress response process; it is the 'wear and tear' on the body that arises from chronic, prolonged or persistent activation of allostatic effectors and a breakdown of the regulatory feedback mechanisms" (Wallace and Harville, 2013, p. 1025).

women across lines of race, ethnicity, social class, education, country of origin, language, ability, and region.

The concept of reproductive justice provides a useful framework to shape the discussion of ethnicity, racism, and birth settings. The reproductive justice framework and movement were started by a group of 12 Black women to address major gaps in reproductive health and rights frameworks that failed to recognize and address the circumstances of women of color and other groups that have often been marginalized and oppressed (Ross, 2017). The reproductive justice framework describes reproductive rights as human rights (Ross and Solinger, 2017). The framework further defines reproductive rights as (1) the right to have children under the circumstances of one's choosing, (2) the right to not have children using the methods of one's choosing, and (3) the right to raise one's children in safe and healthy environments (Ross, 2017). In this way, it centers on access rather than individual choice (Sister Song, n.d.; Ross and Solinger, 2017).

The concept of birthing justice emerged to extend the reproductive justice framework to childbearing. Similar to reproductive justice overall, birthing justice starts from the position that the movement for birthing rights and care options has failed to recognize and address the circumstances of traditionally marginalized and underserved groups, which compound the childbearing challenges faced by more advantaged families (Oparah et al., 2018). Thus, birthing justice is predicated on the idea that while individual choice is necessary, it is not sufficient for just and equitable access and opportunity (Sister Song, n.d.). Research shows, for example, that home birth is on the rise among well-educated, wealthy, and White women (Boucher et al., 2009; MacDorman and Declercq, 2019). However, out-of-pocket costs or locale may put certain birth settings out of reach for socially or financially disadvantaged populations. In such an environment, a reproductive justice framework poses the question, "Do all women really have 'choice' of birth setting?" Accordingly, reproductive and birth justice platforms not only advocate for traditional reproductive and birth rights, but also provide a framework that focuses attention on the social, political, and economic inequalities among different communities that contribute to infringements of these rights and constrain choice (Oparah and Bonaparte, 2015).

The birthing justice framework and movement recognize that many disadvantaged women receive substandard maternal care. In particular, they note that the history and current reality of Black women's receipt of facility-based care in the United States includes lack of access, segregated wards, denial or delays in receiving needed care, biased treatment, and substandard care (Oparah and Bonaparte, 2015). Further, many women of color, women with disabilities, immigrant women, people of varied gender identities and sexual orientations, and other groups lack access to birth options, to quality

TABLE 4-1 Pregnancy and Birth Outcomes by Race, Ethnicity, and Hispanic Origin, 2017

Race and Hispanic Origin	All	Non-Hispanic White	African American/ Black	Alaskan Indian/ American Native	Asian
Demographic					
Age (years) of mother at first birth	26.8	27.6	24.9	23.3	30.3
Births to unmarried mothers (%)	39.8	28.5	69.5	69.1	11.8
Mother born in the 50 states or District of Columbia (%)	76.9	93.2	83.1	98.9	17.8
Maternal education (%)					
High school diploma or higher	86.7	92.8	86.1	78.0	93.2
Bachelor's degree or higher	32.3	41.8	17.3	8.4	64.2
Initiation of prenatal care (%)					
First trimester	77.3	82.4	66.6	63.4	81.1
Late or no prenatal care	6.3	4.5	10.2	12.6	5.1
Health insurance for delivery (%)					
Medicaid	43.0	30.5	65.9	67.3	25.0
Private insurance	49.1	63.1	27.7	19.5	65.2
Self-pay	4.1	3.0	3.0	1.8	6.8
Other	3.8	3.4	3.4	11.4	2.9
Infant birth outcomes (%)					
Preterm gestational age (<37 weeks)	9.9	9.1	13.9	11.9	8.5
Low/very low birthweight	9.7	8.1	16.8	9.7	9.7
Interventions					
Cesarean birth	32.0	30.9	36.0	28.5	33.2
Low-risk[a]	26.0	24.9	30.4	22.8	27.8
Induction of labor	25.7	28.9	23.9	26.7	20.5
Pregnancy-related mortality per 10,000 births	—	13.0	42.8	32.5	14.2
Infant mortality rate per 1,000 live births	5.8	4.7	11.0	9.2	3.8

[a]Low-risk cesarean birth rate is the number of singleton, term (37 weeks or more of gestation based on the obstetric estimate), cephalic cesarean deliveries to women having a first birth per 100 women with singleton, term, cephalic deliveries.
SOURCES: Martin et al. (2018b); Centers for Disease Control and Prevention (2019a); Ely and Driscoll (2019).

Native Hawaiian or Other Pacific Islander	Hispanic Origin					
	All Hispanic	Mexican	Puerto Rican	Cuban	Central/ South American	Other/ Unknown Hispanic
24.9	24.8	24.2	24.7	27.4	26.5	24.8
48.7	52.2	50.2	64.2	52.5	50.5	52.9
36.7	52.0	55.1	71.5	43.7	16.9	68.0
77.3	72.1	70.6	82.9	91.4	61.6	79.5
9.7	13.5	10.5	15.8	28.1	18.4	15.7
52.5	72.3	72.0	76.0	82.2	67.7	74.6
19.6	7.7	7.9	6.1	4.2	9.3	7.0
56.2	60.2	61.7	60.1	52.7	54.7	61.6
28.6	28.5	27.1	34.1	43.1	26.9	29.8
6.3	6.7	6.7	1.4	1.6	12.9	3.5
8.9	4.7	4.5	4.4	2.7	5.5	5.1
10.5	9.6	9.4	11.2	9.1	9.1	10.2
8.9	8.7	8.2	11.4	8.6	8.1	9.7
31.0	31.8	30.4	33.9	45.8	31.3	33.9
26.8	25.6	24.0	27.5	39.2	26.0	26.6
17.5	21.6	21.1	24.2	22.6	20.5	22.8
—	11.4	—	—	—	—	—
7.6	5.1	5.1	6.5	4.0	4.5	—

care, and to care well suited to their needs (Oparah and Bonaparte, 2015, p. 6; Howell et al., 2016; Prather et al., 2018).

In the following section, we consider the birthing justice framework of access with the reality of medical and obstetric risk factors, patterned by the social determinants of health.

STRUCTURAL INEQUITIES AND BIASES

In its conceptual model, the committee recognizes that structural inequities and biases are historically rooted and deeply embedded in policies, laws, governance, and culture, such that power and resources are distributed differentially across characteristics of identity (race, ethnicity, gender, class, sexual orientation, and others), all of which influence health outcomes. Thus, any discussion of risk assessment, choice, and equity in birth settings and birth outcomes must encompass the historical problem of disparate outcomes influenced by structural racism. Disparities and inequities in U.S. health care are well documented across a myriad of chronic medical conditions and mental health disorders (see, e.g., Braveman et al., 2005; Institute of Medicine, 2003). Racism and discrimination—both in the health care system and in everyday life—have a well-documented impact on the health of marginalized communities. The adverse impacts of racism can be manifested in lower-quality health care; residential segregation and lack of affordable housing; acts of state-inflicted violence, punitive policing, and mass incarceration; or the accumulation of daily stressors resulting from micro- and macro-level aggressions, unconscious and conscious bias, and discrimination. They can thereby influence the health outcomes of pregnant people and their infants, causing considerable racial/ethnic disparities in pregnancy-related outcomes (Dominguez et al., 2008).

Moreover, these disparities persist regardless of socioeconomic status (Collins and Hammond, 1996). For example, Black women in the United States had the greatest risk of pregnancy-related mortality from 2011 to 2015, with a mortality ratio of 42.8 per 100,000 live births, followed by AIAN women at 32.5 (Centers for Disease Control and Prevention, 2019a), while the ratio for non-Hispanic White women was 13.0. As discussed earlier in this chapter, non-Hispanic Black women have higher rates of preterm labor (13.9%), low/very low fetal birthweights (16.8%), and infant mortality (11 per 1,000 live births) compared with non-Hispanic White women (refer to Table 4-1). Neither material conditions nor adverse maternal and child outcomes by race and ethnicity have changed significantly over the past four decades (Zambrana et al., 1999). These disparities in outcomes likely arise through a number of mechanisms. Below, we detail inequitable treatment in the health care system, the health effects of racism and discrimination, inequitable allocation of resources, and racism as risk.

Inequitable Treatment in the Health Care System

In the health care system, racism frequently manifests in differences in care. Individuals from racial/ethnic minority groups and of lower socio-economic status tend to receive lower-quality health care than their White and high-status counterparts, even when issues of access are addressed (Agency for Health Research and Quality, 2018; Howell and Zeitlin, 2017; Fiscella and Sanders, 2016; Institute of Medicine, 2003; Anderson et al., 2003). This discrepancy has been documented throughout the health care system (Anderson et al., 2003), including in maternity care (McLemore et al., 2018; Braveman et al., 2010).

Over the past two decades, researchers have documented forms of disrespect and abuse in maternity care (Abuya et al., 2015; Okafor et al., 2015; Sando et al., 2016; Ishola et al., 2017). The term "obstetric violence" was introduced into the discourse on maternal experiences of birth in Latin America in the early 1990s, and was used to help shape discussions of disrespect and abuse within the larger frameworks of structural and gendered violence (Sadler et al., 2016). The term is intended to convey the assertion that the acts it denotes are inadequately captured by other terms such as "maternal dissatisfaction" or "negative birth experiences."

Until relatively recently, mistreatment during labor and birth was assumed to be a problem unique to the global south and/or low-resource systems. Today, however, it is better understood that various forms of disrespect and abuse can also occur in high-resource countries, including the United States, and that rates and types of mistreatment vary by birth setting and by maternal race/ethnicity (Childbirth Connection, 2013; see also Chapter 3). The Listening to Mothers III survey found, for example, that approximately one in five Black and Hispanic women experience mistreatment from hospital-based care providers due to their race, ethnicity, cultural background, and/or language. Compared with 8 percent of White mothers, 19 percent of Hispanic mothers and 21 percent of Black mothers reported poor treatment while hospitalized to give birth (Childbirth Connection, 2013, p. 5). In an article published in 2018, anthropologist Dana-Ain Davis analyzes the birth stories of Black women in the United States. Participants' narratives describe multiple forms of racism encountered over the course of care, leading Davis to argue that the term "obstetric racism" (as opposed to obstetric violence) better captures the particularities of Black women's experiences of prenatal, intrapartum, and postpartum care. Black women see obstetric racism as a threat to positive birth outcomes. In response, some attempt to mitigate their risk of obstetric racism by utilizing midwives and doulas and avoiding the hospital when home and birth center birth services are available (Davis, 2018).

In the hospital setting, racial/ethnic minority patients are reported to experience the most palpable discrimination and lack of clinical attention, and often face the worst clinical outcomes (Sperlich et al., 2017). Women of color have contributed their own stories of mistreatment, bias, and discrimination in the maternity care system. For example, in a recent survey of 2,700 women from a nonrepresentative sample, one-third of women of color who had given birth in a hospital setting reported being mistreated by staff, compared with fewer than one-sixth of White women (Vedam et al., 2019). Mistreatment ranged from violations of physical privacy to being threatened or refused treatment by birth attendants.

In addition to these types of blatant and intentional acts of discrimination, racism may impact the quality of care through implicit bias or poor cross-cultural communication, which itself is a form of bias and discrimination. The way providers perceive their patients' ability to manage pain is influenced by the patient's perceived race and ethnicity and gender, and physicians and other members of the care team may better understand and pick up on implicit cues from patients who share their racial and gender identities (Institute of Medicine, 2003). This could help explain the disparities in epidural use in the United States: White women have the highest rate of epidural use (68.6%), followed by Black women (62.1%), Asian women (61.8%), Native Hawaiian and Other Pacific Islander women (52.8%), Hispanic women (47.7%), and AIAN women (42.1%). Although medical researchers have interpreted differences in epidural use by ethnicity and perceived race as an issue of access, limited research has been performed on the tertiary factors that may contribute to these discrepancies, including patient–provider communication, perceived pain tolerance among members of minority groups, and increased pressure from physician recommendations around whether pain medication is needed (Morris and Schulman, 2014). Patient–provider trust may also play a role. The relationship between patients and providers is often mediated by provider attitudes regarding socioeconomic status, race, and ethnicity. Low-income women are less likely to develop patient–provider trust and communication, increasing the risk for adverse birth outcomes (Sheppard et al., 2004). Provider concordance may play a role as well. There is evidence to suggest that patients in racially concordant relationships are more satisfied with their care and communication (Cooper et al., 2003). However, because of the relative dearth of obstetricians and midwives of color, there is not a robust literature examining the impact of racial concordance on pregnancy care. This raises the critical need to diversify the maternity care workforce, which is discussed at greater length in Chapter 7.

Health Effects of Racism and Discrimination

Racism has also been hypothesized to impact pregnancy and birth outcomes through greater exposure to chronic stress (Giscombé and Lobel, 2005; Nuru-Jeter et al., 2008). Although chronic stress can cause health problems in people of all racial/ethnic backgrounds, racial/ethnic minority individuals may experience unique stressors, such as racial discrimination, or common stressors, such as economic adversity and trauma, at higher rates. For example, in addition to stress related to racial discrimination, low-income women of color may experience stress related to limited economic security, limited childcare availability, the cost of health services, inadequate family and social support, the need to continue working during pregnancy to support the family financially, and other psychological stressors, all of which contribute to negative health outcomes (Dominguez et al., 2008; Lobel et al., 1992; Hogue and Bremner, 2005). Further, the communal impact of mass incarceration, state-imposed violence, policing, and detainment on pregnancy outcomes remains unclear and warrants further research.

Such chronic stress can lead to greater wear and tear, or *weathering*, on the body and brain as environmental factors "get under the skin," a concept known as *allostatic load* (Geronimus, 2002; Seeman et al., 1997; McEwen and Seeman, 1999). As these daily stressors build up and allostatic load increases, cellular aging speeds up, heightening vulnerability to stress-related health conditions, such as diabetes (Alhusen et al., 2016; Rubin, 2016). The higher allostatic load caused by racism is hypothesized to degrade the reproductive health of people of color, making it more difficult for individuals to enter pregnancy healthy. In effect, chronically high levels of interpersonal and systemic discrimination and prejudice can adversely impact pregnancy morbidity, health behaviors, and childbirth outcomes of these target groups (Giurgescu and Misra, 2018; Provenzi et al., 2018; Lima et al., 2018). Evidence suggests that this reflects the embodiment of stress resulting from structural inequity and the physiologic response to systemic racism (see, e.g., Geronimus, 1992; Lobel et al., 1992; Domingez et al., 2008).

Inequitable Allocation of Resources

In addition to the daily stressors due to experiencing racism, the inequitable distribution of societal resources and attention may negatively impact a woman's chances of entering pregnancy and childbirth healthy. This inequitable distribution is the result of a long history of legal (and other) mistreatment of members of relevant social groups. Many women of color and with low incomes have limited education; lower health literacy and knowledge of birth options, including less access to shared decision making; and less access to quality resources such as housing, a living wage, employment, and social services. Thus these women experience the cumulative impact of multiple and chronic stressors. Racial discrimination can be one mechanism by which access to material resources and services that promote health, such as prenatal care, is reduced (National Academies of Sciences, Engineering, and Medicine, 2019). For example, AIAN, Native Hawaiian, and non-Hispanic Black women are least likely to receive prenatal care in the first trimester and most likely to receive late or no care compared with non-Hispanic White women. They are also most likely to rely on Medicaid as their principal source of payment for birth services, followed by Latina women (refer to Table 4-1).

Racism as Risk

As a result of inequitable treatment; chronic stressors, weathering, and intergenerational trauma; and inequitable distribution of resources, women of color enter into their reproductive lives, and ultimately their pregnancies, at risk for adverse pregnancy outcomes. The label "Black," for example, although a social construct and not a marker of genetic difference, has served as a risk factor for almost all poor obstetric outcomes, when in fact, it is racism, not race, that increases Black women's risk. While compounding social disadvantages with financial disadvantage means that low-income women of color face health challenges, it is critically important that membership in a specific perceived racial/ethnic group not be used to over-determine a given patient's risk assessment such that it alone constrains the birth setting or maternity care provider options made available. Thus while properly assessing medical risk and monitoring for medical and/or obstetric complications among women of color is critical, ethnicity or perception of race alone should not determine level of risk. In fact, there is evidence to suggest that socially and financially disadvantaged women may thrive in midwifery models of care across all birth settings (Raisler and Kennedy, 2005; Huynh, 2014; Hill et al., 2018; Hardeman et al., 2019). The woman-centered philosophy of care that characterizes these models affirms agency among women of color, and group prenatal care models offer needed social support. Thus these models likely mitigate the harmful impact of medical models that have historically failed to trust the competence and capabilities of women, particularly Black women, including the experiences of disregard and disrespect described by many Black women in traditional care (Huynh, 2014; Vedam et al., 2019; Yoder and Hardy, 2018; Davis, 2018).

The available evidence is inadequate to determine health outcomes among women of color associated with home and birth center births or with hospital births that follow the midwifery model of care. Until more data are available to guide policy, there may be important opportunities to integrate midwifery models of care and doulas (dedicated support persons for laboring women) for labor support into hospital-based delivery settings. Doing so would enable women of color, particularly those with elevated medical, social, or obstetric risk factors, to still garner the benefits of woman-centered midwifery models of care and labor support.

In summary, racism and racial discrimination, whether manifested in the health care system, through chronic stress, or in reduced access to services, has tangible impacts on the lives of women of color and their families, impacts that are seen in racial/ethnic disparities in adverse birth outcomes.

SOCIAL DETERMINANTS OF HEALTH

The medical and obstetrical risk factors discussed in Chapter 3 must be understood in the context of the social determinants of health, the "upstream factors that shape behavior and influence health" (National Academies of Sciences, Engineering, and Medicine, 2019, p. 81). The word "determinants" in this context should be interpreted as mutable influencing factors, factors that can be changed through social and economic actions. These upstream factors are related to social identity and structural inequity. A previous National Academies report, *Communities in Action: Pathways to Health Equity,* states:

> The dimensions of social identity and location that organize or "structure" differential access to opportunities for health include race and ethnicity, gender, employment and socioeconomic status, disability and immigration status, geography, and more. Structural inequities are the personal, interpersonal, institutional, and systemic drivers—such as, racism, sexism, classism, able-ism, xenophobia, and homophobia—that make those identities salient to the fair distribution of health opportunities and outcomes. Policies that foster inequities at all levels (from organization to community to county, state, and nation) are critical drivers of structural inequities. The social, environmental, economic, and cultural determinants of health are the terrain on which structural inequities produce health inequities. These multiple determinants are the conditions in which people live, including access to good food, water, and housing; the quality of schools, workplaces, and neighborhoods; and the composition of social networks and nature of social relations (National Academies of Sciences, Engineering, and Medicine, 2017, pp. 100–101).

When discussing the social determinants of health, it is important to consider a life-course perspective. The relationship between social factors and health is not one of a series of discrete steps, but rather an integrated continuum of exposures, experiences, and interactions over a lifetime

(Mullings and Wali, 2001; Fine and Kotelchuck, 2010; Braveman et al., 2005). In addition, using an intersectional community-driven lens helps explain the individual, community, environmental, and policy spheres influencing adverse health outcomes across populations and over time.

While there is a growing body of literature on the social, economic, and environmental determinants of health and their impacts on health outcomes, establishing causality is challenging because the evidence is often in the form of cross-sectional analyses, and the pathways to health outcomes are not always clearly delineated. This may be due, in part, to the complexity of the mechanisms involved and the long time periods required to observe outcomes (Braveman and Gottlieb, 2014; Braveman et al., 2011; Marmot et al., 2010; National Academies of Sciences, Engineering, and Medicine, 2017). That said, new methods and frameworks are emerging in the literature to better understand causality amidst complex exposures.

In pregnancy and childbirth, the social determinants of health may be reflected in a woman's knowledge of prenatal care (individual); the amount of support she receives from her family, friends, and community (social); experiences with racism and other social and environmental stressors (social); the way she is treated by her care provider (institutional); and the policies and practices of her insurer (systemic). The committee's approach to understanding the social determinants of health in maternity care is illustrated in its conceptual framework (Figure 1-7 in Chapter 1). The figure shows the social determinants—such as housing, transportation, and education—that influence experiences in the maternity care system for women and infants. It also illustrates how structural inequities and biases, such as institutional racism, underlie the social determinants of health for women from marginalized populations. Although the committee's conceptual framework focuses primarily on the prenatal and intrapartum periods, it is important to note that the social determinants of health affect women's well-being throughout their lives, not just during pregnancy and childbirth.

Of course, each level of influence may occur simultaneously and interact with other levels (National Research Council, 2006). The disadvantages that members of historically marginalized social groups confront in the contemporary United States are not isolated; rather, they tend to cluster and are intergenerational, impacting life-course social and economic opportunities and health outcomes. In other words, people who are at a disadvantage in terms of, for example, socioeconomic status are also at a disadvantage in terms of educational attainment, where they live, where they work, and where they play—all of which impact health outcomes. Furthermore, these disadvantages are not ahistorical; rather, they are part of a long history of legal (and other) mistreatment of members of the relevant social groups.

A vast literature documents a host of social determinants of health associated with poor pregnancy outcomes (Chisholm et al., 2017; Blumenshine et al., 2010; Lu and Halfon, 2003; Lobel et al., 1992; Collins et al., 1993). These social determinants impact a woman's health and the health and well-being of her child, possibly for years to come. We detail the specific influences of interpersonal relationships and social support, transportation, employment status, and housing below.

Interpersonal Relationships and Social Support

Intimate Partner Violence

Nationwide, an estimated 2 percent of U.S. women experience violence in a given year, and one in four women experience violence in their lifetime (Tjaden and Thoennes, 2000). Black women, low-income women, and young women (ages 20–34) are at the greatest risk of abuse from intimate partners (Aizer, 2011). Some studies suggest that violence may start or escalate during pregnancy or the postpartum period, with prevalence rates of intimate partner violence during pregnancy estimated to range from 3.9 to 8.3 percent (Brownridge et al., 2011).

Intimate partner violence both before and during pregnancy is associated with a host of negative maternal and infant outcomes, including maternal and fetal injury, elevated maternal stress, inadequate gestational weight gain and nutrition, substance use, and elevated risk of low-birthweight and preterm birth, among others (American College of Obstetricians and Gynecologists, 2012; Alhusen et al., 2015). The health effects of violence on pregnant women can be direct and immediate (such as injuries associated with blunt trauma to the maternal abdomen) and indirect and downstream (such as exacerbation of chronic illnesses and delayed initiation of prenatal care) (Alhusen et al., 2015). Assaults serious enough to require hospitalization during pregnancy are associated with an average decrease in birthweight of 163 grams (Aizer, 2011).

Women experiencing intimate partner violence during pregnancy need additional support from their health care providers and referrals to community resources (American College of Obstetricians and Gynecologists, 2012). Moreover, having a trusting relationship with care providers during pregnancy may mitigate the adverse effects of violence for both the woman and her infant (Alhusen et al., 2015). Accordingly, women who experience intimate partner violence may be better served in birth settings that allow for greater relationship building between providers and the women they serve.

Moreover, the experience of violence or trauma earlier in life can impact the health of women during pregnancy. Posttraumatic stress disorder, a manifestation of previous traumatic stress, has been associated with increased odds of low birthweight, preterm birth, and pregnancy complications (Seng et al., 2001, 2011; Sperlich et al., 2017). Women with trauma histories and their partners may benefit from trauma-informed approaches to maternity care (Sperlich et al., 2017).

Social Support

The support of family, partners, friends, and systems during pregnancy and childbirth is associated with a host of positive maternal and infant health outcomes. Providing social support during pregnancy to women who need it may reduce the risk of such adverse birth outcomes as preterm birth, low birthweight, and postpartum depression (Collins et al., 1993). A recent Cochrane review found that programs offering additional social support to women at risk of having a low-birthweight infant reduced the risk of hospitalization during pregnancy and cesarean birth. Such programs also slightly reduced the risk of low birthweight and preterm birth among at-risk women (East et al., 2019).

One of the most typical sources of social support during pregnancy is partners, friends, and family members. Among family members, female relatives such as mothers, grandmothers, and sisters can provide needed material and emotional support. However, for some, these sources of support may be disrupted by larger societal trends, such as the rise of mass incarceration. Over the past 50 years, incarceration in the United States has increased on a large scale, and the effects have been felt most acutely in low-income Black and Latino communities (National Research Council, 2014). Women from communities with high rates of incarceration may lose access to important sources of social and material support during pregnancy if they or their loved ones are incarcerated. In an analysis of data from the Pregnancy Risk Assessment Monitoring System (PRAMS), Wildeman (2012) found that having an incarcerated father substantially increased the odds of infant mortality for his offspring, although this relationship was modified by whether the parent was abusive (see the above section on intimate partner violence for a more detailed discussion of the effect of violence on pregnancy outcomes). Another analysis of PRAMS data, conducted by Dumont and colleagues (2014), found that women who had an incarcerated partner or were incarcerated themselves in the year prior to birth were less likely to begin prenatal care in the first trimester or receive at least nine prenatal visits and were more likely to experience stressful events (e.g., homelessness or job loss). In short, women who experience incarceration are at greater social risk, which can translate to greater clinical risk for themselves and their infants.

For women with greater social risk, providing sources of support, whether through a doula, a community health worker, friends, family members, or a group prenatal care model, may be an effective intervention, regardless of setting. Providing low-income women with doulas has been shown to contribute to positive health outcomes, improved patient–provider relationships, improved adherence to medical advice, and increased satisfaction (Wint et al., 2019; Hardeman and Kozhimannil, 2016). One program in New York City pairs low-income Black and Latina women with a certified doula (Thomas et al., 2017). In addition to providing direct labor support during the intrapartum period, the doulas provide case management services (e.g., screening for depression, food insecurity, and intimate partner violence and making referrals to services when necessary) and prenatal education over the course of seven home visits (three prenatal and four postpartum). Women who received these enhanced doula services had lower rates of preterm birth and low birthweight compared with women in the same neighborhood who did not receive those services (Thomas et al., 2017). (See Chapter 5 for additional discussion of outcomes and doula services.)

Community health workers can also serve as a source of social support as well as outreach, education, and informal counseling for pregnant people (American Public Health Association, 2019). In the Safe Start program in Philadelphia, for example, community health workers engaged pregnant women with high clinical risk factors in care navigation. Women in the program had substantially lower odds of inadequate prenatal care, inpatient admission, and emergency room visits, and higher odds of attending their postpartum visit and using contraception postpartum (Srinivas et al., 2019). In addition, group prenatal care models, such as CenteringPregnancy, have been shown to reduce stress and psychosocial risk factors among women with the highest levels of self-rated stress (Ickovics et al., 2011).

Transportation

For decades, transportation has been identified as a potential barrier to accessing prenatal care, especially for low-income and rural women (Institute of Medicine, 1985, 1988). When transportation is limited, unavailable, unaffordable, or difficult to use, women have greater difficulty accessing prenatal care (Heaman et al., 2015). For women in rural areas, the time and distance needed to travel to prenatal care visits may be challenging, particularly if women need to access specialty care in urban areas far from home (Leighton et al., 2019). In urban areas, transportation challenges such as traffic congestion, accessibility of public transit, and ease of using public transit while pregnant or with small children may also create barriers to accessing prenatal care (Heaman et al., 2015; Institute of Medicine, 1988). Disruptions to public transit service may create accessibility challenges as well. For example, in spring 1992, the drivers of the public transit system serving Allegheny County, Pennsylvania, engaged in a 4-week labor strike, causing severe service disruptions (Evans and Lien, 2005). During this time, researchers documented a decrease in the number of prenatal care visits among pregnant women in the area. Women who relied most heavily on public transportation—city residents and Black women—had the greatest reduction in prenatal visits. Among these women, researchers identified lower average birthweights, shorter gestations, and higher rates of smoking during pregnancy (Evans and Lien, 2005).

However, transportation, like the other social determinants of health, is modifiable. Programs that aim to provide available, reliable, and affordable transportation to pregnant people show some promise in increasing use of prenatal care. In a novel pilot program in Columbus, Ohio, pregnant women and new mothers can request on-demand transportation to health clinics, grocery stores, and other important locations using a mobile application similar to popular ridesharing services (The City of Columbus, 2019).

Employment Status

Among social determinants, the workplace and related social policies play a major role in maternal well-being and ability to care for infants (National Partnership for Women & Families, 2018a), as well as reproductive health at a population level. During adolescence, for example, having access to positive educational, social, and employment opportunities can promote healthy growth and development (National Academies of Sciences, Engineering, and Medicine, 2019). These opportunities can also help prevent pregnancy and childbearing during the teenage years (Romero et al., 2016). Although teen pregnancy rates have decreased substantially since the 1990s, rates remain high for youth of color, who are more likely to live in communities with limited educational and employment opportunities, a key social determinant of teenage pregnancy (Romero et al., 2016; National Academies of Sciences, Engineering, and Medicine, 2019).

Specific to pregnancy and childbirth, access to paid parental leave and paid sick days promotes maternal and infant health during pregnancy and through early life. While such access is slowly expanding in the United States (National Partnership for Women & Families, 2018b), it is not available to a large segment of the workforce (Bureau of Labor Statistics, 2019).

In addition, access to workplace protections and exposure to harmful occupational situations is unevenly distributed in the United States, with low-wage, part-time, shift, and self-employed workers, among whom Black women are disproportionately represented, being much less likely to have workplace protections and benefits compared with their more advantaged counterparts (National Partnership for Women & Families, 2018c; Office of the Assistant Secretary for Planning and Evaluation, 2014; Presser,

2003). Indeed, rotating shift work, night shift work, and long work hours themselves pose pregnancy risks (Cai et al., 2019). Moreover, economic security is an important contributor to health and well-being, especially during pregnancy, and women in general experience lower pay relative to their male counterparts, with women of color shouldering greater burdens than White women (National Partnership for Women & Families, 2019a).

Housing

Housing, which includes "the availability or lack of availability of high-quality, safe, and affordable housing for residents of varying income levels," as well as the environments that surround it, has been widely recognized as a social determinant of health (National Academies of Sciences, Engineering, and Medicine, 2017, p. 140). Stable, affordable housing is hypothesized to affect health through several possible mechanisms, including freeing up family resources to afford health expenditures or nutritious food, reducing the stress associated with unstable housing, and improving the safety and quality of the indoor environment, among others (Maqbool et al., 2015). In the United States, access to stable, affordable, and safe housing has historically been limited for African Americans and other racial/ethnic minority groups by discriminatory practices. Housing instability has no one definition but is thought to encompass having difficulty paying housing costs, spending greater than 50 percent of household income on housing, frequent moves, overcrowding, or living temporarily with relatives or friends (Kushel et al., 2006). One estimate places the prevalence of homelessness among pregnant women at 4 percent nationwide, based on data from the PRAMS (Richards et al., 2011).

In studies of reproductive-age women, homelessness and housing instability have been associated with adverse neonatal outcomes. In one study of 613 low-income pregnant women and teenage girls receiving prenatal care in New York City, housing instability was independently associated with low birthweight, even after controlling for clinical, behavioral, and demographic factors (Carrion, 2015).

Other studies of pregnant women who experienced homelessness show a relationship between maternal homelessness and maternal and infant health outcomes. Richards and colleagues (2011), using data from the PRAMS, found that women experiencing homelessness, as compared with women with stable housing, were significantly less likely to receive prenatal care in the first trimester or receive a well-baby checkup. Moreover, the infants of women experiencing homelessness had significantly longer hospital stays and lower birthweights compared with those women with stable housing. A study of nearly 4,000 women experiencing homelessness in Toronto, Canada, found that women who experienced homelessness had an almost three times greater risk of preterm birth and an almost seven times greater risk of low birthweight (Little et al., 2005). The authors note that these increased risks occurred within a setting where health care is universally available (Little et al., 2005).

Housing may affect the health of pregnant women and their offspring through several mechanisms. Pregnant women experiencing homelessness face substantial barriers to prenatal care (Bloom et al., 2004) and adequate nutrition (Little et al., 2005), both of which may contribute to adverse birth outcomes. In addition, the stress associated with homelessness and housing instability has been associated with a greater risk of low birth-weight and preterm birth (Dunkel-Schetter and Tanner, 2012). The external environment or neighborhood surrounding housing can also impact pregnant people's health (National Academies of Sciences, Engineering, and Medicine, 2017). For example, the neighborhood food environment, which refers to "the availability of food venues such as supermarkets, grocery stores, corner stores, and farmer's markets, including food quality and affordability," can support a person's ability to afford and maintain a healthy diet (National Academies of Sciences, Engineering, and Medicine, 2017, p. 145). Given the importance of nutrition during pregnancy for both maternal and child health, programs and interventions to support women's access to nutritious food, such as the Special Supplemental Nutrition Program for Women, Infants, and Children, can positively impact birth outcomes (National Academies of Sciences, Engineering, and Medicine, 2019).

HEALTH SYSTEM: POLICY AND FINANCING

Operating within the context of structural inequities and biases and social determinants of health is the health system. In this section, we explore the innermost circle of our conceptual model, the health system, and its role in the patterns of women's risk in pregnancy and childbirth. The health system, writ large, includes the geographic distribution of the health care workforce; the certification, licensure, and scope of practice of that workforce; the financing of maternity care services; and the resultant access to services for the population. In maternity care, these features of the health system can contribute to a woman's risk profile in pregnancy and birth. We discuss these features of the health care system in detail below.

Geography and Workforce Distribution

Notable disparities in maternal health by geography persist in the United States. For example, women living in rural communities have greater risks of such poor outcomes as preterm birth and maternal and infant mortality, likely because of lack of access to maternity and prenatal care in their local areas (Grzybowski et al., 2011). These statistics are especially troubling considering that 15 percent of U.S. births are to women living in rural communities (Kozhimannil, 2014).

One driver of the disparities in maternal and neonatal health by geography in the United States is likely the uneven distribution of maternity care facilities and providers throughout the country, which leaves many women without access to prenatal and postpartum care, and without birthing options near home. Many rural—and even some urban—areas lack maternity care providers and hospitals with maternity units. A "maternity care desert," as defined by the March of Dimes, is a county in which maternity care services are limited or absent because of either a lack of services or barriers to a woman's ability to access those services (March of Dimes, 2018a). Women living in these counties have limited access to appropriate preventive, prenatal, and postpartum care. All told, as many as 5 million women live in these maternity care deserts. Figure 4-1 shows the number of hospitals with maternity units by U.S. county.

Closures of hospitals in rural and underserved urban areas may also contribute to disparities in outcomes by geography. These closures are the result of a confluence of factors, including the complex fixed and variable

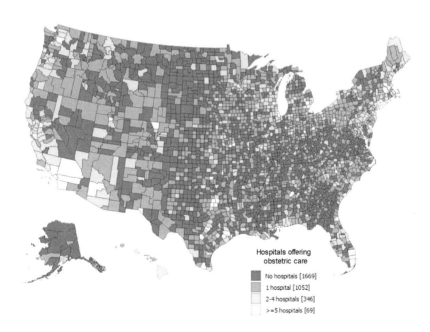

FIGURE 4-1 Access to hospitals offering obstetric care by county, United States, 2016.
SOURCE: March of Dimes (2018a).

costs associated with labor and delivery units, compounded by low patient volumes and low Medicaid reimbursement levels (Hung et al., 2016).

Rural areas have been losing hospitals steadily, with 179 hospitals in rural counties closing between 2004 and 2014. When rural counties are not adjacent to urban areas, the consequences of these closures are clear: an increase in unattended out-of-hospital births, preterm births, and births in hospitals without maternity units (Kozhimannil et al., 2018a). From 2004 to 2014, the total percentage of rural counties in the United States with hospital-based maternity care services declined from 55 percent to 46 percent (Kozhimannil et al., 2018a). All counties experiencing closures of hospital-based maternity units saw significant increases in the number of births occurring in hospitals without a maternity unit. In addition, closures of hospital maternity care units in urban underserved communities often result from high costs and economic pressures. In 2017, for example, the only two maternity care units on the east side of Washington, DC, closed their doors, leaving the predominantly Black and largely low-income population, with limited public transportation services, to find care elsewhere (Itkowitz, 2017). Moreover, hospital closures appear to be associated with decreased use of outpatient prenatal care services, suggesting that when hospitals leave, local prenatal care services follow (Kozhimannil et al., 2018a; Shah, 2018). The lack of access to prenatal care services may be one reason why initiation of prenatal care tends to be later among rural than urban women (American College of Obstetricians and Gynecologists, 2014). Delayed prenatal care has been associated with greater risk of preterm birth, which is of particular concern in rural areas, where the nearest hospital with a neonatal intensive care unit may be hours away (Shah, 2018).

In addition to the lack of available birthing facilities in certain regions of the country, both rural and urban areas are affected by the maldistribution of maternity care providers (see Figure 4-2). In 2016, almost one-half of all counties in the United States were without an obstetrician, and 40 percent had neither an obstetrician nor a certified nurse midwife, largely because they lacked hospitals with maternity services (March of Dimes, 2018a).

Of greatest concern is the relationship between inadequate access to care and the observed increased rates of prematurity following service closures in the more geographically isolated counties. Even after adjusting for maternal age, race/ethnicity, education, and common clinical conditions at the county level, a significant association with increased prematurity remains, with a 0.67 percentage point (95% confidence interval [CI], 0.02–1.33) increase in the year after closure (Kozhimannil et al., 2018a). Particularly concerning is the reduced access to prenatal care among birthing families in the period following service closure. Studies of workforce density have shown that rural counties without hospital obstetric services

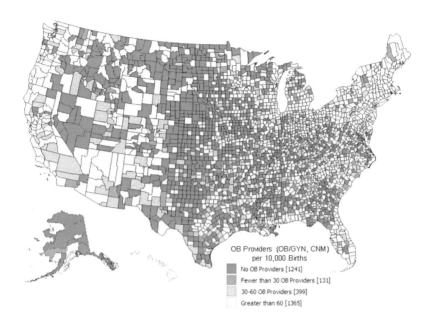

FIGURE 4-2 Distribution of obstetric providers by U.S. county.
SOURCE: March of Dimes (2018a).

are also likely to lack an obstetric workforce, including obstetricians, midwives, and family practice physicians (American College of Obstetricians and Gynecologists, 2014).

Some programs have attempted to address the challenge of providing prenatal care services in rural areas by adapting existing models to suit rural settings. For example, providers of the CenteringPregnancy group prenatal care model in South Carolina found that the program had difficulty engaging and retaining women from rural parts of the state (Centers for Medicare & Medicaid Services, 2019). In response, the program implementers adjusted the CenteringPregnancy model to increase its sustainability among rural programs, which see a lower volume of pregnant women. Program implementers also sought grant funding to support free technical assistance for programs in rural areas. Participants in the program, including rural women, have reduced rates of preterm birth, low birthweight, cesarean sections, and gestational diabetes (Centers for Medicare & Medicaid Services, 2019).

Other systems attempt to address geographic challenges by bringing women to maternity care services. Alaska, for example, has the highest proportion of out-of-hospital births in the country (out-of-hospital births make up 7.9% of all births, compared with 1.6% of births nationwide). Of these births, 5.6 percent occur in birth centers, while 1.9 percent occur in homes. Although the vast majority of births in Alaska are to women living in urban areas, such as Anchorage and Fairbanks, about one-fifth of births are to women who reside outside of these population centers (Alaska Department of Health and Social Services, 2019). If these women have complicated pregnancies or live in remote areas that lack any birthing facilities, they must travel—often long distances—to reach hospitals and specialists equipped to care for them and their newborns (Association of State and Territorial Health Officials, 2015).

Alaska's perinatal regionalization system attempts to address the state's geographic challenge by transporting women to settings with appropriate care. In remote areas, healthy women leave their home communities between 34 and 36 weeks of pregnancy to deliver safely at a regional medical center. Women with more urgent needs for care may travel by ambulance, helicopter, or fixed-wing aircraft to reach appropriate care, and are accompanied by a perinatal transport team that consists of a neonatal nurse practitioner and a registered nurse (Association of State and Territorial Health Officials, 2015). Women who require ongoing treatment from perinatal and neonatal specialists may be transferred by air ambulance to Anchorage, or may move there early in their pregnancy to receive care (Association of State and Territorial Health Officials, 2015). Although this system is successful in bringing women to needed care, it can impose psychosocial and cultural costs on women. For example, Indigenous women may highly value giving birth on their ancestral lands and dislike having to leave their home communities to give birth (Kornelsen et al., 2010; see also the Chapter 3 discussion of preferences in birth setting).

Solutions for addressing the challenges of the women's health care workforce have been proposed. Increasing the number of advanced practice providers working in maternity care is a common recommendation across multiple sources. For example, the American College of Obstetricians and Gynecologists (ACOG) estimates that having nurse practitioners, certified nurse midwives, and physician assistants join OB/GYN practices would meet the demands of women in the future (Rayburn, 2017). Moreover, it may be beneficial to create models that expand family physicians' participation in maternity care and provision of laborist care within hospital and micro-hospital settings, as well as provide midwifery care for low-risk women in home and birth center settings (Avery et al., 2018).

Another potential solution is to increase the number of midwives and freestanding birth centers in rural areas, thereby lowering costs while providing quality care (Centers for Medicare & Medicaid Services, 2019). Rural areas that have experienced the closure of hospital maternity units have had increased out-of-hospital births and births in hospitals without maternity care units (Kozhimannil et al., 2018a). Collaboration between rural home/birth center providers and local hospitals is critical so that coordinated and seamless transfers can occur when necessary. In addition, family physicians play an important role in providing health care in rural areas (Goldstein et al., 2018), including providing the majority of hospital-based maternity care services in those areas (Young, 2017). Despite their importance to rural communities, however, family physicians may face challenges in obtaining hospital privileges to perform cesarean births and building collaborative relationships with other maternity care providers (Eden and Peterson, 2018). Moreover, rural hospital closures may limit their ability to provide full-scope maternity care services.

There is also concern over the lack of diversity in the maternity care workforce. ACOG found in 2017 that 58.7 percent of obstetricians were female, and the majority of them were White, while Black and Hispanic obstetricians currently in the workforce were underrepresented relative to the general population (Rayburn, 2017). This finding reflects the lack of diversity within the maternity care workforce as a whole. For example, 61 percent of all nurse practitioners are non-Hispanic White, as are more than 80 percent of certified nurse midwives in California (Spetz et al., 2018). Limited data on the demographic distribution of licensed doulas are available, but it is widely acknowledged that this profession is disproportionately represented by White women (Lantz et al., 2005). The lack of physicians, nurses, and allied health professionals of color is a long-standing workforce issue in maternity care and health care generally (Xue and Brewer, 2014).

Workforce Certification, Licensure, and Scope of Practice

In addition to the workforce distribution issues discussed above, recent analyses have identified concerns about the supply of maternity care providers—specifically obstetricians—available to meet demand in the United States. Although obstetricians are just one type of provider of maternity care in the United States, they are the focus of the majority of data collected on maternity care providers. Accordingly, the gap in the obstetrician workforce is the most available means of estimating the projected gaps in maternity care providers as a whole. A 2016 report from the National Center for Health Workforce Analysis highlights the future of providers of women's health services, noting that the numbers of both obstetricians and family physicians in the United States are declining. Factors contributing to this decline include early retirement from obstetrics, changing practice patterns (e.g., part-time practices), growing subspecialization, and the increasing value placed on work–life balance (Rayburn, 2017). According to the Health Resources and Services Administration's (HRSA's) Health Workforce Simulation Model (2016), the number of obstetricians is expected to decrease by about 4 percent (from 41,720 to 40,230 full-time equivalents [FTEs]), while total demand is expected to increase by 8 percent (from 41,720 to 45,160 FTEs), based on the assumption that the current rates of retirement and workforce participation will hold over the next decade. Notably, ACOG similarly anticipates large numbers of retirements given that in 2009, on average, male OB/GYNs retired from the obstetrics portion of their practice at age 52 and female OB/GYNs at age 44. Retirements may also be prompted by financial and work–life balance concerns within the workforce (Rayburn, 2017). Additionally, the number of family physicians providing maternity care has declined. The proportion of U.S. family physicians reporting providing maternity care declined from 23.3 percent in 2000 to 9.7 percent in 2010, and those who reported providing such care spent an average (aggregated over 2000 to 2010) of 10 percent of their time doing so (Tong et al., 2012).

Given these trends, the United States will increasingly need to rely on other advanced practice providers for maternal health services, including certified nurse midwives, certified midwives, certified professional midwives, physician assistants, and women's health nurse practitioners. Although evidence on certified midwives and certified professional midwives is more limited, their skills are needed to close the workforce shortages that the United States faces. However, an important barrier exists to increasing the supply of those providers with respect to their ability to be credentialed in some jurisdictions and have practice privileges in some facilities. As noted in Chapter 2, states are responsible for licensing health care professionals and for dictating where they can practice, what services they can provide, and whether they are required to be supervised. The wide variation in regulation, certification, and licensing for nonphysician providers across the United States impedes access to high-quality maternal care for all women, as these providers could prove invaluable in addressing workforce shortages and the maldistribution of other providers if the health care system facilitated their growth and practice. For example, if certified nurse midwives and nurse practitioners were permitted to practice to the full extent of their education and training in all jurisdictions, they could greatly alleviate the shortage of maternity care providers, and could improve access to care for women across the country (see, e.g., Institute of Medicine, 2011; Buerhaus, 2018).

Further limiting access is that not all states license birth centers. Currently, this is the case in nine states (see Figure 4-3). Licensing statutes in those states that have them are generally written with great specificity, designed to ensure that planned births in birth centers are limited, to the extent feasible, to healthy, low-risk women, and that midwives provide care that keeps their clients healthy and continually assess and identify problems early so they can be properly and promptly addressed (American Public Health Association, 1982).

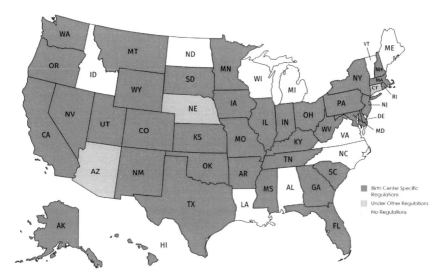

FIGURE 4-3 Birth center licensure and regulation in the United States, by state.
SOURCE: American Association of Birth Centers (2019). Used with permission of the American Association of Birth Centers. Created with Mapchart.net.

Maternity Care Financing

As discussed in Chapter 2, sources of financing for maternity care may include commercial insurance (with some out-of-pocket costs), Medicaid, and self-payment, among others. The type of financing strongly influences a woman's choice of care provider and her access to various types of care. Women covered by Medicaid, a program designed to support low-income individuals, are particularly constrained by financing, as they are unlikely to have the resources to pay for care unless it is covered under the Medicaid program. While women with private insurance may, in theory, have additional options, many are often constrained by the types of providers and settings that are reimbursed under their plans and similarly may be unable to pay for services that are not covered.

Thus a woman's choice of and access to providers and facilities are largely dependent on whether and how her care is financed and the type of coverage she has. Most women with private insurance choose providers and facilities that are covered by their plans, and women with Medicaid use providers who accept Medicaid (Holgash and Heberlein, 2019). In both Medicaid and private insurance, there is variation in what maternity care services are covered and to what extent (Kaiser Family Foundation, 2017, 2007). Timing of entry into prenatal care is also influenced by financing. Medicaid eligibility is dependent on whether a state has expanded Medicaid and whether it has "presumptive" Medicaid. If a state has expanded Medicaid, women with low incomes may already have coverage before pregnancy and may continue to have coverage afterward. If a woman relies on pregnancy-related Medicaid, she cannot receive coverage until after she is pregnant, may experience a delay in access to services if her state does not have presumptive eligibility, and may lose her coverage 2 months after giving birth. If a woman is uninsured and applies for Medicaid or if the state lacks a presumptive eligibility policy, it may take 45 days for Medicaid to go into full effect, which can delay entry into prenatal care. Among policy proposals to strengthen childbearing women's access to health care are legislative provisions to expand access to Medicaid to a full year after birth and to make pregnancy a special enrollment period when a woman can buy into marketplace insurance coverage outside of the annual enrollment period.

Payment is also an issue with respect to incentives for more intervention. For example, Medicaid and other payers generally reimburse hospitals at a higher level for cesareans, although some states (e.g., Minnesota) have leveled vaginal and cesarean provider payment. In addition, payment, especially by Medicaid, may not cover the facility fee for birth, so that home and birth center settings, unable to cover their marginal costs, are unable to accept a large proportion of Medicaid patients. This is the case despite documented cost savings and reduction in preterm birth, among other benefits for Medicaid beneficiaries in birth centers, in comparison with similar women receiving maternity care in typical Medicaid care settings (Hill et al., 2018) and for home versus hospital birth overall (Wax et al., 2010). Moreover, the lowest-reimbursed providers are often those outside of a hospital—in birth centers and home birth settings attended by midwives, whose model of care is among the most labor-intensive (see Chapter 2).

Access to Prenatal and Birth Care

Timely and appropriate prenatal care is important for supporting the health of women and their offspring during pregnancy and at birth. By engaging women early in pregnancy, providers are able to conduct screenings; assess risks; and provide psychosocial, cultural, and educational support to women and their families, with the objective of improving health for women and their babies. While a causal relationship has not been established (Gadson et al., 2017), delayed entry into prenatal care and/or underutilization of these services has been associated with several adverse maternal and neonatal outcomes, including maternal mortality, preterm birth, and low birthweight (Moaddab et al., 2018). Thus, access to affordable, culturally appropriate prenatal care is an important component of the maternity care system. In addition, the cultural competence of care needs to be considered. A recent report from the National Academies, *Vibrant and Healthy Kids*, calls for providing prenatal care and education services that are culturally and linguistically appropriate to promote uptake (National Academies of Sciences, Engineering, and Medicine, 2019).

For some women, access to prenatal care is limited. Black women, AIAN women, women of low socioeconomic status, rural women, and immigrant women all face systemic barriers to accessing early and adequate prenatal care (see Table 4-1 presented earlier; see Box 4-1 for discussion of the challenges to accessing materity care among immigrant women). These barriers include lack of available services, lack of insurance coverage or funds to cover prenatal care visits, and experiences of racism in the health care system, among others (Slaughter-Acey et al., 2019; Swartz et al., 2017; Gadson et al., 2017; Mazul et al., 2017). As discussed earlier in this chapter, other social determinants of health, such as transportation and lack of social support, can also create barriers to accessing prenatal care (Mazul et al., 2017; Heaman et al., 2015).

BOX 4-1
Maternal Health among Immigrant Women

The foreign-born population of the United States is a diverse group, including naturalized U.S. citizens, permanent residents, temporary migrants (e.g., foreign students), unauthorized migrants, and humanitarian migrants (e.g., refugees and asylees) (U.S. Census Bureau, 2019). Today, about 17 percent of U.S. women of childbearing age are foreign-born (U.S. Census Bureau, 2018), and nearly a quarter of U.S. births in 2014 were to foreign-born women (Livingston, 2016). Among foreign-born women, the birth rate per 1,000 women is 84.2, compared with 58.3 among U.S.-born women (Livingston, 2016). While just over 50 percent of native-born U.S. women are mothers, mothers represent 71 percent of foreign-born women (U.S. Census Bureau, 2017).

Given their higher fertility rate, foreign-born women are an important population for maternity care and other services. However, immigrant women may face barriers to accessing public services. The Personal Responsibility and Work Opportunity Reconciliation Act of 1996 (PRWORA)—also known as welfare reform—imposed restrictions on authorized immigrants' access to public programs, including the Supplemental Nutrition Assistance Program (SNAP), Temporary Assistance for Needy Families, and Medicaid (National Academies of Sciences, Engineering, and Medicine, 2019). Although the restrictions on pregnant women's and immigrant children's access to Medicaid have since been removed (National Immigration Law Center, 2010), barriers remain for access to

continued

BOX 4-1 Continued

other public services. Moreover, unauthorized immigrants are not permitted to use public services such as Medicaid or SNAP.

In addition to restrictions on their access to public services in some states, foreign-born women may face exposure to violence and stress due to their immigration status and racial/ethnic identity. An analysis of birth outcomes among native-born White women and Latina foreign- and native-born women before and after a large-scale immigration raid in Pottsville, Iowa, for example, found that foreign-born women had higher risk of low birthweight in the aftermath of the raid, while the risk remained the same for domestic-born White women (Novak et al., 2017).

Foreign-born women in the United States are an underserved group in prenatal care (Acevedo-Garcia and Stone, 2008; Fuentes-Afflick et al., 2006). Immigrant and refugee women are less likely to initiate prenatal care as early as their native-born counterparts, even in situations where health care coverage is universal (Kentoffio et al., 2016). This suggests that immigrant women face barriers to accessing care beyond insurance coverage. Rather, cultural barriers, such as a lack of culturally sensitive care, combined with linguistic barriers and discrimination in the health care system, also play a role in limiting immigrant women's access to care (Kentoffio et al., 2016; United Nations Population Fund, 2006). For refugee women in particular, lack of interpretation services, mistrust of the health care system, and limited social and financial support for accessing health care services may create additional barriers (United States Committee for Refugees and Immigrants, n.d.).

Despite these barriers, some studies have shown that foreign-born status can have a protective effect against adverse birth outcomes among Latinx and Black immigrant women (Giuntella, 2016; Acevedo-Garcia et al., 2007). For instance, using linked birth certificate data, Giuntella (2016) found that infants born to Latina immigrant women had a lower incidence of low birthweight and higher average weight at birth compared with infants born to U.S.-born White women in two U.S. states, a phenomenon that has been replicated in other studies of immigrants (Ramraj et al., 2015). However, Giuntella also found substantial differences by the woman's country of origin. Babies born to mothers of Mexican and Cuban origin had a lower incidence of low birthweight compared with U.S.-born White women, while the incidence was higher among babies born to Puerto Rican women. Moreover, Giuntella showed that this protective effect diminishes over time, with subsequent generations of Latinx immigrants having a greater risk of low birthweight relative to their U.S.-born counterparts (Giuntella, 2016).

Enhanced prenatal care services, such as those tested in the Strong Start for Mothers and Newborns initiative, may be one method for increasing access to prenatal care and reducing disparities in birth outcomes. Box 4-2 provides a detailed description of the Strong Start initiative and recent outcomes.

BOX 4-2
Strong Start for Mothers and Newborns Initiative

The Strong Start for Mothers and Newborns initiative was designed to compare three models of enhanced prenatal care to determine whether, and if so to what extent, these models affect preterm birth rates and other poor maternity care outcomes (Hill et al., 2018). The program engaged 27 awardees and 211 provider sites across 32 states, which were selected through an application process. Almost 46,000 women selected the site and model of prenatal care of their choice: (1) centering or group prenatal care; (2) maternity health home care; and (3) midwife-led, freestanding birth center care. The national evaluation of Strong Start was a rigorous, multifaceted effort that included case studies, focus groups, client surveys, and clinical data. Outcome data were then linked with Medicaid claims data to examine and compare costs associated with the three care models from pregnancy through the first year of the newborn's life.

Strong Start participants were Medicaid or Children's Health Insurance Program (CHIP) beneficiaries. The birth center sample captured more diversity relative to previous birth center study populations, with 12 percent Black and 23 percent Hispanic/Latina; lower education levels; and higher rates of medical and social risk factors, such as depression, anxiety, tobacco use, and obesity (Alliman et al., 2019). Nevertheless, the birth center group had lower rates of psychosocial risk and fewer medical factors than participants in the other two care model groups. Logistic regression and risk reduction analyses attempting to control for these baseline differences showed that the birth center group had reduced rates of preterm birth and low birthweight and decreased racial/ethnic disparities compared with national rates. For preterm birth (defined in the program evaluation as any birth at less than 37 weeks gestation) in the birth center care group, rates were similar among Black (5%), Hispanic/Latina (5%), and White (4%) participants, while rates of low birthweight (defined as neonatal birthweight less than 2,500 grams) were lower than national rates but more disparate for Black (6%), Hispanic/Latina (4%), and White (3%) participants (Hill et al., 2018). For the same time period in the United States as a whole, preterm birth rates varied significantly by race for Black (13.8%), Hispanic/Latina (9%), and White (9%) participants. Disparities for low-birthweight births in the United States showed similar patterns for Black (13.7%), Hispanic/Latina (7.3%), and White (7%) participants (Martin et al., 2018a).

The Strong Start initiative performed a separate analysis using birth certificate and Medicaid claims data to identify two comparison groups of women with similar risk profiles living in the same counties who received usual prenatal care versus birth center prenatal care. In the comparison group analysis, participants receiving enhanced prenatal care were matched by risk profile with Medicaid beneficiaries in the same counties receiving usual or nonenhanced prenatal care. Comparative analyses demonstrated significant improvements for women in birth center care compared with usual care for a range of outcomes, including preterm birth (6.3% vs. 8.5%, p <.01), low birthweight (5.9% vs. 7.4%, p <.05), average gestation age (39 weeks vs. 38.6 weeks, p <.01), cesarean birth (17.5% vs. 29%,

continued

BOX 4-2 Continued

p <.01), vaginal birth rate for women with a previous cesarean (24.2% vs. 12.5%, p <.05), and infant emergency department visits through the first year of life (0.86 vs. 0.99, p <.01). However, the lack of randomization, standardization of within-group care processes, and documentation of fidelity of implementation makes it difficult to ascertain the factors that might account for the differences in outcomes.

Average cost savings to Medicaid for each mother–baby dyad with birth center prenatal care was $2,010 for the time period from pregnancy through the end of the first year. Cost savings were driven by lower cesarean rates and shorter hospital stays, as well as fewer emergency department visits during the first year after the birth (Hill et al., 2018).

In an analysis limited to the birth center Strong Start data, Alliman and colleagues (2019) found that the 6,424 Medicaid enrollees using birth center care experienced preterm birth rates of 4.4 percent and low-birthweight rates of 3.7 percent, compared with U.S. rates of 9.9 percent and 8.2 percent, respectively. The total cesarean rate was 12.3 percent, with a primary cesarean rate of 8.7 percent (Alliman et al., 2019). However, these results were not tested for statistical significance. The breastfeeding initiation was 92.9 percent compared with a national rate of 83.1 percent (Alliman et al., 2019). In the birth center arm of Strong Start, eligible women participated in birth center prenatal care and experienced these improved outcomes even if they elected hospital delivery (Alliman et al., 2019).

Summary

The structure, policies, and financing of the health care system all influence the health outcomes of pregnant people and newborns. These features of the health system can contribute to a woman's risk profile in pregnancy and birth, her ability to access and choose birth settings, and the quality of care she receives in those settings. In the presence of systemic barriers—whether financial, social, or regulatory—the choice made is often constrained and made in the absence of available alternatives.

Finding 4-1: Birthing facilities and maternity care providers are unevenly distributed across the United States, leaving many women without access to prenatal, birthing, and postpartum care and choices among options near home.

Finding 4-2: Women living in rural communities and underserved urban areas have greater risks of poor outcomes, such as preterm birth and maternal and infant mortality, in part because of lack of access to maternity and prenatal care in their local areas.

Finding 4-3: Access to midwifery care is limited in some settings because some types of midwives are not licensed in some states and do not have admitting privileges in some medical facilities, but this varies across the country. The wide variation in regulation, certification, and licensing of maternity care professionals across the United States is an impediment to access to all birth settings.

Finding 4-4: Access to all types of birth settings and providers is limited because of the lack of universal coverage for all women, for all types of providers, and at levels that cover the cost of care.

CONCLUSION

This chapter has reviewed the many systems-level social and environmental factors that can influence a woman's health status, readiness for pregnancy, access to and use of prenatal and intrapartum care, and access to choices surrounding that care. Risk during pregnancy and childbirth is not simply the result of medical and obstetrical risk factors. Rather, these individual-level risk factors are often the result of a series of systems-level factors, such as structural inequalities and biases (in both the health system and society at large), policy and financing features of the health system, and the social determinants of health. These upstream factors, the conditions and context within which an individual lives, shape a woman's health and the health and well-being of her child. These negative or positive social influences can change a woman's risk profile in pregnancy and in childbirth.

Moreover, these systems-level factors can confer their own risk on pregnant women. As an example, inequities in maternal and newborn outcomes, in particular for Black and AIAN women, can be traced to structural inequities and biases including racism, which both increases stress during pregnancy and influences how a woman is treated. Delayed prenatal care in the face of provider shortages, for example, can increase a woman's risk for a host of adverse pregnancy outcomes, without changing her individual medical and obstetrical risk. This in turn influences her willingness to seek maternity care and other aspects of access to care. Understanding the role that nonclinical factors play in determining clinical risk is essential for developing risk-appropriate models of care.

CONCLUSION 4-1: Systems-level factors and social determinants of health such as structural racism, lack of financial resources, availability of transportation, housing instability, lack of social support, stress, limited availability of healthy and nutritious foods, lower level of education, and lack of access to health care (including mental health

care) are correlated with higher risk for poor pregnancy outcomes and
inequity in care and outcomes.

These systemic risk factors are felt at the individual and population
levels. For individual women, systemic risk factors hamper access and
contribute to medical, obstetrical, and social risks. At the population level,
these systemic factors translate into disparities in maternal and neonatal
outcomes along lines of race, class, and geography. Other social determinants of health also influence both access and outcomes, including housing,
employment status, health literacy and education, transportation, location
of services, and location of maternity care professionals. Policy regarding
access and financing can strongly impact women's ability to get adequate
maternity care.

As a result, women's options will be limited by the availability of different types of birth settings and maternity care providers within or near their
community, including hospital resources and within-hospital options. Availability is particularly challenging in rural areas and in some inner cities.
A woman's choices are further limited by health insurance and Medicaid
restrictions; economic circumstances; access to transportation; and cultural
and linguistic factors, such as language barriers with providers and her
perception of how she will be received and treated.

Understanding and differentiating the risk stratification conferred by
individual- and systems-level risk as well as access to choices of birth settings for pregnant people in the United States is one key aspect of analyzing health outcomes by birth setting. In the next chapter, we turn to this
consideration, as well as other data and methodological considerations for
understanding birth settings research.

5

Issues in Measuring Outcomes
by Birth Settings:
Data and Methods

Inherent in the charge to the committee (refer to Box 1-1 in Chapter 1) was the question of the state of the knowledge base for systems of care for childbirth and how that knowledge base can be strengthened in ways that optimally bridge knowledge and decisions about policies and practices. This chapter addresses that question—an important one because such decisions will be most sound when they draw on a robust and comprehensive body of relevant information.

To that end, the first section of this chapter provides an overview of the strengths and limitations of data used to study clinical outcomes with respect to birth settings, including vital statistics and birth registry data. Next, the chapter examines methodological issues relevant for birth settings research; the types of questions that are salient in making decisions about policy and practice; and how, ideally, the different types and sources of high-quality evidence could best be used in concert to answer those questions. These questions require methods that make it possible to measure outcomes that move beyond traditional clinical variables and include perceptions of racism, disrespect and unequal treatment, women's experiences of care, human-centered design, and patient-reported outcomes. Finally, we conclude with a discussion of two tools for grading the quality of evidence typical in this field.

DATA SOURCES

In this section, we discuss the strengths and limitations of the data sources commonly used when conducting research on birth settings. These data come primarily from the National Vital Statistics report, managed by the Centers for Disease Control and Prevention (CDC), and birth registries, which use an intention-to-treat model (i.e., models indicating intended birth setting) to track outcomes for women and infants. We discuss each of these data sources in turn below.

Of course, additional data sources could be used for research in this area. Such sources include linked birth certificate and hospital data, which add more valid information on many morbidities, as well as insurer data. The committee does not discuss these data sources in detail, however, because of the need to focus on those data sources that are most valuable for comparing outcomes across birth settings. Hospital discharge data, by definition, include only information on hospital births, and do not include information on birth center or home births. Thus, linked birth certificate and hospital discharge data are not a good data source for understanding variations in birth characteristics or outcomes by birth setting.

Vital Statistics Data

Vital statistics data from birth certificates provide information on each of the approximately 3.9 million births occurring in the United States each year, by place of birth (birth setting) and sociodemographic and limited medical characteristics (Centers for Disease Control and Prevention, 2017b; Martin et al., 2018a). These data have the benefit of being population based, reducing selection bias. Two types of data are potentially available from vital statistics: (1) information on the number and characteristics of birth, by birth setting (hospital, home, birth center); and (2) information on birth outcomes, including infant mortality, preterm births, and low birthweight, by birthplace. The strength of these data lies in providing a complete count of births by important characteristics, including birth setting. However, these data also have significant limitations regarding their use for birth settings research (Centers for Disease Control and Prevention, 2017b).

The question on the birth certificate on place of birth reports *exclusively* on the birth setting at the time of birth (Centers for Disease Control and Prevention, 2017b), and not on the intended setting at the onset of labor, potentially leading to misclassification bias. As a result, women who planned a home or birth center birth but were transferred to a hospital during labor and delivery are reported as hospital births in vital statistics data (MacDorman and Declercq, 2019), and identification of individuals who intended a home or birth center birth has been challenging. Instead, most researchers agree that analysis indicating intended birth setting (based on birth registry data, discussed below) is the methodologically most robust method for analyzing data by birth setting (Scarf et al., 2018). That is, as elaborated below, it is essential that studies evaluate outcomes based on intended place of delivery and not actual place of birth.

Studies show that in the United States, approximately 11 percent of planned home births result in intrapartum transfers (Cheyney et al., 2014a) and that 16 percent of birth center births require movement to a higher level of care (Stapleton et al., 2013). It is important to note that complications in planned home or birth center births that occur prior to or during transfer to a hospital can lead to bias in estimates of outcomes. The result is that the number of planned home and birth center births reported in vital statistics data is an underestimate by the number of intrapartum transfers. The example of cesarean section makes this clear: when studies examine outcomes by actual rather than intended place of birth, the cesarean rates for planned home and birth center births appear to be zero, as cesareans occur only after transfer to a hospital. As a result, all cesareans are misattributed to a hospital sample when in reality they may have started as planned home or birth center births (MacDorman and Declercq, 2019). In addition, the outcomes of patient transfer may differ from those of births that occurred in their planned setting. Although most transfers are nonemergent and occur for such reasons as failure to progress and need for anesthesia (Vedam et al., 2014a), some are emergencies, and not being able to attribute these outcomes back to the intended place of birth could significantly bias estimates of outcomes by birth setting against hospitals.

For births that occur at home, moreover, information is available on the planning status of the birth (i.e., planned or unplanned home birth, or unknown whether planned) for all states except California, which accounts for one out of every eight U.S. births (Centers for Disease Control and Prevention, 2017b; MacDorman and Declercq, 2019). This means that planned and unplanned home births in California are combined in the overall home birth category. As a result, significant bias can occur when analyzing birth outcomes, since outcomes for unplanned home births are often less favorable given that the setting is unprepared for the birth (MacDorman and Declercq, 2019). Even in Oregon, the only state where planning status and intended location are both recorded on the birth certificate, it is impossible to distinguish between birth center or planned home births and planned unassisted births (or births without a trained attendant) (Snowden et al., 2015), which are known to have significantly higher rates of mortality than midwife-attended home births (Vogel, 2011).

On the other hand, there are also several biases in these studies favoring home births. First, some of the "unintended" home births may in fact be misclassified as noncertified midwife births in states where their practice is unregulated. In addition, home to hospital or birth center to hospital transfers and their outcomes accrue to the hospital. Moreover, as hospitals take care of all risk categories of women, the expected outcomes for hospital birth should be worse than the outcomes for low-risk women in home and birth center settings. Some studies mitigate against this bias by choosing low-risk populations giving birth in hospitals and hospital births attended by midwives as the reference group.

For some biases, the direction is unclear. Studies on the effects of different types of midwives on outcomes, for example, are hampered by lack of data regarding who assumes care of the mother–infant dyad after transfer to the hospital. Data on death with congenital anomalies are difficult to interpret given that often studies lack granularity on the type of anomaly, and its lethality. Furthermore, fetal death, if divergent across groups, might contribute to selection bias of a healthier birth cohort for home births. These potential misclassification biases were discussed extensively by the committee; however, the committee was unable to reach consensus on the direction of bias given limitations in the availability of variables that would allow quantification of the number of planned unassisted births. Additional research and data are needed to better understand this question.

Additional limitations of birth certificate data for epidemiologic analysis have been widely discussed in the literature, and include the inability of birth certificates to provide information on clinical intentions, as well as concerns about the completeness, validity, and reliability of the reporting of specific data items (DiGuiseppe et al., 2002; Ananth, 2005; Cahill and Macones, 2006; Schoendorf and Branum, 2006; Cheyney et al., 2014a).

Data quality measures are generally good for most sociodemographic items reported on the birth certificate, as well as for place of birth, source of payment for the delivery, and basic medical variables such as birthweight, period of gestation, and mortality (DiGuiseppe et al., 2002; Zollinger et al., 2006; Vinikoor et al., 2010; Martin et al., 2013; Deitz et al., 2015). Although more recent studies are needed, studies based on older data suggest that the 5-minute Apgar score is reasonably well reported in vital statistics data (DiGuiseppe et al., 2002; Zollinger et al., 2006). In contrast, other studies have found that some items on birth certificates (such as attempted labor induction) are undercounted (Deitz et al., 2015; DiGuiseppe et al., 2002; Li et al., 2017; Martin et al., 2013; Vinikoor et al., 2010; Zollinger et al., 2006).

Other, more detailed medical variables, particularly those based on a checkbox on the birth certificate, may be less well reported. Data on hypertension and diabetes are of moderate to fair quality, with a tendency toward being underreported, although the quality of reporting of these data varies significantly by state (Ananth, 2005; Martin et al., 2013; Dietz et al., 2015). Regarding neonatal seizures and serious neurologic dysfunction, a recent study by Li and colleagues (2017) compares South Carolina birth certificate data from the 2003 birth certificate revision with hospital discharge and Medicaid data (Li et al., 2017). The authors found sensitivity rates for birth certificate reporting of neonatal seizures or serious neurologic dysfunction of 7 percent and 0 percent for hospital and planned home births, respectively. Thus, despite improvements across revisions, U.S. birth certificates underreport or falsely report seizures, especially among home births.[1] The authors conclude that "birth certificates alone should not be used to measure neonatal seizures or serious neurologic dysfunction." Multiple sources of data, such as discharge summaries and Medicaid claims data, are needed to supplement birth certificate data to obtain an accurate understanding of seizure prevalence in all three U.S. birth settings. Despite these concerns, this variable has been used in studies on birth setting, given the concern over hypoxic ischemic encephalopathy in the out-of-hospital setting, where immediate access to surgical delivery may not be available (see, e.g., Cheng et al., 2013; Tilden et al., 2017).

The reliability of Apgar score = 0 for birth settings research has also been widely questioned. For example, Watterberg (2013) found large differences in reporting of Apgar score = 0 between physicians and home birth midwives, and they suggest that Apgar score <4 is a more robust measure for birth settings research.

In addition, some data items may be reported differently depending on the birth setting. For example, midwives in home and birth center settings may file birth certificates 10 days or more postpartum, while birth certificates for hospital births are typically filed 1–3 days following birth, depending on the mode of delivery (Zollinger et al., 2006; Li et al., 2017). This means that out-of-hospital midwives reporting on complications in the early postpartum period may report conditions over a longer period of time relative to hospital clerks. In addition, an analysis of vital statistics data conducted by Grünebaum and colleagues (2015a) found that midwives attending planned births in out-of-hospital settings assigned a significantly higher proportion of Apgar scores of 10 compared with midwives or physicians in the hospital setting, suggesting a bias toward higher Apgar scores outside of hospitals.

Taken together, these limitations mean that an analysis of birth outcomes by birth setting based on U.S. vital statistics data alone cannot be recommended. Yet these types of analyses are common in the literature (see Chapter 5).

---

[1] Sensitivity, positive predictive values, false positive rates, and kappa values for neonatal seizure recording were, respectively, 7 percent, 66 percent, 34 percent, and 0.12 for the 2003 revision of birth certificates (547,177 hospital births from 2004 to 2013), and 5 percent, 33 percent, 67 percent, and 0.09 for the 1998 revision (396,776 hospital births from 1996 to 2003). Among 660 planned home births between 2004 and 2013 and 920 home births between 1996 and 2003, values were 0, 0, 100 percent, and –0.002, respectively (Li et al., 2017, p. 1047).

Birth Registry Data

Another data source for studies on outcomes by birth setting is birth registries that, by design, collect data indicating intended birth setting. These data also can be used to attribute outcome to provider type and level of care over the course of pregnancy, birth, and ideally early childhood (Stapleton, 2011; Cheyney et al., 2014b; Caughey and Cheyney, 2019).

In the United States, there are two birth registries: one curated by the Midwives Alliance of North America's (MANA's) Division of Research, called the MANA Statistics Project (MANA Stats) (Cheyney et al., 2014b); and another curated by the American Association of Birth Centers (AABC), called the Perinatal Data Registry (PDR; formerly called the Uniform Data Set, or UDS) (Stapleton, 2011). These datasets were validated by sampling a percentage of courses of care and comparing midwives' entries into the registry with the medical record. The MANA Stats validation study found that variables were accurately entered by participants, as evidenced by the perfect or near perfect agreement among pre- and postreview variables (kappas ranging from 0.98 to 1.00; see Cheyney et al. 2014b), suggesting that any errors in this dataset are primarily random and not systematic for the outcomes assessed. Similarly, the validation study for the PDR (formerly UDS) found 97.1 percent agreement between the medical record and data entered into the online system (see Stapleton et al., 2013).

The MANA Stats and PDR datasets are the largest databases on midwife-led births occurring primarily in home or birth center settings in the United States. Both datasets are open to all practitioners attending births in all settings and include records from certified nurse midwives (CNMs), certified midwives (CMs), certified professional midwives (CPMs), and licensed midwives (LMs), as well as doctors of osteopathy (DOs), naturopathic doctors, and doctors of medicine (MDs). Records are submitted online voluntarily and capture perinatal and birth data, with nearly 200 variables collected across the prenatal and postnatal care periods (Cheyney et al., 2014b). Similarly, the PDR registry is a voluntary, online, comprehensive registry that contains perinatal data for use in AABC member centers (Stapleton, 2011).

In addition to MANA Stats and the PDR, some state or multistate networks, such as Perinatal Quality Collaboratives (PQCs), collect data on women and infants in order to improve perinatal care. PQCs are currently active in 32 states, 13 of which are actively working with the CDC (Henderson et al., 2018; see also Chapter 7). In addition, the American College of Obstetricians and Gynecologists (ACOG) is currently piloting a birth registry for maternal care that would allow providers and institutions to measure outcomes for and the quality of care they provide to women and infants (American College of Obstetricians and Gynecologists, n.d.).

A limitation of registry-based studies is that, unlike vital statistics, they are not population based, limiting their generalizability. In addition, participation in these registries is voluntary. The MANA Stats registry includes records from an estimated 20–30 percent of actively practicing CPMs (who attend most of the home births in the United States), with a substantially lower proportion of CNMs (who attend more hospital births) contributing. It captures about 20 percent of home births that occur in the United States annually (Cheyney et al., 2014b). As for birth centers, only 41 percent belong to the AABC, and less than 80 percent of members participate in the PDR online registry (Stapleton et al., 2013). These registries capture data primarily on home and birth center births, and thus, lack the ability to capture outcomes across concurrently collected hospital data. Finally, while many states have a PQC available, those states that are not part of the National Network of Perinatal Quality Collaboratives (NNPQC) created by the CDC are not obligated to share their information with other states, and participation of institutions within the state PQC is often voluntary (Henderson et al., 2018). Taken together, these limitations mean that an analysis of birth outcomes by birth setting based on U.S. registry data alone is not recommended, though these studies may be useful for describing within-group variation. For example, registry data may be useful in studying within-group maternal risk factors and birth outcomes (e.g., see Bovbjerg et al., 2017) or for the analysis of physiologic processes (such as length of third stage) that are less sensitive to selection bias. These limitations are similar to those inherent in vital statistics data. In summary, multiple data sources may have complimentary value in understanding the quality of care and outcomes associated with various birth settings.

Confounding Factors

In addition to the sources of bias associated with vital statistics and birth registry data, studies on birth settings are subject to potential confounding. As discussed in Chapters 3 and 4, differences exist in the demographic, cultural, social, and clinical characteristics among women who choose home or freestanding birth center births versus hospital births, and these differences have not been systematically measured (Caughey and Cheyney, 2019). Women choosing home or birth center birth may also differ in their desire to have an unmedicated vaginal birth or may be healthier overall than hospital patients, such that their need for medical interventions is reduced. Furthermore, many studies lack the statistical power to reliably evaluate rare outcomes (such as perinatal or maternal mortality), although most studies are adequately powered for common outcomes such as cesarean birth and neonatal intensive care unit (NICU) admissions (Caughey and Cheyney, 2019).

As a result, adequate data are not currently available with which to make comparisons across birth settings for the rarest of events, such as maternal mortality, where it would be necessary to control for maternal risk factors, provider type, and planned place of birth—impossible given the very small number of cases reported in the literature (e.g., the literature has reported just one maternal death following a home birth). In addition, the overall low number of home and birth center births in the United States (less than 2% of all births), the fragmentation of datasets (the PDR and MANA Stats, e.g., each separately collect data on a percentage of home and birth center births, and these datasets have yet to be merged), and the infrequency of mortality mean that samples are commonly combined—intrapartum and neonatal mortality or home and birth center, for instance. This improves power, but reduces the ability to attribute specific outcomes to specific birth settings and distinct provider types while controlling for confounders. Even with the collapsing of categories, confidence intervals are still often quite wide and estimates unstable. These are significant considerations that limited the committee's ability to nuance comparisons of outcomes by birth setting in many instances. These challenges are discussed in more detail in the following chapter.

Summary

Vital statistics data are informative, but the inability to track intended place of birth or the planning status of home births in California's records limits their utility in birth settings research. And while birth registry data allow indication of intended birth setting, the reporting of these data is generally voluntary, and the data are not collected nationally or across all birth settings.

Finding 5-1: Vital statistics and birth registry data each have limitations for evaluating birth outcomes by setting, provider types, and intentionality.

STUDY DESIGN AND METHODOLOGIES

The utility of evidence is maximized when it is appropriately matched to the needs of those who will be using it, which can vary depending on the context and the primary purpose of the user. High-quality information is needed by communities, community leaders, maternity care providers, funders, and policy makers at the local, state, and federal levels. Decision makers and researchers can be called upon to generate and use evidence to inform decisions that apply at different levels of a system and even across different systems. In maternity care, the system at issue may be the health care or public health or social service system, and the level may be national, regional, or local. Decision makers typically have a range of questions when attempting to address an important issue. In addition to information that describes the scope of the issue and research or evaluation evidence about the effectiveness of actions they might consider to address it, they frequently seek information with direct relevance to their local context. Such information may be related to implementation; costs; sustainability; specific characteristics of the community; and other factors that could impede or facilitate the success of an intervention, program, or policy (Institute of Medicine, 2010). Decision makers also need to contend with the interrelated nature of factors that affect the issue they hope to address. Evidence needs may vary accordingly, and an issue is typically best addressed when examined from multiple perspectives and with multiple forms of evidence.

Evidence that is useful to inform decisions about policies and practices related to maternity care may come from a variety of disciplines and sources of evidence using a diversity of methods. The following is one way of categorizing study designs and sources of evidence that can be useful for addressing questions relevant to maternity care research and decision making (Institute of Medicine, 2010):

- observational studies,
- qualitative research and analysis,
- mixed-methods studies,
- evidence synthesis methods,
- experimental studies, and
- quasi-experimental studies.

Across these categories, it is important to emphasize that each of these types of evidence has its own inherent quality standards, as detailed below. The value of any source as the "best" evidence is relative, depending on the decision-making context and the type of issue being addressed. It is counterproductive to expect any one type of evidence to be the best fit for all uses (Flay et al., 2005). To understand how an intervention works, for example, qualitative designs can be the most valuable and appropriate (MacKinnon, 2008). And to assess practitioner implementation or organizational adoption of a new practice, it can be useful to carry out longitudinal studies of quality improvement and of how organizational policies are implemented and enforced. The quality of any type of evidence synthesis hinges on consistency in identifying and appraising the quality of the research evidence included and in the care taken in secondary interpretation of findings across diverse studies.

Trade-offs are involved in considering the utility of any single type of evidence available to answer questions about such complex, multilevel public health issues as maternal and infant health. Typically, no one study or type of evidence is sufficient to support decisions, and therefore the use of multiple types of evidence is often the best approach (Mercer et al., 2007). For situations in which the evidence is inadequate, incomplete, and/or inconsistent, the best available evidence can be interpreted through processes that bring tacit knowledge and the experience of professionals and other stakeholders to bear (Institute of Medicine, 2010). Table 5-1 provides a summary of research designs, types, and strengths and weaknesses of five common study designs.

TABLE 5-1 Typology of Research Designs

Experimental Studies	
	Syntheses encompass meta-analyses that use statistical methods to pool results from a sample of existing experimental and/or quasi-experimental studies, and systematic reviews that provide organized summaries of a body of research addressing a focused question, whether using the same or multiple methodologies.
Types	Randomized controlled trials (RCTs)
Strengths and Weaknesses	RCT studies have the strengths of being able to measure the effectiveness of interventions and minimize bias. However, feasibility issues, ethical constraints, and variables that cannot be controlled make this design inapplicable for many studies (Institute of Medicine, 2008). RCTs are less well suited to studying effects of large-scale social programs and policies (West et al., 2008).
Quasi-Experimental Studies	
	A design similar to experimental except the researcher cannot draw a causal conclusion because there is less than complete control over the variables in the study.
Types	Nonrandomized experimental studies (uncontrolled before-and-after studies, time-series designs, controlled before-and-after studies) (Grimshaw et al., 2000)
Strengths and Weaknesses	Quasi-experimental designs can be used when randomization is not feasible or ethical or when a sample size is too small for randomization. They have weaknesses similar to those of experimental designs, including regression effects (when the results overestimate or underestimate the effect of a treatment) and confounding[a] (Goodwin, 2005; Harris et al., 2006).
Observational Studies	
	The researcher assesses variables and relationships among them, but does not manipulate those variables or introduce any intervention. A large proportion of studies on birth settings have used study designs that fall into this category.

TABLE 5-1 Continued

Types	Cross-sectional or longitudinal survey research, ethnographic studies, secondary analysis of existing databases, trend analysis, cohort and case-control studies, predictive studies, archival studies, census studies, monitoring and surveillance studies, ecological studies, implementation tracking, policy analysis
Strengths and Weaknesses	Observational studies have the benefit of allowing researchers to examine multiple outcomes. Weaknesses of observational studies include missing data, selection bias, confounding bias, and information bias (Boyko, 2013).

Qualitative Studies

	Qualitative researchers collect detailed information from individuals or groups and have the ability to use these responses to formulate grounded theory about a topic (Johnson and Onwuegbuzie, 2004).
Types	Ethnographic studies, focus group or key informant interviews, direct observation, content or documentary analysis, case studies, logic modeling or program theory analysis, process and implementation monitoring
Strengths and Weaknesses	Qualitative research designs allow researchers to assess the experiences and perceptions of respondents at a much richer level than is possible with quantitative methods. Questions and data-gathering techniques can be appropriately expanded or modified in response to what is learned as data are collected. A weakness of qualitative methods is that subjectivity can occur not only in the design and in the interpretation of the findings, but also in the role of the researcher as an instrument of the research process (Institute of Medicine, 2010).

Mixed-Method Studies

	Mixed-methods approaches are suitable for interpreting information across the boundaries of quantitative assessments, such as the prevalence of a condition, the statistical significance of an effect, or cost considerations, and assessments of the nature, process, or meaning of a condition, intervention, or outcome (O'Cathian, 2009; Wisdom et al., 2012).
Types	Complementary methodologies, typically including both qualitative and quantitative approaches to data gathering and analysis
Strengths and Weaknesses	Mixed-methods approaches allow researchers to conduct more in-depth analyses because some of the weaknesses present in both qualitative and quantitative research can be compensated. Weaknesses of mixed-methods approaches include added workload and the fact that using both methods will not completely erase the already known weaknesses found in qualitative and quantitative designs independently (Johnson and Onweugbuzie, 2004).

[a]Confounding is defined as "distortion of the association between an exposure and an outcome due to the influence of another variable that is also associated with both" (Snowden et al., 2018, p. 724).

The most commonly used study design for birth settings is observational studies, because they have the benefit of allowing researchers to examine multiple outcomes (Boyko, 2013). Observational studies are case-control studies, cohort studies, or cross-sectional studies. Each of these study designs comes with strengths and weaknesses. Case-control and retrospective cohort studies allow researchers to study events and characteristics that were present in the past, while cross-sectional and prospective cohort studies allow researchers to study an event occurring in the future. Cohort studies have the advantage of examining multiple outcomes and can be used to calculate rates of exposure, but they require a large sample size, which can be difficult when studying rare outcomes, and they are susceptible to selection bias. Existing records can be used to measure multiple outcomes for case-control studies, which makes them easier to conduct. Unfortunately, they may contain recall bias and are difficult to validate while also not allowing control of extraneous variables (Song and Chung, 2010). Finally, cross-sectional study designs can be used to measure outcomes between groups, but are unable to measure the cause and effect of outcomes and do not require groups to be equivalent (Goodwin, 2005; Song and Chung, 2010). For more in-depth information on birthing experiences, researchers utilize mixed-methods designs or qualitative research. Mixed methods allow researchers to obtain evidence after the implementation of policies or programs to measure the intended or unintended effects.

Randomization and experimental controls are rarely used when studying birth settings and maternal and neonatal outcomes because it would be difficult to find women who would agree to be randomized to one or another birth setting (Hendrix et al., 2009). In addition, many randomized controlled trials (RCTs) used to study effects of intrapartum practices are limited to assessing outcomes that can be measured during the intrapartum phase of care and provide little meaningful information about additional outcomes of interest after this period (Institute of Medicine, 2008). This point is made clear by outcomes measured in the larger, more impactful RCTs included in a Cochrane systematic review of studies of the effects of intrapartum care. Just 16 percent of those RCTs made *any* measure of the infant after hospital discharge (Teune et al., 2013). Randomization has the potential to reduce selection bias, but this bias cannot be eliminated completely (Jadad and Enkin, 2008). When a study is designed, it is important to look at the characteristics of the participants and also the characteristics of those who do not wish to participate or are not eligible. Those who choose to participate may not be representative of the target population and thus may have an impact on the validity of the findings (Carmichael and Snowden, 2019).

Moreover, recent discourse on RCTs (and most prospective research), particularly in the health field, have noted the historic underrepresentation of people of color and people of low socioeconomic status in health care trials. Although there is an imperative to increase enrollment of those women, it is also important to acknowledge that medical mistrust, mistrust of research, and access to engagement in care remain barriers that disproportionally impede participation of low-income people and people of color in prospective research (Geller et al., 2011).

ASSESSING THE QUALITY OF EVIDENCE

Decision makers are often faced with an abundance of data and information that they must sift through to obtain the knowledge they seek. This process requires consistency in how the quality of available evidence is assessed. Although it can appear simplest to use a hierarchy among the types of evidence, in reality no single gold standard of evidence can be used to answer all types of questions; rather, what constitutes the "best" evidence depends on the question being asked, and how the evidence aligns with the user's needs and interests and how relevant it is to the question at hand and its context. The quality of the evidence also needs to be judged according to established criteria and standards that are appropriate to the type of evidence. Each of the different sources of evidence described above can be linked to appropriate criteria for judging the quality of evidence, which can be found in the literature, although in all cases, high-quality evidence avoids bias, confounding, measurement error, and other threats to validity whenever possible (Institute of Medicine, 2010; Mercer et al., 2007). This section describes two common tools used for grading the quality of evidence in the birth settings literature: the Birth Place Research Quality (ResQu) Index and the Grading of Recommendations, Assessment, Development, and Evaluation (GRADE) approach. To facilitate the discussion of health outcomes by birth setting that appears in Chapter 5, the committee identified relevant literature and, using the ResQu Index and the GRADE approach, assessed the quality rating of each identified article. Chapter 6 summarizes the most recent literature available on outcomes by birth settings.

The committee chose to use both GRADE and the ResQu index because while GRADE is ubiquitous, and thus a highly accessible way of evaluating study quality, we also felt it was advisable to apply a scoring system that had been specifically designed for birth settings research, given the nature of our statement of task. Interestingly, this approach enabled us to see the impact on quality ratings when models indicating intended birth setting are weighted (ResQu Index) over RCT design (GRADE). Taken together, these tools enabled us to see and nuance the relative strengths and weaknesses of each study.

ResQu Index

Recognizing varying standards for assessing the quality of study designs used to investigate outcomes by birth setting, the limitations of existing datasets for examining these outcomes, and the challenges of comparing outcomes across states or regions, an international panel of experts developed and validated the ResQu Index (Vedam et al., 2017). The ResQu Index allows researchers to evaluate the strength of studies related to birth settings and accounts for items that are critical to birth settings research but less relevant to other epidemiological studies, such as use of models indicating intended birth setting. This tool is used to assess study rigor based on 27 criteria specific to evaluating the effects of birth setting on maternal, fetal, and neonatal outcomes. These criteria are grouped into five categories: (1) quality of design, (2) definition of sample, (3) measurement of outcomes, (4) comparability of cohorts, and (5) accuracy of interpretation and reporting.[2] Each criterion is scored, with a higher value indicating higher quality, and a summary score is then calculated to rate the quality of a study as high (scores of 75% and above), moderate (65–74%), or weak/low (less than 65%). Strengths of the ResQu Index include permitting re-

---

[2]Each category contains subcategories that are scored with a rubric based on the information provided within the article. The criteria for quality of design include the following: provides a clear statement of the research question/objective; defines and describes each birth setting clearly (e.g., provider, facilities, location); indicates type of study design; defines key terms (e.g., low risk, outcome, mortality, morbidity, postpartum hemorrhage [PPH]) consistently, transparently, and appropriately (e.g., National Institute for Health and Care Excellence [NICE], American College of Obstetricians and Gynecologists [ACOG], or country-specific guidelines); and indicates ethics approval. The criteria for definition of sample (if relevant) include the following: distinguishes between planned home births with skilled attendants and free or unplanned births, includes sample size calculation, and uses reliable method of sampling and recruitment for each cohort. The criteria for measurement of outcomes include the following: gathers outcome data from reliable sources (e.g., medical records, registration data); identifies planned birth setting at time in pregnancy that is appropriate to selected outcome measures; provider type (for birth) is indicated, measured, and adjusted for in analysis; uses cohort size with appropriate power for selected outcomes being measured; uses reliable method to indicate changes of birth setting; indicates timing of transfer between birth settings in labor or postpartum period; applies reliable and appropriate statistical methods to compare outcomes between cohorts; and reports and minimizes missing data. The criteria for comparability of cohorts include the following: uses cohorts with comparable obstetric and sociodemographic characteristics; retains women in original birth setting cohort for analysis (intention to treat); provides consistent inclusion criteria; and controls for confounders, including sociodemographic and health profile. The criteria for accuracy of interpretation and reporting include the following: presents results of statistical comparisons clearly and effectively; bases discussion and conclusions on reported data; addresses impact of size of cohorts for each outcome measured; addresses impact of incomplete data; addresses impact of retrospective data; addresses effect of level of service integration between home, birth center, and hospital; and addresses impact of local/regional standards, policies, and protocols (Vedam et al., 2017).

searchers to exclude criteria rarely applicable to birth settings research, such as randomization and blinding, and facilitating collaboration among evaluators. In addition, comparisons of the interrater consistency and consensus of scores from different scorers showed considerable similarity in rating.

Development of quality assessment instruments inevitably involves subjective assessment particularly related to the selection and weighting of features. While careful attention was paid to multidisciplinary input and attempts were made to maximize content validity and consistency for this index, the relative emphasis on various study qualities is debatable; differential weighting would produce different scores. Application of the ResQu Index is, as with other all scales, subject to some individual interpretation. In addition, the ResQu Index was not designed to evaluate qualitative studies. The nature of its design in fact means that no qualitative study could be rated highly even though the developers themselves acknowledge that questions about safety and maternal experience by birth setting cannot and should not be answered by quantitative or statistical approaches alone (Vedam et al., 2017).

GRADE Approach

GRADE provides guidelines for grading the quality of evidence in health care literature. The grading process entails assessing the design, limitations, inconsistency, indirectness, imprecision, and publication bias of a study. The reviewer then summarizes the quality rating for each outcome and the estimate of the effect (e.g., risk ratio, odds ratio, or hazard ratio). The confidence in an estimate of the effect is used when the reviewer decides if the recommendations from the study can be supported based on the provided evidence (Guyatt et al., 2008; Meader et al., 2014). An important limitation to using the GRADE approach when reviewing birth settings research is that observational studies start as low-quality evidence because they are deemed to fail to develop and apply appropriate eligibility criteria, to have flawed measurement of both exposure and outcome, to fail to adequately control confounding, and to have incomplete follow-up (Schünemann, 2013).

CONCLUSION

Data and methodological limitations make the study of birth settings challenging. Decision makers need research and evidence that appropriately match their needs, but these needs vary greatly by context, and not all evidence is fit-for-purpose. Vital statistics and birth registry data each have limitations for evaluating birth outcomes by setting, provider types, and intentionality (Finding 5-1).

Modifications to birth certificate records, such as those adopted by Oregon, to include intended birth setting are important for improving the usefulness of these data for birth settings research. The quality of birth settings research could be greatly improved if all states were to fully adopt this revised and updated version without modification. Additional improvements would include designation of planned attended and planned unassisted home births, and identification of the type of physician or midwife attending the birth.

CONCLUSION 5-1: Modifications to the birth certificate that allow inquiry into birth settings based on models indicating intended birth setting, including planned attended and planned unassisted home births in the United States and intended birth attendants, and development of best practices for use of these expanded data in birth settings research are needed to better understand and assess outcomes by birth settings.

Such changes would allow states to track the rates and associated outcomes of unassisted home births, which have been estimated to be on the rise, particularly in areas where vaginal birth after cesarean, vaginal breech, and vaginal twin births are not available in hospital settings (Holten and de Miranda, 2016). While the committee acknowledges that implementation of changes to birth certificate records is often slow, as evidenced by the prolonged time period required to see general use of the 2003 modification of the birth certificate, these changes are imperative to allow the conduct of accurate analyses by birthplace. Adoption of these changes at the state level may speed implementation; however, a piecemeal state-by-state approach is unlikely to yield needed, nationally comparable data.

Recognizing the strengths and limitations of the data and methodologies for birth settings research, we turn in the next chapter to examining what the current evidence base can reveal about health outcomes for women and infants by birth setting.

6

Maternal and Newborn Outcomes by Birth Setting

The previous chapter describes the challenges involved in studying the effects of birth settings on maternal and neonatal outcomes in the United States. In addition to the deficiencies in data sources and methodological limitations discussed in that chapter, the literature on birth settings compares a wide array of beneficial and nonbeneficial outcomes across and within settings. Often these studies do not report the same outcomes or use the same definitions or terminology, making it difficult to develop assessments or to draw useful conclusions across the existing body of literature (Khan, 2019). In addition, the overall small number of U.S. women giving birth in home and birth center settings (under 2%) compared with hospital settings (about 98%) complicates many studies of outcomes by setting (MacDorman and Declercq, 2019). The reason is that infrequent events such as maternal and infant death, while of great interest to the committee, tend to have unstable estimates with wide confidence intervals as a result of relatively small sample sizes for home and birth center subgroups.

Aspects of care during the childbearing year are also variable and dependent on such factors as the health of the mother and infant, models of prenatal and intrapartum care, the type of birth attendant, practice standards, and facility policies across and within birth settings and regions. Furthermore, as discussed in Chapter 2, the definition of what constitutes a birth center varies across the literature, both nationally and internationally, and most U.S. data sources cannot reliably track movement across birth settings or accurately attribute outcomes to the intended provider or place of birth (i.e., an intention-to-treat model). Where possible, the committee differentiates between outcomes for home births and outcomes for birth center births; however, some studies combine these births as "planned, out-of-hospital births" for analysis, which makes it impossible to compare the two (see, e.g., Snowden et al., 2015; Bovbjerg et al., 2017).

With these caveats in mind, this chapter provides a framework for understanding outcomes by birth setting and reviews the available research on maternal and newborn health outcomes for low-risk women for all three U.S. birth settings—home, birth center, and hospital—as well as data on outcomes by provider type where available. It then reviews studies of outcomes by birth setting internationally. Finally, the chapter concludes with a discussion of how interprofessional collaboration influences outcomes across and within birth settings. Where possible, we highlight the broad spectrum of outcomes that are of interest for this report and point to gaps in data and understanding that need to be filled by further research.

Importantly, we note that the literature reviewed focuses on outcomes by birth setting for low-risk women. As discussed in Chapter 3, maternal or fetal condition may have a significant influence on the choice of birth setting, as women who have medical or obstetric risk factors or comorbidities or are pregnant with fetuses at risk for complications are likely to give birth in a hospital. Conversely, healthy low-risk women living in regions with access to home and birth center birth will be overrepresented in these settings. In the same way, hospital level will influence the sample studied; for example, very high-risk women and fetuses are overrepresented in tertiary care facilities. These differences make direct comparisons across settings difficult. In the absence of adequate data to control for risk level and demographic differences, accurate comparisons are impossible.

UNDERSTANDING MATERNAL AND INFANT OUTCOMES

Miller and colleagues (2016) describe a continuum of global maternity care wherein two patterns result in excess of morbidity and mortality. The authors refer to these extremes as "too little, too late" (TLTL) and "too much, too soon" (TMTS). TLTL is used to describe care in which inadequate staffing, training, infrastructure, supplies, and medications (Austin et al., 2014, p. 2176) result in care that is withheld, below an evidence-based standard, or simply unavailable until it is too late. Severe morbidity and mortality result from this pattern of care. The converse system, TMTS, is characterized by routine overuse of interventions and the medicalization of healthy, uncomplicated pregnancies and births. Miller and colleagues (2016) argue that TMTS care often includes the unnecessary use of nonevidence-based interventions (e.g., continuous electronic fetal monitoring), as well as the overuse of interventions that can be lifesaving but are potentially harmful when applied routinely, without medical indication (e.g., cesarean section). In these systems, overintervention drives morbidity.

As facility births have increased globally, so has the recognition that TMTS systems can produce harm, increase costs, and concentrate disrespect and abuse in childbirth (Freedman and Kruk, 2014; World Health Organization, 2014; International Confederation of Midwives, White Ribbon Alliance, International Pediatric Association, and World Health Organization, 2015; Miller and Lalonde, 2015). While TMTS systems are typically associated with high-resource nations and TLTL with low- and middle-resource ones, because of inequality, these extremes often coexist within a single nation as a result of inequality.

When preventable maternal (or fetal) death and severe morbidity occur in U.S. hospitals, these outcomes may result either from TMTS (as in the case of morbidity associated with higher-than-ideal cesarean rates) or from TLTL (as with unrecognized hemorrhage). When preventable death and suffering occur at home or in birth centers, these outcomes are likely the result of TLTL. In its review of the literature, the committee identified a number of maternal and infant outcomes of interest related to these TMTS and TLTL concepts. These outcomes include maternal and infant mortality and morbidity indicators, which have been the traditional focus of birth settings research, as well as psychosocial outcomes, including several measures of dignity in the childbirth process, such as bodily autonomy, maternal agency, respectful care, and empowerment. The committee chose to review as many of these outcomes as possible because, taken together, they provide a broader understanding of what "safety" and a "healthy mother, healthy baby, and healthy family" mean to childbearing families and to members of the care team. In short, this broader perspective recognizes that the *experience* of care cannot be separated from clinical outcomes; it is not a complement or secondary consideration, but an important aspect of ensuring high-quality childbirth care (World Health Organization, 2018). Moreover, the experience of care and the outcome of care are closely associated. Although the committee recognizes the importance of patient experience in childbirth care, the literature on women's experiences in the maternity care system is limited. That literature is discussed in detail below.

Thus, in the discussion that follows, we examine the relationship between what we are calling intervention-related morbidity and birth setting, including outcomes and interventions reported in the literature, such as infection, induction, augmentation, postpartum hemorrhage, and genital tract tearing. We recognize that some of these interventions are necessary, unavoidable regardless of setting, or the result of maternal request. Nonetheless, because the desire to avoid unnecessary interventions is a primary reason families choose home and birth center births and because lower rates of these morbidities are also desirable from cost savings and quality-of-care perspectives, we review them in detail below. These morbidity outcomes are widely reported in the field, and thus are the focus of our review. However, we wish to emphasize that a broader conception of maternal morbidity is warranted. A more comprehensive view of morbidity would acknowledge the experiences of women and encompass such disorders as postpartum depression and anxiety, disrespect, unconsented care, coercion, and other forms of mistreatment that are starting to be documented in the United States (Vedam et al., 2019). These experiences impact not only the health of the person following childbirth but also that of the infant and family.

Additionally, the literature on health outcomes by birth setting would benefit from disaggregation of outcomes by race/ethnicity, socioeconomic status, and sexual orientation and gender identity, where possible. While the current literature on outcomes largely does not address differences by race and ethnicity or other subpopulations, as noted in Chapters 3 and 4, traditionally marginalized groups often accrue a disproportionate share of clinical and social risk factors for adverse outcomes during pregnancy and birth. In the sections below, we report variations in outcomes by subpopulations where available, but underscore the general paucity of evidence in this area and the need for future research to grapple with potential variation in outcomes by subpopulations, particularly for historically marginalized groups. Given the difficulty of studying outcomes by birth setting for the reasons outlined above, as well as the tendency toward confirmatory bias noted by Roome and colleagues (2016),[1] the committee, whose membership is diverse professionally, grappled with multiple tensions. Ultimately, we believe this was a strength because it led us to better understand multiple perspectives and viewpoints in a way that reflects the wide range of views and preferences held by U.S. women regarding place of birth. In general, we concluded that each setting—home, birth center, and hospital—offers a set of risks and benefits that accrue to either the pregnant woman or the newborn. And while no setting can fully remove risk from birth, evidence suggests that many risks are modifiable at the level of systems, processes, providers, and policies.

---

[1]Roome and colleagues (2016) reviewed the position statements on home birth for midwifery and obstetric colleges in the United States, the United Kingdom, Canada, Australia, and New Zealand in an effort to examine how the same body of research tends to lead to different positions on the acceptability of birth in the home setting. They found that midwifery organizations tend to support home birth as a viable option for healthy women, whereas physicians' organizations have statements that oppose this option. In 2015, the United Kingdom was the only country reviewed where physician- and midwife-led organizations had issued a joint statement in support of home birth. Roome and colleagues found widely differing stances that they argue reflect traditional midwifery perspectives on childbirth as a physiologic process versus obstetric perspectives, which focus on the potential for pathology. Ultimately, these authors assert that the differences in position statements are largely the by-product of confirmatory bias (i.e., the tendency to process information by looking for, or interpreting, information that is consistent with one's existing beliefs).

FETAL AND NEONATAL OUTCOMES BY U.S. BIRTH SETTING

Neonatal outcomes include neonatal mortality and neonatal morbidity. Death before delivery of the fetus is termed an intrapartum death. Death after birth is termed early neonatal mortality (up to 7 days of life[2]). Death up to 28 days is termed neonatal mortality; death 29 days to 1 year of age, postneonatal mortality; and death up to 1 year of age, infant mortality. The majority of infant deaths occur during the first 7 days of life. This terminology is important as different studies refer to various timepoints and apply the term perinatal mortality inconsistently. Measures of neonatal morbidity include seizures, neonatal intensive care unit (NICU) admissions, hypoxic-ischemic encephalopathy, and low Apgar scores. The rates of neonatal mortality and morbidity across settings vary depending on the population studied and the parameters set by the researchers (e.g., whether researchers excluded congenital anomalies, or restricted the population to low-risk mothers).

As discussed in Chapter 3, unforeseen emergencies related to either the birth process or an unrecognized condition of the newborn may require immediate skilled intervention, including cesarean delivery or neonatal resuscitation. In these cases, the ability to access higher-level care without delay is critical for the safety of the fetus or newborn. Risk for the newborn in a home or birth center birth setting and in hospitals without these capabilities may be mitigated through various strategies, including selection of low-risk mothers; referral to an obstetric or maternal–fetal medicine provider for pregnancy complications; minimization of transfer times in case of a need to transfer; barrier-free transfer to a hospital for birth complications; collaborative professional models of care; formal training of skilled practitioners; and professional regulation, oversight, and accountability (see Chapter 7).

Several studies of health outcomes for newborns in home and birth center settings have been conducted in the United States. Hospital births attended by midwives are generally used as the baseline against which these birth settings are compared, and some studies report comparisons by provider type across and within setting as well. U.S. studies use registry and birth certificate data. The findings from these studies are shown in Tables 6-1 and 6-2.

---

[2] Causes of death in this group refer to failure to resuscitate or consequences of severe hypoxic ischemic encephalopathy (see Chapter 3).

TABLE 6-1 Rate and Percentage of Neonatal Mortality by U.S. Birth Setting

Study	Data Source/Sample Size
Neonatal Mortality (neonatal death reported as 0 to 27 or 28 days)	
Bovbjerg et al., 2017 (ResQu: high, GRADE: low)	MANA 2.0 dataset (2004–2009) and 4.0 dataset (2012–2014) 47,394 out-of-hospital births
Grünebaum et al., 2014 (ResQu: low)	CDC linked birth/infant death dataset (2006–2009) 12,709,881 hospital physician 1,096,555 hospital midwife 39,523 freestanding birth center midwife 61,993 home midwife 28,119 home other
Grünebaum et al., 2016 (ResQu: low)	CDC linked birth/infant death dataset (2006–2009) 1,096,555 hospital CNM 18,389 home CNM 43,604 home uncertified midwife
Grünebaum et al., 2017a (ResQu: low, GRADE: fair)	CDC linked birth/infant death dataset (2009–2013) 1,077,197 hospital midwife 11,779,659 hospital physician 96,817 intended home births
Grünebaum et al., 2017b (ResQu: low, GRADE: poor)	CDC linked birth/infant death dataset (2008–2012) 1,363,199 hospital midwife 14,447,355 hospital MD 95,657 home midwife
Malloy, 2010	CDC linked birth/infant death dataset (2000–2004) 1,237,129 hospital CNM births 17,389 hospital other midwife births 13,529 home CNM births 42,375 home other midwife births 25,319 birth center CNM births
Snowden et al., 2015 (ResQu: high, GRADE: good)	Oregon birth, infant death, and fetal death certificates (2012–2013) 75,923 hospital births 3,203 out-of-hospital births 601 planned out of hospital but birthed at hospital
Thornton et al., 2017 (ResQu: high, GRADE: poor)	AABC (2006–2011) 8,776 planned birth center births 2,527 planned hospital births

Inclusion/ Exclusion Criteria	Birth Setting	Mortality %	Mortality Rate per 1,000 Live Births
Planned home or birth center births	Planned home and birth center births	—	1.98
Singleton, vertex, term (≥37 weeks and weight of ≥2,500 g) without congenital malformations	Hospital births with midwife	—	0.32
	Hospital births with MD	—	0.55
	Freestanding birth center births with midwife	—	0.59
	Home midwife	—	1.26
	Home other	—	1.87
Singleton, term (≥37 weeks), ≥2,500 g, nonanomalous	Hospital births with CNM	—	0.32
	Home births with CNM	—	1.00
	Home births with uncertified midwife	—	1.37
Singleton, term (≥37 weeks), weight ≥2,500 g, nonanomalous	Hospital births with midwife	—	0.31
	Hospital births with MD	—	0.51
	Home births	—	1.21
Singleton, term (≥37 weeks), birth weight ≥2,500 g	Hospital births with CNM	—	0.35
	Hospital births with MD	—	0.60
	Home births with midwife	—	1.28
Singleton, term (37–42 weeks), vaginal births	Hospital births with CNM	—	0.5
	Hospital births with other midwife	—	0.4
	Birth center births with CNM	—	0.6
	Home births with CNM	—	1.0
	Home births with other midwife	—	1.8
Singleton, term (≥37 weeks), cephalic, nonanomalous	Hospital births	0.06	—
	Planned home births	0.05	—
	Planned birth center births	0.24	—
Received prenatal care in birth center, singleton, ≥37 weeks, admitted in spontaneous labor	Hospital births	0.04	—
	Birth center births	0.03	—

continued

TABLE 6-1 Continued

Study	Data Source/Sample Size
Tilden et al., 2017 (ResQu: high, GRADE: fair)	U.S. birth and death records (2007–2010) 106,823 hospital births 3,147 out-of-hospital births

Early Neonatal Mortality (early neonatal death reported as 0 to 6, 7, or 8 days)

Bachilova et al., 2018 (ResQu: high, GRADE: poor)	CDC linked birth/infant death certificates (2011–2013) 71,704 planned home births
Cheyney et al., 2014a (ResQu: high, GRADE: poor)	MANA 2.0 dataset (2004–2009) 16,924 planned out-of-hospital births
Cox et al., 2015 (ResQu: high, GRADE: poor)	MANA 2.0 dataset (2004–2009) 1,052 TOLAC planned out-of-hospital births 12,092 out-of-hospital births
Grünebaum et al., 2014 (ResQu: low)	CDC linked birth/infant death dataset (2006–2009) 12,709,881 hospital physician 1,096,555 hospital midwife 39,523 freestanding birth center midwife 61,993 home midwife 28,119 home other

Late Neonatal Mortality (late neonatal death reported as 7 to 27 days)

Cheyney et al., 2014a (ResQu: high, GRADE: poor)	MANA 2.0 dataset (2004–2009) 16,924 planned out-of-hospital births

Inclusion/ Exclusion Criteria	Birth Setting	Mortality %	Mortality Rate per 1,000 Live Births
Single, term (≥37 weeks), vertex, nonanomolous, delivered by VBAC	Hospital births	0.08	—
	Out-of-hospital births	0.13	—
Planned home births, ≥34 weeks, nonanomolous	Planned home births	—	1.5
Planned home births not transferred to another provider prior to labor	Planned home births	—	0.88
Planned out-of-hospital birth not transferred to another provider prior to labor, multiparous women without a history of cesarean delivery Early neonatal death by days not specified	VBAC out-of-hospital births	—	0.95
	Out-of-hospital births	—	0.41
Singleton, vertex, term (≥37 weeks and weight of ≥2,500 g) without congenital malformations	Hospital births with midwife	—	0.14
	Hospital births with MD	—	0.29
	Freestanding birth center births with midwife	—	0.46
	Home midwife	—	0.93
	Home other	—	1.65
Planned home births not transferred to another provider prior to labor	Planned home births	—	0.41

continued

TABLE 6-1 Continued

Study	Data Source/Sample Size
Cox et al., 2015 (ResQu: high, GRADE: poor)	MANA 2.0 dataset (2004–2009) 1,052 TOLAC planned out-of-hospital births 12,092 out-of-hospital births

NOTES: AABC = American Association of Birth Centers; CDC = Centers for Disease Control and Prevention; CNM = certified nurse midwife; GRADE = Grading of Recommendations, Assessment, Development, and Evaluation; MANA = Midwives Alliance of North America; ResQu = Birth Place Research Quality; TOLAC = trial of labor after cesarian; VBAC = vaginal birth after cesarean.

Inclusion/ Exclusion Criteria	Birth Setting	Mortality %	Mortality Rate per 1,000 Live Births
Planned out-of-hospital births not transferred to another provider prior to labor, multiparous women without a history of cesarean delivery Late neonatal death by days not specified	VBAC out-of-hospital births	—	0.95
	Out-of-hospital births	—	0.17

TABLE 6-2 Rate and Percentage of Neonatal Morbidity by U.S Birth Setting

Study	Data Source/ Sample Size	Inclusion/Exclusion Criteria
Bovbjerg et al., 2017 (ResQu: high, GRADE: low)	MANA 2.0 dataset (2004–2009) and 4.0 dataset (2012–2014) 47,394 out-of-hospital births	Planned home or birth center births
Cheng et al., 2013 (ResQu: moderate)	CDC birth certificate data (2008) 12,039 planned home births 2,069,714 planned hospital births	Singleton, term (37–42 weeks), vertex, planned birth center and home births
Cheyney et al, 2014a (ResQu: high, GRADE: poor)	MANA 2.0 dataset (2004–2009) 16,924 planned out-of-hospital births	Planned home births not transferred to another provider prior to labor

Birth Setting	Outcome	Morbidity %	Morbidity Rate per 1,000 Live Births
Planned home and birth center births	Apgar 5 min <4	0.5	-
	Apgar 5 min <7	1.5	-
	Neonatal hospitalization first 6 weeks	7.4	-
	NICU admission first 6 weeks	2.8	-
Hospital births Planned home births by CNM	**Apgar 5 min <4**		
	Hospital births	0.24	-
	Home births CNM	0.19	-
Planned home births by other midwives	Home births other midwife	0.27	-
	Apgar 5 min <7		
	Hospital births	1.17	-
	Home births CNM	1.06	-
	Home births other midwife	2.63	-
	Ventilator support >6 h		
	Hospital births	0.27	-
	Home births CNM	0.18	-
	Home births other midwife	0.23	-
	NICU admissions		
	Hospital births	3.03	-
	Home births CNM	0.37	-
	Home births other midwife	0.64	-
Planned home births	**Apgar 5 min <7**		
	Planned home births	1.5	-
	NICU admission in the first 6 weeks		
	Planned home births	2.8	-

continued

TABLE 6-2 Continued

Study	Data Source/ Sample Size	Inclusion/Exclusion Criteria
Cox et al., 2015 (ResQu: high, GRADE: poor)	MANA 2.0 dataset (2004–2009) 1,052 TOLAC planned out-of-hospital births 12,092 out-of-hospital births	Planned out-of-hospital births not transferred to another provider prior to labor, multiparous women without a history of cesarean delivery
Grünebaum et al., 2013 (ResQu: low)	CDC birth certificate data (2007–2010) 12,663,051 hospital physician 1,118,578 hospital midwife 42,216 freestanding birth center midwife 67,429 home midwife	Singleton, term (≥37 weeks), ≥2,500 g

Birth Setting	Outcome	Morbidity %	Morbidity Rate per 1,000 Live Births
TOLAC out-of-hospital births	**Apgar 5 min <4**		
	TOLAC out-of-hospital births	1.0	-
	Out-of-hospital births	0.4	-
	NICU admission		
	TOLAC out-of-hospital births	4.2	-
	Out-of-hospital births	2.0	-
	Infant hospitalization in first 6 weeks		
	TOLAC out-of-hospital births	17.0	-
	Out-of-hospital births	7.8	-
Hospital MD	**Apgar 5 min = 0**		
Hospital midwife	Hospital MD	-	0.16
	Hospital midwife	-	0.09
Freestanding birth center midwife	Freestanding birth center midwife	-	0.55
Home midwife	Home midwife	-	1.63

continued

TABLE 6-2 Continued

Study	Data Source/ Sample Size	Inclusion/Exclusion Criteria
Malloy, 2010	CDC linked birth/infant death dataset (2000–2004) 1,237,129 hospital CNM births 17,389 hospital other midwife births 13,529 home CNM births 42,375 home other midwife births 25,319 birth center CNM births	Singleton, term (37–42 weeks), vaginal births

Birth Setting	Outcome	Morbidity %	Morbidity Rate per 1,000 Live Births
Hospital births with CNM	**Apgar 5 min <4**		
Hospital births with other midwife	Hospital births CNM	-	0.7
	Hospital births other midwife	-	0.6
Birth center births with CNM	Birth center births CNM	-	0.5
	Home births CNM	-	5.5
Home births with CNM	Home births other midwife	-	2.3
Home births with other midwife	**Injury at birth**		
	Hospital births CNM	-	3.1
	Hospital births other midwife	-	1.5
	Birth center births CNM	-	0.9
	Home births CNM	-	2.4
	Home births other midwife	-	1.7
	Mechanical ventilation <30 min		
	Hospital births CNM	-	15.1
	Hospital births other midwife	-	20.8
	Birth center births CNM	-	10.2
	Home births CNM	-	10.8
	Home births other midwife	-	15.6
	Mechanical ventilation >30 min		
	Hospital births CNM	-	2.7
	Hospital births other midwife	-	2.6
	Birth center births CNM	-	1.4
	Home births CNM	-	2.0
	Home births other midwife	-	3.9

continued

TABLE 6-2 Continued

Study	Data Source/ Sample Size	Inclusion/Exclusion Criteria
Snowden et al., 2015 (ResQu: high, GRADE: good)	Oregon birth, infant death, and fetal death certificates (2012–2013) 75,923 hospital births 3,203 out-of-hospital births 601 planned out of hospital but birthed at hospital	Singleton, term (≥37 weeks), cephalic, nonanomalous
Thornton et al., 2017 (ResQu: high, GRADE: poor)	AABC (2006–2011) 8,776 planned birth center births 2,527 planned hospital births	Received prenatal care in birth center, singleton, ≥37 weeks, admitted in spontaneous labor

Birth Setting	Outcome	Morbidity %	Morbidity Rate per 1,000 Live Births
Hospital birth	**Apgar 5 min <4**		
Planned home birth	Hospital births	0.4	-
	Planned home births	0.3	-
Planned birth center birth	Planned birth center births	0.6	-
	Apgar 5 min <7		
	Hospital births	1.9	-
	Planned home births	1.2	-
	Planned birth center births	2.5	-
	NICU admission		
	Hospital births	3.0	-
	Planned home births	0.8	-
	Planned birth center births	1.1	-
	Ventilation		
	Hospital births	3.3	-
	Planned home births	2.5	-
	Planned birth center births	4.5	-
Hospital birth	**Apgar 5 min <7**		
Birth center birth	Hospital births	0.51	-
	Birth center births	0.80	-
	Neonatal composite		
	Hospital births	0.44	-
	Birth center births	0.44	-
	Newborn ventilation <10 min		
	Hospital births	2.26	-
	Birth center births	3.05	-

continued

TABLE 6-2 Continued

Study	Data Source/ Sample Size	Inclusion/Exclusion Criteria
Tilden et al., 2017 (ResQu: high, GRADE: fair)	U.S. birth and death records (2007–2010) 106,823 hospital births 3,147 out-of- hospital births	Single, term (≥37 weeks), vertex, nonanomolous, delivered by VBAC

NOTE: AABC = American Association of Birth Centers; CDC = Centers for Disease Control and Prevention; CNM = certified nurse midwife; GRADE = Grading of Recommendations, Assessment, Development, and Evaluation; MANA = Midwives Alliance of North America; NICU = neonatal intensive care unit; ResQu = Birth Place Research Quality; TOLAC = trial of labor after cesarian; VBAC = vaginal birth after cesarean.

Birth Setting	Outcome	Morbidity %	Morbidity Rate per 1,000 Live Births
Hospital	**Apgar 5 min <4**		
Out of hospital	Hospital	0.4	
	Out of hospital	0.73	
	Apgar 5 min <7		
	Hospital	2.68	
	Out of hospital	4.42	
	Ventilator support		
	Hospital	0.29	
	Out of hospital	0.38	
	NICU admission		
	Hospital	3.10	
	Out of hospital	1.11	
	Birth injury		
	Hospital	0.10	
	Out of hospital	0.03	

Systematic Reviews

Two important systematic reviews have examined neonatal outcomes for home and birth center settings as compared with hospital settings: Phillippi and colleagues (2018) and Wax and colleages (2010). We discuss each study in detail below.

Phillippi and colleagues (2018) conducted a systematic review of 17 studies on neonatal outcomes; all of the studies evaluated neonatal mortality, and some also evaluated neonatal morbidity. Collectively, the studies included outcomes for the neonates of a total of 84,500 women admitted to a birth center in labor, including outcomes after transfer. The review found that in no study with a hospital comparison group was there a higher rate of neonatal mortality in the birth center group, and that nulliparous women and women older than 35 had a higher risk of poor neonatal outcomes in both birth centers and hospitals. In any studies that included births with a gestation more than 42 weeks, a higher risk of neonatal mortality was found for those pregnancies (Phillippi et al., 2018). All of these studies demonstrated selection of a favorable medical, obstetric, and social risk profile among women choosing home and birth center settings.

Wax and colleagues (2010) published a systematic review of birth outcomes for planned home and hospital births, which included all English-language, peer-reviewed publications from high-resource countries available at the time that reported fetal and neonatal outcomes by birth setting. Neonatal outcomes for planned home births included lower rate of low birthweight (less than 10% for gestational age or less than 2,500 grams) (1.3% vs. 2.2%; odds ratio [OR] 0.60; confidence interval [CI] 0.50–0.71), compared with the hospital sample. The neonatal mortality rate was nearly twice as high in planned home births as compared with planned hospital births (0.20% vs. 0.09%; OR 1.98; CI 1.19–3.28), and nearly three times as high when only nonanomalous infants were included in the analysis (0.15% vs. 0.04%; OR 2.87; CI 1.32–6.25). It is important to note that when sensitivity analyses were performed, which removed older studies and excluded those that had used matching, there was no significant difference in prematurity and neonatal death between the two birth settings (Wax et al., 2010).

Birth Registry Studies

A number of studies use birth registries, allowing for analysis on an intention-to-treat basis. As discussed in Chapter 4, however, they are limited in that reporting to registries is not mandatory. This means that findings come from samples rather than complete populations, and thus may not be generalizable. Moreover, because these studies are descriptive in nature, none has an explicit comparison group. Four descriptive studies using registry data—by Cox and colleagues (2015; 1.24/1,000 for women without a history of cesarean [ResQu: high, GRADE: poor]),[3] Cheney and colleagues (2014a; 0.85/1,000 [ResQu: high, GRADE: poor]),[4] Johnson and Daviss (2005; 1–2/1,000 [ResQu: moderate, GRADE: poor]), and Stapleton and colleagues (2013; 0.47/1,000 [ResQu: high, GRADE: poor])—have documented low rates of perinatal mortality at home and in birth centers for healthy, low-risk women in the United States using birth registry data. Thornton and colleagues (2017 [ResQu: high, GRADE: poor]), similarly using registry data, compared midwife-led birth center and hospital groups and found no difference in the neonatal outcome composite[5] (0.44% for both groups).[6]

Vital Statistics Studies

A number of other frequently cited studies report fetal and neonatal outcomes by birth setting using vital statistics. In 2012, the state of Oregon added new variables to the birth certificate (intended place of birth and the type of intended provider at the onset of labor), allowing Snowden and colleagues (2015) to use an intention-to-treat approach to examine outcomes by birth setting. The authors limited analyses to data from Oregon collected over the 2-year period following the change to the birth certificate, yielding a sample of 75,923 hospital births and 3,203 home and birth center births.

---

[3] The study by Cox and colleagues (2015), who used the same data registry, describes neonatal outcomes for women (n = 1,052) who planned a vaginal birth after cesarean (VBAC) at home with midwives who were contributing data to the Midwives Alliance of North America Statistics Project (MANA Stats) 2.0 data registry between 2004 and 2009. Five neonatal deaths (4.75/1,000) occurred in the prior cesarean group compared with 1.24/1,000 in multiparas without a history of cesarean (p = 0.015).

[4] Cheyney and colleagues (2014a) found elevated rates of fetal intrapartum and neonatal mortality in a home birth sample (n = 16,924) when clients with higher-risk factors such as breech, twins, labor after cesarean section with no prior vaginal birth, gestational diabetes, and preeclampsia were included in the sample. Low Apgar scores (<7) occurred in 1.5 percent of newborns, and postpartum neonatal transfers were infrequent, occurring in only 0.9 percent of births. In terms of postnatal outcomes, 86 percent of newborns were breastfeeding exclusively at 6 weeks of age. Excluding lethal anomalies, the intrapartum, early neonatal, and late neonatal mortality rates were 1.30, 0.41, and 0.35 per 1,000, respectively, when higher-risk births were included, for a combined perinatal death rate of 2.06 per 1,000. When the sample was limited to low-risk women (term, singleton, vertex, no previous cesarean), the intrapartum mortality rate dropped to 0.85/1,000.

[5] The neonatal outcome composite consisted of severe prenatal outcomes: intrapartum and newborn mortality, hypoxic neurologic injury, Apgar score <4 at 5 minutes, seizures, persistent pulmonary hypertension, positive pressure ventilation >10 minutes, and meconium aspiration syndrome.

[6] Thornton and colleagues (2017), using Perinatal Data Registry data, used exclusion criteria to form low-risk groups admitted to birth centers (n = 8,776) and those that chose hospital admission (n = 2,527).

Looking at singleton, term, nonanomalous births, this study found poorer outcomes at home and in birth centers—specifically, a perinatal mortality rate of 3.9 per 1,000 in home birth and birth center births compared with 1.8 per 1,000 in hospital births, and a neonatal mortality rate of 1.6 per 1,000 in home birth and birth center births compared with 0.6 per 1,000 in hospital births (Snowden et al., 2015).

Malloy (2010) conducted a retrospective cohort study measuring infant outcomes by setting and birth attendant using linked birth and death files from 2000 to 2004. The samples included hospital births attended by a certified nurse midwife (CNM), hospital births attended by another type of midwife, birth center birth attended by a CNM, home births attended by a CNM, and home births attended by another type of midwife. The neonatal mortality rate (measured as 0–27 days after birth) was 0.5/1,000 live births for hospital-CNM, 0.4/1,000 for hospital-other midwife, 0.6/1,000 for birth center-CNM, 1.0 for home-CNM, and 1.8/1,000 for home-other midwife. Births at home with a CNM or other midwife had a higher risk of neonatal death compared with hospital births with a CNM (2.02/1,000, CI 1.18–3.45; 3.63/1,000, CI 2.89–4.67, respectively). Home births attended by any midwife had a greater risk of a low 5-minute Apgar score <4 (home-CNM 7.83/1,000, CI: 6.09–10.1; home-other midwife 3.39/1,000, CI 2.70–4.24) compared with CNM-attended hospital deliveries.

Other studies also used vital statistics data (see, e.g., Cheng, 2013[7] [ResQu: moderate]; Grünebaum et al., 2013,[8]

---

[7]The study by Cheng and colleagues (2013) used 2008 vital statistics data from 27 states, which included the 2003 revision of the birth certificate that delineates the location of a birth as hospital, freestanding birth center, or home, and further as accidental, intended, or unknown if intended. Although the 2003 revision of the birth certificate includes information about where the birth took place and the planned status of that birth, it does not take into account intention-to-treat. Thus, the data do not account, for example, for planned home births that were transferred to hospitals. The authors compared outcomes of neonates whose mothers had planned home births and those who delivered in hospitals, and found that, compared with hospital births, more planned home births had 5-minute Apgar scores below 4 and a lower rate of NICU admission; they do not report neonatal mortality.

[8]In their 2013 study, Grünebaum and colleagues used birth certificate data from the CDC's National Center for Health Statistics to examine deliveries by physicians and midwives in and out of the hospital between 2007 and 2010 for a national sample of nearly 14 million singleton term births. Term was defined as 37 weeks or more gestation and a birthweight of 2,500 g or more. The majority of term singleton births (91%; n = 12,663,051) were physician-attended hospital births; midwife-attended hospital births constituted 8 percent of births (n = 1,118,678), 0.3 percent were midwife-led freestanding birth center births (n = 42,216), and 0.5 percent (n = 67,429) were midwife home deliveries. Grünebaum and colleagues (2013) found that, compared with hospital births attended by physicians or midwives, home births and births in freestanding birth centers attended by midwives had a significantly higher risk of a 5-minute Apgar score of 0 and neonatal seizures or serious neurologic dysfunction. This risk was greater for nulliparous women. In addition, women who gave birth at home with

2014,[9] 2015b[10] [ResQu: low]; Bachilova et al., 2018[11] [ResQu: low, GRADE: poor]; and Wasden et al., 2017[12] [ResQu: low]). Collectively,

a midwife attending were significantly more likely to have macrosomic infants (birthweight greater than 4,000 g); see Tables 5-1 and 5-2. The distinction between causality and correlation should be noted here. Birth settings would not cause higher birthweight, but home births could be correlated with higher birthweight for multiple reasons, such as waiting until the natural onset of labor rather than undergoing induction (see, e.g., Zhang et al., 2010).

[9] The 2014 study by Grünebaum and colleagues used the CDC-linked birth and infant death dataset from 2006–2009 for early and total neonatal mortality for nearly 14 million singleton, vertex, and term births without congenital anomalies. This dataset included births attended by midwives and physicians in the hospital and midwives at home and in birth centers. The authors used midwife-attended home births as a proxy for planned home births. Compared with deliveries by hospital midwives, home births were more likely to be postterm, and mothers were more likely to have macrosomic infants. Midwife-attended home births also had a significantly higher total neonatal mortality risk relative to deliveries attended by midwives in the hospital, and the risk of neonatal mortality increased for postterm births and nulliparous women. Similar results were observed for early neonatal mortality. The excess total neonatal mortality for midwife-attended home births compared with midwife-attended hospital births was estimated at 0.93 per 1,000 births, and the excess early neonatal mortality at 0.79 per 1,000 births. In birth center births, excess total neonatal mortality was reported as .26 per 1,000 births, and excess early neonatal mortality as .32 per 1,000 births (Grünebaum, 2014).

[10] The 2015 study by Grünebaum and colleagues used a national sample of about 12 million deliveries from 2010–2012 CDC-linked vital records to analyze the frequency of four perinatal risk factors—breech presentation, prior cesarean delivery, twins, and gestational age 41 weeks or longer—that were associated with planned midwife-attended home births in the United States and compare them with deliveries performed in the hospital by CNMs. (Home births attended by others were excluded; only planned home births attended by midwives were included.) Compared with CNM-attended hospital births, all four risk factors were significantly higher among midwife-attended planned home births, and three were significantly higher for planned home births attended by midwives not certified by the American Midwifery Certification Board.

[11] The 2018 study by Bachilova and colleagues used CDC-linked vital records for 2011–2013 to conduct a 3-year retrospective cohort study of 71,704 planned home births in the United States. The authors found an overall early neonatal mortality rate of 1.5 per 1,000 planned home births, with significantly elevated risk in some subgroups. The risk of early neonatal death was significantly higher among nulliparous women (adjusted odds ratio [aOR] 2.71; 95% CI 1.71–4.31), women with previous cesarean births (aOR 2.62; 95% CI 1.25–5.52), nonvertex presentations (aOR 4.27; 95% CI 1.33–13.75), plural births (aOR 9.79; 95% CI 4.25–22.57), preterm births (34– <37 weeks gestation) (aOR 4.68; 95% CI 2.30–9.51), and births at ≥41 weeks gestation (aOR 1.76; 95% CI 1.09–2.84). The authors conclude that early neonatal deaths occur more commonly when certain risk factors are present and that more careful patient selection may reduce adverse neonatal outcomes among planned home births.

[12] Wasden and colleagues (2017) used vital statistics data from New York City as their control group to identify the risk of HIE (hypoxic ischemic encephalopathy) compared with infants who received head cooling for HIE at a New York City institution. Demographics, obstetric information, location of birth, and intended location of birth were obtained from the vital records for both the cases and controls. A total of 69 infants underwent head cooling for HIE and were matched with 276 normal controls. After adjusting for pregnancy characteristics and mode of delivery, the odds of having an infant requiring treatment for HIE was 44 (95% CI 1.7–256.4) for out-of-hospital births compared with infants without HIE, regardless of

these authors found worse neonatal outcomes for completed home births, including higher rates of neonatal mortality (Grünebaum and colleagues only), low 5-minute Apgar scores, and neonatal seizures. However, these studies were unable to track outcomes using an intention-to-treat model, and the impact of misclassification on the reliability of findings from studies based on vital statistics has not been conclusively studied. Similarly, as discussed in Chapter 4, it is difficult to ensure that all of the home births in a study sample were planned and attended because of variability in birth certificates from state to state whereby some accidental home births cannot be distinguished from planned ones (California), and planned, unassisted home births (also called "freebirths") cannot be readily distinguished from those that are attended by a trained midwife (all states).

Comparative Risk of Neonatal Mortality and Morbidity

U.S. studies show elevated rates of neonatal mortality in home births compared with hospital births; see Tables 6-3 and 6-4. The relative risk to the infant may be two-fold, with absolute risks of about 1.2/1,000 versus 0.6/1,000 for home and hospital, respectively. The literature is not conclusive as to the magnitude of these rates because the available data make it difficult to distinguish between planned and unplanned or accidental home births, attended and intentionally unassisted births (also called "freebirths"), and provider type, if present.

Finding 6-1: Statistically significant increases in the relative risk of neonatal death in the home compared with the hospital setting have been reported in most U.S. studies of low-risk births using vital statistics data. However, the precise magnitude of the difference is difficult to assess given flaws in the underlying data. Regarding serious neonatal morbidity, studies report a wide range of risk for low-risk home versus hospital birth and by provider type. Given the importance of understanding these severe morbidities, the differing results among studies are of concern and require further study.

Research is critically needed to further evaluate neonatal outcomes among home and freestanding birth centers. Vital statistics studies of freestanding birth center outcomes show an increased risk of poor neonatal outcomes. Studies conducted in the United States using an intention-to-treat

---

intended place of birth. For those who did plan a home birth, the odds of having an infant with HIE were 21 (95% CI 1.7–256.4) compared with infants not requiring treatment for HIE. The authors conclude that out-of-hospital births were associated with increased odds of having an infant requiring treatment for HIE.

approach have demonstrated that births in birth centers and hospitals have similar to slightly elevated rates of neonatal and perinatal mortality.

> *Finding 6-2: Vital statistics studies of low-risk births in freestanding birth centers show an increased risk of poor neonatal outcomes, while studies conducted in the United States using models indicating intended place of birth have demonstrated that low-risk births in birth centers and hospitals have similar to elevated rates of neonatal mortality. Findings of studies of the comparative risk of neonatal morbidity between low-risk birth center and hospital births are mixed, with variation across studies by outcome and provider type.*

Moreover, giving the interrelationship of midwife credentialing with birth settings, its mediating effect on perinatal outcomes cannot be ascertained with confidence from the current literature.

MATERNAL OUTCOMES BY U.S. BIRTH SETTING

Overuse and associated intervention-related maternal morbidity have been well documented in U.S. hospitals. Over the past several decades, cesarean birth rates have increased to 31.9 percent (Hamilton et al., 2019), which is higher than the generally recognized level at which lifesaving maternal and neonatal benefits outweigh the risks. Potential complications of cesarean births include a greater incidence of both maternal and infant outcomes including hemorrhage, infection, and admission to the intensive care unit; longer hospital stays; reduced breastfeeding success; and infant respiratory problems. A Healthy People 2020 goal is to reduce the nulliparous, vertex, term, singleton (NVTS) cesarean rate to 23.9 percent (Office of Disease Prevention and Health Promotion, 2019).

As discussed in Chapter 2, hospitals across the United States vary widely in terms of rural or urban setting, level of care, resources available, and staffing models. Researchers have examined some of these differences and how they impact maternal outcomes, including interventions during birth and morbidities. Kozhimannil (2014) looked at differences between urban and rural hospitals, and found that rates of non-indicated cesarean birth and non-indicated labor induction were not dramatically different between the two in 2010 (16.9% and 17.8% for cesarean birth and 16.5% and 12% for induction, respectively). However, the rates of cesarean birth rose in both types of hospital between 2002 and 2010, and the rate of non-indicated labor induction rose disproportionately faster in rural compared with urban hospitals. Snyder and colleagues (2011) compared the rates of labor intervention in university and community hospitals across Ohio. They found that women giving birth in community hospitals were more likely

TABLE 6-3 Comparative Risk of Neonatal Mortality by Birth Setting

Study	Data Source/Sample Size	Inclusion/Exclusion Criteria
Total Neonatal Mortality		
Grünebaum et al., 2014 (ResQu: low)	CDC linked birth/infant death dataset (2006–2009) 12,709,881 hospital physician 1,096,555 hospital midwife 39,523 freestanding birth center midwife 61,993 home midwife 28,119 home other	Singleton, vertex, term (≥37 weeks and weight of ≥2,500 g) without congenital malformations Neonatal death reported as 0–27 days
Grünebaum et al., 2016 (ResQu: low)	CDC linked birth/infant death dataset (2006–2009) 1,096,555 hospital CNM 18,389 home CNM 43,604 home uncertified midwife	Singleton, term (≥37 weeks), ≥2,500 g, nonanomalous Neonatal death reported as 0–27 days
Grünebaum et al., 2017b (ResQu: low, GRADE: poor)	CDC linked birth/infant death dataset (2008–2012) 1,363,199 hospital midwife 14,447,355 hospital MD 95,657 home midwife	Singleton, term (≥37 weeks), birthweight ≥2,500 g
Malloy, 2010	CDC linked birth/infant death dataset (2000–2004) 1,237,129 hospital CNM 17,389 in-hospital other midwife 13,529 home CNM 42,375 home other midwife 25,319 birthing center CNM	Singleton, term (37–42 weeks), vaginal births Neonatal death reported as 0–27 days
Snowden et al., 2015 (ResQu: high, GRADE: good)	Oregon birth, infant death, and fetal death certificates (2012–2013) 75,923 hospital 3,203 out-of-hospital 601 planned out-of-hospital but birthed at hospital	Singleton, term (≥37 weeks), cephalic, nonanomalous Neonatal death reported as 0–28 days Infant death after reclassification of hospital transfers as planned out-of-hospital
Tilden et al., 2017 (ResQu: high, GRADE: fair)	U.S. birth and death records (2007–2010) 106,823 hospital 3,147 out-of-hospital	Single, term (≥37 weeks), vertex, nonanomolous, delivered by VBAC

Type of Birth	RR (95% CI)	Adj. OR (95% CI)
Hospital midwife (ref)	1.00	—
Hospital MD	1.69 (1.52–1.88)	—
Freestanding birth center midwife	1.81 (1.19–2.75)	—
Home midwife	3.87 (3.03–4.95)	—
Home other	5.75 (4.31–7.68)	—
Hospital with CNM	0.33 (0.21–0.53)	—
Home with CNM (ref)	1.00	—
Home with uncertified midwife	1.41 (0.83–2.38)	—
Hospital with CNM (ref)	1.00	—
Hospital with MD	1.71 (1.6–1.9)	—
Home with midwife	3.62 (3–4.4)	—
Hospital with CNM (ref)	—	1.00
Hospital with other midwife	—	0.79 (0.37–1.66)
Birth center with CNM	—	1.54 (0.94–2.54)
Home with CNM	—	2.02 (1.18–3.45)
Home with other midwife	—	3.63 (2.89–4.67)
Hospital (ref)	—	1.00
Out-of-hospital	—	1.68 (0.77–3.66)
Hospital (ref)	—	1.00
Out-of-hospital	—	2.10 (0.73–6.05)

continued

TABLE 6-3 Continued

Study	Data Source/Sample Size	Inclusion/Exclusion Criteria
Early Neonatal Mortality		
Grünebaum et al., 2014 (ResQu: low)		Singleton, vertex, term (≥37 weeks and weight of ≥2,500 g) without congenital malformations Early neonatal death reported as 0–6 days

NOTE: CDC = Centers for Disease Control and Prevention; CNM = certified nurse midwife; GRADE = Grading of Recommendations, Assessment, Development, and Evaluation; ResQu = Birth Place Research Quality; VBAC = vaginal birth after cesarean.`

Type of Birth	RR (95% CI)	Adj. OR (95% CI)
Hospital midwife (ref)	1.00	—
Hospital MD	2.04 (1.73–2.39)	—
Freestanding birth center midwife	3.26 (2.01–5.31)	—
Home midwife	6.60 (4.88–8.93)	—
Home other	11.73 (8.45–16.28)	—

TABLE 6-4 Comparative Risk of Neonatal Morbidity by Birth Setting

Study	Data Source/Sample Size	Inclusion/Exclusion Criteria
Cheng et al., 2013 (ResQu: moderate)	CDC birth certificate data (2008) 12,039 planned home 2,069,714 planned hospital	Singleton, term (37–42 weeks), vertex, planned birth center and home
Grünebaum et al., 2013 (ResQu: low)	CDC birth certificate data (2007–2010) 12,663,051 hospital physician 1,118,578 hospital midwife 42,216 freestanding birth center midwife 67,429 home midwife	Singleton, term (≥37 weeks), ≥2,500 g

Birth Setting	Outcome	RR (95% CI)	Adj. OR (95% CI)
Hospital	**Apgar 5 min <4**		
Planned home by CNM	Hospital (ref)	—	1.00
	Home CNM	—	0.69 (0.26–1.83)
Planned home by other midwives	Home other midwife	—	1.62 (1.01–1.83)
	Apgar 5 min <7		
	Hospital (ref)	—	1.00
	Home CNM	—	0.77 (0.52–1.16)
	Home other midwife	—	2.92 (2.49–3.42)
	Ventilator support >6 h		
	Hospital (ref)	—	1.00
	Home CNM	—	0.73 (0.33–1.63)
	Home other midwife	—	0.91 (0.53–1.54)
	NICU admissions		
	Hospital (ref)	—	1.00
	Home CNM	—	0.13 (0.07–0.23)
	Home other midwife	—	0.24 (0.18–0.34)
Hospital MD	**Apgar 5 min = 0**		
Hospital midwife	Hospital MD (ref)	1.00	—
	Hospital midwife	0.55 (0.45–0.68)	—
Freestanding birth center midwife	Freestanding birth center midwife	3.56 (2.36–5.36)	—
Home midwife	Home midwife	10.55 (8.62–12.93)	—

continued

TABLE 6-4 Continued

Study	Data Source/Sample Size	Inclusion/Exclusion Criteria
Malloy, 2010	CDC linked birth/infant death dataset (2000–2004) 1,237,129 hospital CNM 17,389 hospital other midwife 13,529 home CNM 42,375 home other midwife 25,319 birthing center CNM	Singleton, term (37–42 weeks), vaginal

Birth Setting	Outcome	RR (95% CI)	Adj. OR (95% CI)
Hospital with CNM	**Apgar 5 min <4**		
Hospital with other midwife	Hospital CNM (ref)	—	1.00
	Hospital other midwife	—	0.78 (0.42–1.46)
Birth center with CNM	Birth center CNM	—	0.80 (0.45–1.42)
	Home CNM	—	7.83 (6.09–10.1)
	Home other midwife	—	3.39 (2.70–4.24)
Home with CNM	**Injury at birth**		
Home with other midwife	Hospital CNM (ref)	—	1.00
	Hospital other midwife	—	0.47 (0.31–0.70)
	Birth center CNM	—	0.36 (0.23–0.55)
	Home CNM	—	0.84 (0.58–1.22)
	Home other midwife	—	0.59 (0.46–0.76)
	Mechanical ventilation <30 min		
	Hospital CNM (ref)	—	1.00
	Hospital other midwife	—	1.33 (1.18–1.51)
	Birth center CNM	—	0.79 (0.69–0.92
	Home CNM	—	0.74 (0.61–0.89)
	Home other midwife	—	1.08 (0.98–1.18)
	Mechanical ventilation 30 min		
	Hospital CNM (ref)	—	1.00
	Hospital other midwife	—	0.98 (0.73–1.33)
	Birth center CNM	—	0.66 (0.47–0.94)
	Home CNM	—	0.83 (0.55–1.25)
	Home other midwife	—	1.63 (1.38–1.94)

continued

TABLE 6-4 Continued

Study	Data Source/Sample Size	Inclusion/Exclusion Criteria
Snowden et al., 2015 (ResQu: high, GRADE: good)	Oregon birth, infant death, and fetal death certificates (2012–2013) 75,923 hospital 3,203 out-of-hospital 601 planned out of hospital but birthed at hospital	Singleton, term (≥37 weeks), cephalic, nonanomalous Adjusted odds ratio after reclassification of hospital transfers as planned out-of-hospital
Thornton et al., 2017 (ResQu: high, GRADE: poor)	AABC (2006–2011) 8,776 planned birth center 2,527 planned hospital	Received prenatal care in birth center, singleton, ≥37 weeks, admitted in spontaneous labor

Birth Setting	Outcome	RR (95% CI)	Adj. OR (95% CI)
Hospital (ref)	**Apgar 5 min <4**		
Out-of-hospital	Hospital (ref)	—	1.00
	Out-of-hospital	—	1.56 (0.98–2.47)
	Apgar 5 min <7		
	Hospital (ref)	—	1.00
	Out-of-hospital	—	1.31 (1.04–1.66)
	NICU admission		
	Hospital (ref)	—	1.00
	Out-of-hospital	—	0.71 (0.55–0.92)
	Ventilation		
	Hospital (ref)	—	1.00
	Out-of-hospital	—	1.36 (1.14–1.62)
Hospital	**Apgar 5 min 3–7**		
Birth center	Hospital (ref)	—	1.00
	Birth center	—	1.51 (0.80–2.85)
	Neonatal composite		
	Hospital (ref)	—	1.00
	Birth center	—	1.13 (0.60–2.13)
	Newborn ventilation <10 min		
	Hospital (ref)	—	1.00
	Birth center	—	1.31 (0.97–1.79)

continued

TABLE 6-4 Continued

Study	Data Source/Sample Size	Inclusion/Exclusion Criteria
Tilden et al., 2017 (ResQu: high, GRADE: fair)	U.S. birth and death records (2007–2010) 106,823 hospital 3,147 out-of-hospital	Single, term (≥37 weeks), vertex, nonanomolous, delivered by VBAC
Wasden et al., 2017 (ResQu: low)	Hospital database linked with New York City vital records 69 cases of HIE 276 matched controls	≥36 weeks and one of the following: Apgar ≤5 at 10 min resuscitation including endotracheal intubation or bag/mask ventilation at 10 min Acidosis, defined as either umbilical cord arterial pH <7 or any postnatal arterial pH <7 within 60 min of birth Base deficit ≥16 mmol/L in an umbilical cord sample or any blood sample obtained within 60 min of birth (i.e., arterial or venous blood)

NOTE: AABC = American Association of Birth Centers; CDC = Centers for Disease Control and Prevention; CNM = certified nurse midwife; GRADE = Grading of Recommendations, Assessment, Development, and Evaluation; HIE = hypoxic ischemic encephalopathy; NICU = neonatal intensive care unit; ResQu = Birth Place Research Quality.

Birth Setting	Outcome	RR (95% CI)	Adj. OR (95% CI)
Hospital	**Apgar 5 min <4**		
Out-of-hospital	Hospital (ref)	—	1.00
	Out-of-hospital	—	1.77 (1.12–2.79)
	Apgar 5 min <7		
	Hospital (ref)	—	1.00
	Out-of-hospital	—	1.62 (1.35–1.96)
	Ventilator support		
	Hospital (ref)	—	1.00
	Out-of-hospital	—	1.36 (0.75—2.46)
	NICU admission		
	Hospital (ref)	—	1.00
	Out-of-hospital	—	0.40 (0.29–0.57)
	Birth injury		
	Hospital (ref)	—	1.00
	Out-of-hospital	—	0.78 (0.58–1.04)
Out-of-hospital with HIE	**HIE**		
Planned home with HIE	Neonates w/o HIE	—	1.00
Neonates without HIE	Out-of-hospital w/HIE	—	44 (4.5–424.0)
	Planned home w/HIE	—	21 (1.7–256.4)

to be induced at 37 weeks (1.7 adjusted odds ratio [aOR]), at 38 weeks (1.8 aOR), and at 39–42 weeks (2.0 aOR) compared with women in university hospitals. However, rates of cesarean birth did not differ between the two types of hospitals. Fingar and colleagues (2018) looked at rates of severe maternal morbidity across multiple kinds of hospitals. They found the outcome to be more prevalent in safety net hospitals, minority-serving hospitals, teaching hospitals, public (compared with privately owned) hospitals, and hospitals in the Northeast and South.

Much of the research examining hospital-specific rates of intervention and morbidity consists of studies that compare hospital births with home or birth center births in order to draw conclusions about differences among settings. Because of their goal of making comparisons, these studies usually adjust the population studied to match the lower-risk profiles of women who give birth at home or in a birth center; for example, a study might look only at births that are singleton, vertex, and full-term. Thus, the rates gleaned from the hospital data cannot be used as representative of the rates for all hospital births, only of the rates for low-risk women in hospital settings. Recognizing this limitation of studies that compare home and birth center births with hospital births, these studies have consistently found higher rates of maternal intervention and morbidity in planned hospital births. We review this literature—systematic reviews, studies using birth registry data, and studies using vital statistics data—in detail below; the results are summarized in Table 6-5.

Systematic Reviews

Wax and colleagues (2010) published a systematic review of the literature on health outcomes following planned home and hospital births that provided data on morbidity in the home setting as well. The authors included all English-language, peer-reviewed publications from high-resource countries available at the time that reported maternal, fetal, and neonatal outcomes by birth setting. In alignment with the committee's findings, these authors note that it is impossible to evaluate maternal mortality by birth setting, as these data are not reported in the literature, or small sample sizes do not allow for meaningful analysis. However, they were able to compare planned home and hospital births for a broad range of general morbidity and intervention-related morbidity indicators. They found that planned home births were associated with fewer maternal interventions, including epidural analgesia (9.0% vs. 22.9%; OR 0.24; CI 0.22–0.25); electronic fetal heart rate monitoring (13.8% vs. 62.6%; OR 0.10; CI 0.09–0.10); episiotomy (7.0% vs. 10.4%; OR 0.26; CI 0.24–0.28); operative delivery (3.5% vs. 10.2%; OR 0.26; CI 0.24–0.28); and cesarean birth in healthy, low-risk mothers (5.0% vs. 9.3%; OR 0.42; CI 0.39–0.45). Women who planned home births were also less likely to experience 3rd- and 4th-degree tears 1.2% vs. 2.5%; OR 0.35; CI 0.33–0.45); infection (0.7% vs. 2.6%; OR 0.27; CI 0.19–0.39); postpartum hemorrhage/bleeding (4.9% vs. 5.0%; OR 0.66; CI 0.61–0.71); vaginal lacerations (7.9% vs. 22.4%; OR 0.85; CI 0.78–0.93); and retained placenta (1.2% vs. 1.6%; OR 0.65; CI 0.51–0.83). This association between reduced morbidity and home birth settings may be attributable both to home birth models of care and to the fact that healthy women who are highly motivated to avoid interventions are proportionately overrepresented in home birth samples.

Vital Statistics Studies

More recent research on maternal outcomes by birth setting has largely upheld the findings of the Wax and colleagues (2010) systematic review. Using vital statistics data, Cheng and colleagues (2013 [ResQu: moderate]) found lower rates of interventions in the home compared with births in the hospital setting, including operative vaginal birth (0.1% vs. 6.2%; aOR 0.12; CI 0.08–0.17), labor induction (1.4% vs. 25.7%; aOR 0.19; CI 0.18–0.22), augmentation of labor (2.1% vs. 22.2%; aOR 0.29; CI 0.27–0.31), and use of antibiotics in labor (2.6% vs. 15.2%; aOR 0.40; CI 0.37–0.42). Three studies of birth center outcomes also used vital statistics data (MacDorman and Declercq, 2016[13]; Li et al., 2017[14]; Stephenson-Famy et al., 2018[15]).

---

[13] MacDorman and Declercq (2016 [ResQu: moderate, GRADE: poor]) examined trends in out-of-hospital births (n = 59,674) that occurred between the years of 2004 and 2014. Data for this study came from 47 states and Washington, DC, using birth certificate data that had been revised after 2003. Results showed that out-of-hospital births increased by 72 percent over the 10-year period. Compared with women who had hospital births, out-of-hospital births had lower prepregnancy obestity and higher rates of breastfeeding initiation and vaginal birth after cesarean (VBAC). Results were significant at the p <0.05 level.

[14] Li and colleagues (2017 [GRADE: poor]) conducted a population-based cohort study with matched birth certificate data (1996–2013) and Medicaid claims and hospital discharge abstracts in South Carolina to evaluate the validity of reports of neonatal seizures in infants born at home or in birth centers and then transferred to the hospital (n = 1,233). Their results showed birth certificates were not reliable as a sole source for analyzing the prevalence of neonatal seizures

[15] Stephenson-Famy and colleagues (2018 [ResQu: moderate, GRADE: poor) performed a retrospective cohort study using birth certificate data (2004 to 2011) of women who planned to give birth in a birth center (n = 7,118 planned birth center births). A total of 93 percent of women gave birth at the birth center, and 7 percent gave birth in a hospital setting. Nulliparity was the most significant risk factor for hospital transfer (aOR 7.2; CI 5.3–9.8), followed by maternal age >40 (aOR 3.7; CI 2.1–6.7) and inadequate prenatal care (aOR 3.7; CI 2.7–5.0).

TABLE 6-5 Rate, Percentage, and Comparative Risk of Maternal
Intervention-Related Morbidity by Birth Setting

Study	Data Source/ Sample Size	Inclusion/Exclusion Criteria	Birth Setting
Bovbjerg et al., 2017 (ResQu: high, GRADE: low)	MANA 2.0 dataset (2004–2009) and 4.0 dataset (2012–2014) 47,394 out-of-hospital	Planned home or birth center	Planned home and birth center
Cheng et al., 2013 (ResQu: moderate)	CDC birth certificate data (2008) 12,039 planned home 2,069,714 planned hospital	Singleton, term (37–42 weeks), vertex, planned birth center and home	Hospital Planned home
Cheyney et al., 2014a (ResQu: high, GRADE: poor)	MANA 2.0 dataset (2004–2009) 16,924 planned out-of-hospital	Planned home not transferred to another provider prior to labor	Planned home

Outcome	Morbidity %	Morbidity Rate per 1,000 Live Births	Adj. OR (95% CI)
Cesarean Delivery	5.4		
Vaginal only		—	—
Any genital tract trauma	53.2	—	—
Postpartum hemorrhage >1000 cc	3.4	—	—
Augmentation of Labor			
Hospital	22.2	—	1.00
Planned home	2.1	—	0.29 (0.27–0.31)
Induction of Labor			
Hospital	25.7	—	1.00
Planned home	1.4	—	0.19 (0.18–0.22)
Cesarean Birth	5.2	—	—
Episiotomy	1.4	—	—
1st- or 2nd-degree perineal laceration	40.9	—	—
3rd- or 4th-degree perineal laceration	1.2	—	—
If Intrapartum Transfer			
Oxytocin augmentation	22.0	—	—

continued

TABLE 6-5 Continued

Study	Data Source/ Sample Size	Inclusion/Exclusion Criteria	Birth Setting
Snowden et al., 2015 (ResQu: high, GRADE: good)	Oregon birth, infant death, and fetal death certificates (2012–2013) 75,923 hospital 3,203 out-of-hospital 601 planned out of hospital but birthed at hospital	Singleton, term (≥37 weeks), cephalic, nonanomalous. Odds ratios were calculated for planned out-of-hospital with planned hospital delivery.	Hospital Planned home Planned birth center
Stapleton et al., 2013 (ResQu: high, GRADE: poor)	AABC (2007–2010) 15,574 birth center	Planned birth center, singleton, vertex, live-born infant at ≥37 weeks gestation.	Birth center
Thornton et al., 2017 (ResQu: high, GRADE: poor)	AABC (2006–2011) 8,776 planned birth center 2,527 planned hospital	Received prenatal care in birth center, singleton, ≥37 weeks, admitted in spontaneous labor.	Hospital Birth center

NOTE: AABC = American Association of Birth Centers; CDC = Centers for Disease Control and Prevention; GRADE = Grading of Recommendations, Assessment, Development, and Evaluation; MANA = Midwives Alliance of North America; ResQu = Birth Place Research Quality.

Outcome	Morbidity %	Morbidity Rate per 1,000 Live Births	Adj. OR (95% CI)
Augmentation of Labor			
Hospital (ref)	26.4	—	1.00
Planned home	1.2	—	—
Planned birth center	1.1	—	—
Out-of-hospital	—	—	0.21 (0.19–0.24)
Induction of Labor			
Hospital (ref)	30.4	—	1.00
Planned home	1.3	—	—
Planned birth center	1.9	—	—
Out-of-hospital	—	—	0.11 (0.09–0.12)
Cesarean Delivery			
Hospital (ref)	24.7	—	1.00
Planned home	0	—	—
Planned birth center	0	—	—
Out-of-hospital	—	—	0.18 (0.16–0.22)
Severe Perineal Lacerations			
Hospital (ref)	1.3	—	1.00
Planned home	0.4	—	—
Planned birth center	1.4	—	—
Out-of-hospital	—	—	0.69 (0.49–0.98)
Primary Cesarean			
Birth center	6.0	—	—
Cesarean			
Hospital	4.99	—	1.00
Birth center	4.14	—	0.62 (0.49–0.79)
Postpartum Hemorrhage			
Hospital	4.63	—	1.00
Birth center	6.18	—	1.19 (0.97–1.48)

Birth Registry Studies

As noted above and in Chapter 5, studies using birth registries allow for analysis on an intention-to-treat basis; however, because reporting to registries is not mandatory these results may not be generalizable. In addition, these studies are descriptive and do not have an explicit comparison group. Cheyney and colleagues (2014a [ResQu: high, GRADE: poor]), using data from a national registry, describe outcomes of planned home births in the United States between 2004 and 2009. Among 16,924 women who went into labor intending to give birth at home, 89.1 percent completed their birth at home. The majority of intrapartum transfers from home to hospital were for slow, nonprogressive labors, and only 4.5 percent of the total sample required oxytocin augmentation and/or epidural analgesia. The rates of spontaneous vaginal birth, assisted vaginal birth, and cesarean birth were 93.6 percent, 1.2 percent, and 5.2 percent, respectively (Cheyney et al., 2014a).

Four studies of birth center outcomes use data collected prospectively through the Perinatal Data Registry (PDR), a national, validated, online data collection tool developed by the American Association of Birth Centers (AABC) (Stapleton et al., 2013[16]; Jolles et al, 2017[17]; Thornton et al., 2017[18]; Alliman et al., 2019[19]). An additional study evaluates outcomes of

---

[16]In a descriptive study, Stapleton and colleagues (2013 [ResQu: high, GRADE: poor]) evaluated outcomes of care for more than 15,500 women eligible for birth center admission in labor using the AABC's data registry (called the Uniform Data Set, or UDS, at the time, now the PDR). The authors found a spontaneous vaginal birth rate of 93 percent and a cesarean birth rate of 6 percent; the remaining births were assisted vaginal births (Stapleton et al., 2013). The intrapartum transfer rate after admission to a birth center was 12.4 percent, and of those, 0.9 percent were considered emergency transfers. Intrapartum fetal deaths were 0.47 per 1,000, and neonatal deaths, excluding anomalies, were 0.40 per 1,000.

[17]Jolles and colleagues (2017) analyzed data from Medicaid enrollees whose birth outcomes were recorded in the PDR. This study compared cesarean section rates between similar cohorts of healthy women who chose elective hospitalization versus a birth center birth. The authors found a significantly increased risk of cesarean section among planned hospital births. Cesarean rates for low-risk women admitted to a birth center were 2.7 percent, compared with 9 percent for low-risk women admitted to a hospital.

[18]Using PDR data (Thornton et al., 2017 [ResQu: high, GRADE: poor]), exclusion criteria were used to form low-risk groups admitted to birth centers (n = 8,776) and those that chose hospital admission (n = 2,527). Comparing midwife-led birth center and hospital groups with midwifery care, the authors found a nonsignificant difference in cesarean birth rates (4.14% for birth centers vs. 4.99% for hospitals), a significant difference in breastfeeding initiation rates (94.5% for birth centers vs. 72.8% for hospitals), and no difference in the neonatal outcome composite (0.44% for both groups).

[19]Alliman and colleagues (2019) found that Medicaid beneficiaries (n = 6,424) enrolled in AABC Strong Start birth center sites experienced preterm birth rates of 4.4 percent and low-birthweight rates of 3.7 percent, compared with CDC birth certificate rates (n = 3,945,875) of 9.9 percent and 8.2 percent, respectively. The total cesarean rate was 12.3 percent, with

the Strong Start Initiative—a project developed by the Centers for Medicare & Medicaid Innovation (CMMI) and conducted between 2013 and 2017 (Hill et al., 2018; see Chapter 4). Birth center studies using registry data consistently indicate that women who participate in birth center care experience low cesarean rates (6–12%) and high breastfeeding initiation rates (92–95%) (Jolles et al., 2017; Stapleton et al., 2013; Thornton et al., 2017).

Summary

Maternal outcomes by birth setting are remarkably consistent: low-risk home and birth center births are associated with lower rates of perineal laceration; reduced rates of medical intervention, including cesarean delivery; and higher rates of breastfeeding initiation and exclusive breastfeeding at 6–8 weeks postpartum. Most of the published data are from observational cohort studies, but several of those studies are based on large samples (Bailey, 2017; Hill et al., 2018; Stapleton et al., 2013) or include most or all birth center births in a region or country for a period of time (Birthplace in England Collaborative Group, 2011; Hollowell et al., 2017; Bailey, 2017; Grigg et al., 2017; Sprague et al., 2018).

Lower rates of intervention and higher rates of breastfeeding are at least partially attributable to selection bias, wherein those who choose home or birth center birth are often highly motivated to achieve a physiologic birth and to breastfeed. The precise effect of selection bias on birth center outcomes is not known. However, the balance of evidence also suggests that there is something about the wellness-oriented, individualized, relationship-centered approach of midwifery care across home, birth center, and hospital settings that contributes to lower rates of medical interventions that can be dangerous when overused.

To find reliable comparison groups for lower-risk birth center and home birth participants, some studies used exclusion criteria to compile low-risk groups so that women with no risk factors in each model could be compared. Other studies used regression analysis to control for differing risk levels to achieve more comparable groups for analysis. Overall, birth center outcomes are consistent for low- or lower-risk women for increased odds of spontaneous vaginal birth, decreased risk for cesarean and assisted vaginal birth, increased initiation and continuation of breastfeeding, and similar intrapartum and neonatal outcomes relative to hospital birth outcomes.

---

a primary cesarean rate of 8.7 percent for births at Strong Start birth centers. Breastfeeding initiation was 92.9 percent compared with a national rate of 83.1 percent. In the birth center arm of Strong Start, eligible women participated in birth center prenatal care, and experienced these improved outcomes even if they elected hospital delivery. (Refer to Box 4-1).

Finding 6-3: In the United States, low-risk women choosing home or birth center birth compared with women choosing hospital birth have lower rates of intervention, including cesarean birth, operative vaginal delivery, induction of labor, augmentation of labor, and episiotomy, and lower rates of intervention-related maternal morbidity, such as infection, postpartum hemorrhage, and genital tract tearing. These findings are consistent across studies. The fact that women choosing home and birth center births tend to select these settings because of their desire for fewer interventions contributes to these lower rates.

Intervention-related maternal morbidity also varies greatly across hospital settings. There are promising strategies and approaches to lowering the rates of non–medically indicated, morbidity-related interventions in hospital settings (see Chapter 7 for further discussion of these models).

PATIENT EXPERIENCE AND SATISFACTION BY U.S. BIRTH SETTING

Factors in Maternal Satisfaction and Relationship to Outcomes

Maternal satisfaction across birth settings has typically been highest when women are supported in choosing the birth setting and provider type that align most closely with their value systems, individual pregnancy characteristics, and personal preferences. Multiple studies from Europe and Canada have measured maternal satisfaction (Janssen et al., 2006; Christiaens and Bracke, 2009; Lindgren and Erlandsson, 2010), but no study in the United States has systematically compared maternal satisfaction across birth settings. A systematic review with publications from multiple countries by Hodnett (2002) found the most critical predictors of satisfaction to be individual expectations, the amount of support received from caregivers, the quality of the caregiver–patient relationship, and maternal involvement in decision making.

Several recent studies note high rates of maternal satisfaction when care is received from midwives regardless of location (Sandall et al., 2010; Macpherson et al., 2016), when doula care is provided (Hardin and Buckner, 2004; Kozhimannil et al., 2016; Thomas et al., 2017), by mode of delivery (Bossano et al., 2017; Alderdice et al., 2019), and when care is midwife-led at home and in birth centers (Fleming et al., 2016). For additional discussion of outcomes associated with doula care, see Box 6-1.

In addition, it is known that one-to-one nursing care during labor and birth influences women's satisfaction with their birth experience (Hodnett et al., 2002). Type of nursing care is a major factor in how women perceive the birth experience. Numerous studies informed by the voices of new

BOX 6-1
Influence of Doulas on Outcomes Across Settings

Doulas care for women in every birth setting—home, birth center, and hospital. Some women utilize doula services throughout all phases of childbirth—ante-, intra-, and postpartum—while others use them during only one of the phases.

A Cochrane review on continuous support during labor (which is one portion of what doulas provide) included 26 trials with nearly 16,000 participants. Bohren and colleagues (2017) found that continuous labor support may contribute to several positive outcomes in childbirth, including increased spontaneous vaginal birth; shorter duration of labor; decreased rates of cesarean birth, instrumental vaginal birth, use of any analgesia, and use of regional analgesia; and decreases in low 5-minute Apgar scores and negative feelings about childbirth experiences. No evidence of harms of continuous labor support were noted (Hodnett et al., 2013). A subgroup analysis found that effects of the doula model of labor support were greater than effects of continuous support provided by either a member of the hospital staff or someone from the woman's social network (e.g., sister, friend) (Bohren et al., 2017).

Observational studies published since that systematic review have confirmed the association between doula care and lower cesarean rates (Devereaux and Sullivan, 2013; de Sousa Soares et al., 2016; Kozhimannil et al., 2016). Additional studies have further replicated these findings, noting specifically that doula support that begins during pregnancy and continues through childbirth and the postpartum period is associated with higher rates of breastfeeding initiation and longer duration rates, as well as lower preterm birth rates. Two other positive outcomes noted in the literature are fewer low-birthweight babies and lower rates of postpartum depression (Trotter et al., 1992).

As to why doula support may influence positive outcomes, one hypothesis is the doula's instilling and boosting women's confidence and self-efficacy. By being empowered to believe in the power of their bodies and their innate ability to labor and give birth, women come to know that they are capable of far more than they may previously have thought. Particularly among disadvantaged populations, in whom self-efficacy can be particularly low, doula care has demonstrated great impact (Gruber et al., 2013). Many successful peer doula programs in the United States have been particularly efficacious in working with such populations. Such programs as the East Bay Community Birth Support Project in California, whereby previously incarcerated peers are trained as doulas, not only benefit the pregnant women but also decrease rates of recidivism among the women who become doulas (Stanley et al., 2015). Based on what is known about racial concordance between patients and their providers, peer doula programs that strive to achieve racial and community concordance would go far in advancing the agenda of improving materal–fetal outcomes among women of color.

An important study compared outcomes among Medicaid enrollees who did and did not receive doula care. Differences were noted in that the cesarean rate for the two groups were 22.3 percent and 31.5 percent, respectively. After controlling for various influential factors, odds of cesarean section were 40.9 per-

continued

BOX 6-1 Continued

cent lower for doula-supported births (Kozhimanni et al., 2013). A similar study among women of lower socioeconomic status with disproportionately higher poor baseline health, conducted by the State Department of Health in New York City, found that women paired with doulas had lower rates of preterm birth and low-birthweight babies. Additional studies report similar results (see, e.g., Kozhimannil et al., 2015; Thomas et al., 2017; Thurston et al., 2019).

Potential cost savings to Medicaid programs that include funding for doula care could be substantial (Edwards et al., 2013; Kozhimanni et al., 2013). Doulas influence the bottom-line costs of birth through their positive effect on, among other outcomes, cesarean birth rates, time in labor, use of analgesia/anesthesia, and breastfeeding rates. Researchers looking at the economic impact of doula involvement in births in Wisconsin calculated (from 2010 birth data) an estimated savings of $28,997,754.80 if every low-risk birth (in hospitals) were attended by a professional doula. That figure breaks down to an estimated cost savings of $424.14 per delivery, or $530.89 per *low-risk* delivery (Chapple et al., 2013).

mothers have found that women value support, encouragement, physical presence, explanations, and respect for their need for control (Corbett and Callister, 2000; Tumblin and Simkin, 2001; Hodnett, 2002; Matthews and Callister, 2004; Brown et al., 2009; Lyndon et al., 2017). Labor and delivery nurses have likewise been explicit about how the quality and quantity of their care is affected by inadequate nurse staffing (Simpson et al., 2012, 2016; Simpson and Lyndon, 2017a). In the context of inadequate staffing, nurses report that they are unable to accomplish all aspects of nursing care required because they are balancing the most pressing demands of the clinical needs of their additional patients. Labor support and physical presence at the bedside are the first aspects of care suspended when an obstetric unit is short-staffed (Simpson et al., 2012, 2016), even though multiple studies have shown that these aspects of care are essential to positive birth experiences. Box 6-2 elaborates on nurses' influence on labor and birth outcomes.

Some U.S. women report finding some aspects of their childbirth experience to have been negative or traumatic, including feeling inadequately supported during the perinatal period and having poor-quality relationships/interactions with their care provider. Lack of support—a poor outcome in itself—has been associated with other undesirable psychosocial sequelae, including increased rates of postpartum mood disorders (Bell and Andersson, 2016; Tani and Castagna, 2017), birth trauma (Simpson and Catling, 2016; Hollander et al., 2017; Reed et al., 2017), and cesarean regret (Porter et al., 2007; Burcher et al., 2016).

BOX 6-2
Nurses' Influence on Labor and Birth Outcomes

Research on the influence on patient outcomes of nursing care during labor and birth is challenging, and thus there are limited data available to support these type of definitive links. It is difficult to connect individual aspects of nursing care to patient outcomes in part because of the way nursing care is documented in the electronic medical record and in part because nursing care is not billed as a specific inpatient service, but bundled into the fees charged for the hospital room and bed. Numerous assessment parameters for the mother and fetus are automatically generated from the electronic fetal monitor and transferred into the medical record without requirements for nurse verification. There has been a trend away from narrative nursing notes. Nurses can view data from the fetal monitor and enter data in the medical record remotely from a central station or in another patient's room; thus nursing documentation does not equate to nursing bedside attendance, making that an unreliable factor in measuring the effect of nursing care.

The value of nursing care is diminished by historical hospital billing practices not specifying care by registered nurses, which is inconsistent with the reality that patients are admitted to the hospital only if they need nursing care. Nearly all other aspects of the hospital stay, including but not limited to procedures and tests, can be done on an outpatient basis. Only if patients require around-the-clock nursing care are they deemed appropriate for hospital admission by third-party payers. Lacing billing codes embedded in the electronic medical record for other care-givers hinders the ability to measure nursing care.

Much of the evidence on nurses' influence on maternity outcomes is based on qualitative studies. However, several quantitative studies address nurses' role in whether women have a cesarean or vaginal birth, including two randomized controlled trials (RCTs) (Hodnett et al., 2002; Gagnon et al., 1997). Two recent studies indicate that this issue requires more study (Edmonds et al., 2017; Greene et al., 2019).

In 2002, a multicenter RCT compared one-to-one nursing care during labor with routine care among 6,915 women in the United States and Canada. Nursing care was provided to the intervention group by nurses who had been trained in labor support techniques. No clinical differences in outcomes were found between the groups (Hodnett et al., 2002). More than one-third of women in both groups had labor induction or augmentation with oxytocin, two-thirds in both groups had epidural anesthesia, and three-quarters in both groups had continuous electronic fetal monitoring. The researchers concluded that continuous labor support by nurses did not have an effect on clinical outcomes of women in perinatal units characterized by high rates of routine interventions (Hodnett et al., 2002). However, patient satisfaction was significantly higher among women who received one-to-one nursing care.

Gagnon and colleagues (2007) retrospectively evaluated outcomes of 467 nulliparous women based on how many nurses had provided care during labor. They found an association between number of nurses for each woman during

continued

BOX 6-2 Continued

labor and risk of cesarean birth: the more nurses, the greater the risk. Gagnon and colleagues (2007) suggest a link between continuity of nursing care during labor and risk of cesarean birth.

A recent focus on the rate of cesarean birth in the United States and its association with maternal morbidity and mortality has renewed interest in this topic. Two recent retrospective studies evaluated the role of the labor nurse in influencing mode of birth (Edmonds et al., 2017; Greene et al., 2019). Similar to Radin and colleagues (1993), these more recent studies limited the patient population included in their analysis to women who were nulliparous, term, singleton, and vertex (NTSV). In both recent studies, a cesarean birth was attributed to a labor nurse and differences among nurses evaluated; however, different methods of attribution were used. Edmonds and collagues (2017) attributed the cesarean to the labor nurse circulating for either a vaginal or cesarean birth. This method of attribution has limitations, as the nurse who attends the cesarean birth as the circulator cannot be assumed to have influenced the outcome or cared for the woman in labor; such factors as length of nursing care, quality of care, reason for the decision, decision maker, and patient assignment must be considered. This method of attribution also cannot be generalized, as many birthing hospitals change the nurse assignment for the circulating nurse when a decision for a cesarean is made. Radin and colleagues (1993) used the nurse present for birth as well, but further qualified attribution of the cesarean to the nurse having cared for the woman from at least 6 cm cervical dilation until birth; thus nursing care during labor was included as a potential influencing factor.

Greene and colleagues (2019) attributed cesarean births to nurses using two methods: (1) the nurse who spent the most time with the patient during the first stage of labor, using documentation of maternal vital signs in the medical record as a proxy for nursing care; and (2) the nurse who initiated second-stage labor pushing. Based on these attribution criteria, these authors found differences in cesarean rates among groups of labor nurses. A limitation of their attribution method, however, is that most maternal vital signs are generated automatically by the electronic fetal monitor and simultaneously transferred to the medical record, and do not require bedside attendance by the labor nurse. Therefore, this method can potentially identify the nurse responsible for the woman in labor but cannot assess nursing care or the amount of time the nurse spent at the bedside. As others have found in studies attempting to attribute method of birth to individual physicians, attribution of the cesarean to an individual labor nurse is a complex issue, especially when retrospective data from the electronic health record are used as the data source, and much more study is needed before a generalizable method can be used in clinical practice.

When asked, labor nurses are quick to say they influence outcomes, including women's satisfaction with the birth experience and whether they have a vaginal or cesarean birth (James et al., 2003; Simpson et al., 2006; Sleutel et al., 2007; Edmonds and Jones, 2013; Lyndon et al., 2017; Simpson and Lyndon, 2017a). Nurses have reported routinely offering the following aspects of care to promote a vaginal and avoid a cesarean birth: offering emotional support; providing labor support (including ambulation, frequent repositioning, hydrotherapy, use of a peanut birthing ball, passive fetal descent in second-stage labor, appropriate titration of oxytocin for induction and augmentation of labor); sharing adequate and accurate information about what to expect; advocating on behalf of women; preparing and encouraging women to advocate for themselves; and communicating with physician colleagues on positive aspects of labor progress (Simpson and Lyndon, 2017b). These findings are consistent with those of earlier studies in which labor nurses reported advocating for more time to allow a chance for vaginal birth and using various emotional and physical labor support techniques to promote labor progress (James et al., 2003; Simpson et al., 2006; Sleutel et al., 2007; Edmonds and Jones, 2013; Lyndon et al., 2017; Simpson and Lyndon, 2017b). These aspects of nursing care in the context of labor management guidelines have been shown to be successful in decreasing cesarean births (Bell et al., 2017; Main et al., 2019; Tussey et al., 2015; White VanGompel et al., 2019). New mothers value the emotional and physical support of the nurse and feel that those aspects of nursing care are influential in determining birth outcomes (Lyndon et al., 2017). In one study, women indicated that they assume their labor nurses will be skilled and competent to handle any childbirth emergency in a timely manner and are confident that maternal–fetal assessment is ongoing, so when they evaluated the quality of nursing care, emotional and physical labor support were the primary considerations (Lyndon et al., 2017). Physicians who attended births indicated that the nurse assigned to care for their patient in labor had a great deal of influence on the method of birth (Simpson et al., 2006; Lyndon et al., 2017). Physicians valued emotional and physical support during labor care as key influencing factors.

It is likely that nursing care during labor and birth directly influences patient outcomes; however, measuring it has been challenging. Nurse researchers in the medical-surgical and intensive care unit specialties in the acute care setting have been studying the effect of nursing care on outcomes for many years. They have been able to link nurse staffing with risk of adverse patient outcomes in a variety of acute care settings (Kane et al., 2007; Lucero et al., 2010; Aiken et al., 2012; Ball et al., 2018; Griffiths et al., 2018; Recio-Saucedo et al., 2018). There are likely similar associations between nursing care during labor and birth and maternal–child outcomes; however, studies of these associations have yet to be conducted. In contrast to the study of patients in medical-surgical and intensive care units because of a medical or surgical problem requiring hospitalization, studying nursing care for a generally healthy population of women giving birth in a hospital and attempting to link that care with uncommon adverse outcomes has posed many methodologic challenges that have yet to be overcome.

A recent article by Vedam and colleagues (2019) reports findings from a convenience sample survey, administered by a multidisciplinary team that included service users, that was designed to capture the lived experiences of maternity care among diverse populations and across U.S. births settings. Patient-designed survey items included questions about verbal and physical abuse, failure to meet professional standards of care, autonomy, discrimination, poor rapport with providers, and substandard conditions within the health system. The researchers found that 17.3 percent of women, or one in six, had experienced at least one form of mistreatment during labor and birth (n = 2,138). Forms of mistreatment included loss of autonomy; being shouted at, scolded, or threatened; and having requests for help ignored or refused. Women who transferred to a hospital from a planned home or birth center birth or whose opinion on the best course of action differed from their provider's reported even higher rates of mistreatment. Women's experiences also differed significantly by birth setting, with 5.1 percent of women who gave birth at home reporting mistreatment versus 28.1 percent of women who gave birth in a hospital. A reduced likelihood of mistreatment was associated with giving birth vaginally, giving birth in a community setting (home or birth center birth), and giving birth with a midwife as the primary attendant regardless of location of care. Being White, multiparous, and older than age 30 were associated with lower levels of mistreatment. Mistreatment rates among women of color were consistently higher than those among White women, and this relationship held even when the authors accounted for interactions between race and other characteristics, such as socioeconomic status. Any mistreatment was reported by 27.2 percent of low-income women of color versus 18.7 percent of low-income White women. Regardless of maternal race and ethnicity, having a Black partner was also associated with a higher rate of mistreatment. Experiences of care and perceived vulnerability to obstetric violence or obstetric racism appear to play important roles in shaping maternal decision making around where and with whom to give birth, as well as around what constitutes safety. (See also the discussion of institutional bias and discrimination in Chapter 4.)

Summary

Psychosocial outcomes, including several measures of dignity in the childbirth process, such as bodily autonomy, maternal agency, respectful care, and empowerment, are important. Some studies show that patient satisfaction is higher and reports of disrespectful care are lower among home and birth center births than among hospital births. Recent research has prompted greater understanding that various forms of disrespect and abuse can occur during the childbirth process in the United States and that rates and types of mistreatment vary by maternal race/ethnicity.

Finding 6-4: Some women experience a gap between the care they expect and want and the care they receive. Women want safety, freedom of choice in birth setting and provider, choice among care practices, and respectful treatment. Individual expectations, the amount of support received from caregivers, the quality of the caregiver–patient relationship, and involvement in decision making appear to be the greatest influences on women's satisfaction with the experience of childbirth.

INTERNATIONAL STUDIES OF OUTCOMES BY BIRTH SETTING

The committee examined studies of outcomes by birth setting internationally that could provide comparisons with the United States (see, e.g., Hutton et al., 2009, 2016; Janssen et al., 2009, 2015; Birthplace in England Collaborative Group, 2011; Schroeder et al., 2012; de Jonge et al., 2013, 2015, 2017; Homer et al., 2014; Vedam et al., 2014b; Zielinski et al., 2015; Bolten et al., 2016; Scarf et al., 2016, 2018). The committee chose Australia, Canada, the Netherlands, and the United Kingdom because they are high-resource countries and have relatively robust data on birth settings and outcomes from their vital statistics systems, as well as a range of well-conducted studies. Table 6-6 provides a comparison by country of types of providers, birth settings, and selected outcomes.

Of course, it is important to note the deep differences among countries that shape the types of health care systems in each nation. The committee commissioned a study to identify these differences across the four identified countries (Kennedy et al., 2019). The paper authors note several important commonalities. First, the four countries share a commitment to integration of care across birth providers and systems. In these countries, out-of-hospital birth providers are part of an integrated, regulated maternity care system. For example, in Australia, the Netherlands, and the United Kingdom, almost all vaginal births include at least one midwife in attendance, usually as the only professional present if the birth is without complications. In all four countries, midwives are trained through a post-secondary education program and prepared to handle first-line complications. This integration translates to a second shared feature of maternity care systems in these countries: seamless transfer across settings. Strong systems are in place in all four countries to provide for collaboration, consultation, transfer, and transport when access to an obstetrician is needed.

A third difference Kennedy and colleagues identified is the presence of universal access to primary and maternity care, including access to different (risk-appropriate) provider options during pregnancy and birth. This universal access to care (including preconception care) means women are neither without coverage prior to becoming pregnant nor dropped from health

TABLE 6-6 Comparison of Types of Providers, Birth Settings, and Selected Outcomes, by Country

	Year
Live births (per 1,000 births)	2017
Crude birth rate [b]	2017
Children per woman (ages 15–49)[c]	2017
Gross domestic product (GDP) per capita (US$)[c]	2018
Infant mortality (per 1,000 births)[c]	2017
Neonatal mortality (per 1,000 births)[c]	2017
Perinatal mortality (per 1,000 births) (includes stillbirths)[c]	2017
Fetal death rate/stillbirth (per 1,000 births)	2017
Maternal mortality (per 100,000 births)	2017
% preterm births	2017
% low birthweight	2017
% severe maternal morbidity[j]	2008–2013
% cesarean births	2017
% births delivered by OB	2017
% births delivered by MW	2017
% births delivered by FP/GP	2017
% births in hospitals	2017
% births in birth centers	2017
% births at home	2017
% privately funded birth care	2017
% publicly funded birth care	2017
GINI Index[c]	2013–2017

NOTES: OB = obstetrician; MW = midwife; FP/GP = family physician/general practitioner. The GINI index measures the extent to which the distribution of income or consumption of expenditure among individuals/households within countries deviates from a perfectly equal distribution (Organisation for Economic Co-operation and Development, 2019).

[a]Martin et al. (2018b).
[b]Australian Institute of Health and Welfare (2019).
[c]Organisation for Economic Co-Operation and Development (2019).
[d]Perined (2019).
[e]The World Bank (2019).
[f]Statistics Canada (2019).
[g]Office for National Statistics (2019).
[h]Centers for Disease Control and Prevention (2019a).
[i]Chawanpaiboon et al. (2019).
[j]Lipkind et al. (2019).
[k]Canadian Association of Midwives (2019).

U.S.	Australia	Canada	Netherlands	UK
3385.6[a]	301.1[b]	376.3[c]	165.7[d]	754.8[c]
11.8[e]	12.4[e]	10.3[e]	9.9[e]	11.4[e]
1.77	1.74	1.5	1.62	1.74
62,853	54,144	48,107	56,326	45,505
5.8	3.3	4.5	3.6	3.9
3.9	2.4	3.5	2.7	2.8
5.9	8.1	5.8	4.8	6.3
—	7[b]	7.6[f]	—	4.2[g]
16.9 (2016)[b]	1.6[c]	6.6[c]	1.8[c]	6.5[c]
9.93[a]	8.7[b]	7.9[f]	—	7[i]
8.3[c]	6.7[b]	6.5[c]	6 (2016)[c]	6.9[c]
15.6	8.2	—	—	5
32[a]	34.6[b]	27.7[c]	16.2[c]	27.4[c]
89.2[a]	—	—	—	—
9.9[a]	—	10.8[k]	—	—
—	—	—	—	—
98.4[a]	97[b]	97.9[f]	71.5[d]	—
0.5[a]	2[b]	—	15.1[d]	—
0.1[a]	0.3[b]	2.1[f]	12.7[d]	2.1[g]
49.1[a]	—	—	—	—
43.0[a]	—	—	—	—
41.5 (2016)	35.8 (2014)	34 (2013)	28.2 (2015)	33.2 (2015)

care coverage after they have had their baby, as is the experience of many Medicaid recipients in the United States (Ranji et al., 2019). In addition to these features, all four countries have adopted a practice of respectful care, including respect for maternal autonomy. This culture of respect informs the evidence-based guidelines in place in each country. These guidelines are intended to support clinical decision making for women and their providers and include information on appropriate risk selection and assessment, as well as out-of-hospital birth options. For example, the UK NICE Guidelines for Intrapartum Care (National Institute for Health and Care Excellence, 2017) clearly define the risk factors and situations in which consultation and (or) transfer of a laboring woman is required. Importantly, the guidelines support women's choice in birth setting, reflecting the practice of trusting women to make appropriate decisions for themselves, their babies, and their families (Kennedy et al., 2019).

Australia, Canada, the Netherlands, and the United Kingdom also provide additional social and welfare supports as compared with the United States, as well as increased availability of maternal and paternal maternity benefits. As a result, the level of disparities and inequity among childbearing people and risk propensities are different from those found among childbearing people in the United States. Accordingly, international comparisons are inherently limited, but they do provide insights into how changes in the structure of health care systems might affect birth outcomes.

International Studies of Home Birth Outcomes

When examining international studies of home birth outcomes, it is important to recognize that the context of the maternity care systems in the four countries the committee chose for comparison is very different from that of the current U.S. system, being characterized by universal health coverage and access, standardized high-level midwifery training, regulated risk-based selection of birth setting, and systems for transfer to a higher level of care when needed. Studies from the four comparison countries are often based on local or national registry data, allowing for an intention-to-treat approach to analysis. Although this minimizes selection bias, missing data are often treated as uninformative, an assumption that is likely incorrect (Wiegerinck et al., 2018). Overall, the international studies reviewed by the committee indicate that benefits result from fewer maternal interventions. They also generally find no difference in neonatal death between planned home and hospital birth cohorts. Notable exceptions exist, including infants born to primiparous women, for whom higher rates of perinatal mortality are seen in the United Kingdom (Birthplace in England Collaborative Group, 2011), and several studies from the Netherlands (Evers et al., 2010; Daysal, 2015; Wiegerinck et al., 2018) show both higher perinatal mortality and an effect of distance on outcome. Table 6-7 shows international studies of neonatal outcomes by birth setting; Table 6-8 shows international studies of maternal outcomes by birth setting.

While four large studies from the Netherlands have found no significant differences in intrapartum or neonatal mortality rates for planned home versus planned hospital births (de Jonge et al., 2009 [ResQu: high][20]; van der Kooy et al., 2011 [ResQu: high, GRADE: fair][21]; de Jonge et al., 2015 [ResQu: high, GRADE: fair][22]; and de Jonge et al. (2013 [ResQu: high, GRADE: fair]),[23] the evidence on outcomes by setting in the Netherlands is mixed. Wiegerinck and colleagues (2018 [ResQu: high, GRADE: poor]) compared intrapartum and neonatal mortality in low-risk term women starting labor in midwife-led versus obstetrician-led care (n = 57,396). Perinatal mortality occurred in 30 of 46,764 (0.064%) women in midwife-led care and in 2 of 10,632 (0.019%) women in obstetrician-led care (OR 3.4, 95% CI 0.8–14.3).

In Australia, Kennare and colleagues (2010 [ResQu: moderate, GRADE, poor]) found similar perinatal mortality rates between home births and hospital births (7.9 vs. 8.2 per 1,000 births) using a retrospective population-based design. However, they found a higher intrapartum fetal death rate in the home birth group (1.8 vs. 0.8 per 1,000 births), with significantly lower cesarean (9.2% vs. 27.1%) and episiotomy (3.6% vs. 21.7%) rates for home versus hospital births. Catling-Paul and colleagues (2013 [ResQu: low, GRADE: poor]) examined 12 publicly funded home birth programs in Australia (n = 1,807; 9 of the programs provided information, for a total of 97% of all home births nationally) and found, after excluding babies with fetal anomalies, a neonatal mortality rate of 1.7 per 1,000 births and a 5.4 percent cesarean rate. The largest study to date (n = 258,161, with 0.3% planning a home birth) within the country was a retrospective analysis of public birth data conducted by Homer and colleagues (2014 [ResQu: high,

---

[20]The study compares 529,688 low-risk women with uncomplicated pregnancies who intended to have midwife-led care at the onset of labor (n = 321,307 planned home and n = 163,261 hospital births) (de Jonge et al., 2009 [ResQu: high]).

[21]The study reports a retrospective analysis of intention-to-treat and perfect guidelines approaches (n = 679,952 low-risk women) (van der Kooy et al., 2011). The perfect guideline approach "includes the subset of women within the natural prospective approach population who in retrospect were compliant with the guidelines, which define low risk at the onset of labor and therefore are allowed to choose between a home or hospital birth under supervision of a midwife" (van der Kooy et al., 2011, p. 1039).

[22]The study compares low-risk women planning midwife-led care for home versus hospital births (n = 466,112 planned home births and n = 276,958 planned hospital births) (de Jonge et al., 2015).

[23]The study retrospectively analyzes national perinatal registry and maternal morbidity data, finding no ignificant differences in severe maternal morbidity (admission to intensive care unit [ICU], or hemolysis, levatenzymes, low platelet count [HELLP] syndrome) between home births (n = 92,333) and hospital births (n = 54,419) for low-risk, term, singleton pregnancies.

TABLE 6-7 Rate, Percentage, and Risk of Neonatal Morbidity and
Mortality in Australia, Canada, the Netherlands, and the United Kingdom

Study	Data Source/ Sample Size	Inclusion/Exclusion Criteria	Birth Setting
Birthplace in England Collaborative Group, 2011 (ResQu: high, GRADE: good) England	National Health Service (Apr 2008–Apr 2010) 11,282 planned obstetric unit N = 64,538 16,840 planned home 11,282 planned freestanding midwifery unit 19,706 planned OB unit 16,710 planned alongside midwifery unit Samples were restricted to women who were not missing any potential confounder data. Refer to article for sample sizes.	Women attended by a National Health Service (NHS) midwife during any phase of labor at ≥37 weeks gestation in spontaneous labor. Primary outcome was perinatal mortality and intrapartum-related neonatal morbidities (stillbirth after start of care in labor, early neonatal death, neonatal encephalopathy, meconium aspiration syndrome, brachial plexus injury, fractured humerus or clavicle).	Obstetric unit Home Freestanding midwifery unit Alongside midwifery unit
Catling-Paul et al., 2013 (ResQu: low, GRADE: poor) Australia	12 publicly funded home birth programs (2005–2010) 1,807 home	Planned home at the onset of labor. Hospital transfers excluded.	Home
de Jonge et al., 2009 (ResQu: high) Netherlands	Netherlands Perinatal Registry (2000–2006) 321,307 planned home 163,261 planned hospital 45,120 unknown	Singleton birth, term (37–42 weeks), no risk factors prior to labor.	Planned hospital birth Planned home Unknown intended place

Outcome	Morbidity/ Mortality %	Morbidity/ Mortality Rate per 1,000 Live Births	Risk
Primary Outcome			Adj. OR (95%) CI
Obstetric unit (ref)	—	4.4	1
Home	—	4.2	1.16 (0.76–1.77)
Freestanding midwifery unit	—	3.5	0.92 (0.58–1.46)
Alongside midwifery unit	—	3.6	0.92 (0.60–1.39)
Neonatal Mortality	—	3.3	—
Apgar 5 min <7	0.7	—	—
Respiratory distress	0.4	—	—
Intrapartum and Neonatal Death 0–7 Days			Adj. RR (95%) CI
Hospital (ref)	0.07	—	1
Home	0.06	—	1.0 (0.78–1.27)
Unknown	0.05	—	0.71 (0.45–1.12)
Admission to NICU			
Hospital (ref)	0.20	—	1
Home	0.17	—	1.00 (0.86–1.16)
Unknown	0.25	—	1.33 (1.07–1.65)

continued

TABLE 6-7 Continued

Study	Data Source/ Sample Size	Inclusion/Exclusion Criteria	Birth Setting
de Jonge et al., 2015 (ResQu: high, GRADE: fair) Netherlands	Netherlands Perinatal Registry (2000–2009) 466,112 planned home births 276,958 planned hospital births	Singleton birth, spontaneous labor at ≥37 weeks, no risk factors prior to labor, in midwife-led care at the onset of labor. A combination of intrapartum or neonatal mortality or NICU admission within 28 days of birth.	
Evers et al., 2010 Netherlands	NICU of the University Medical Center in Utrecht (2007–2008) 16,672 nulliparous women 21,063 multiparous women	Singleton or twin birth, ≥37 without congenital malformations.	Nulliparous Multiparous

Outcome	Morbidity/ Mortality %	Morbidity/ Mortality Rate per 1,000 Live Births	Risk
Intrapartum and Neonatal Death <28 days			Adj. OR (95%) CI
Nulliparous home	—	1.02	0.99 (0.79–1.24)
Nulliparous hospital (ref)	—	1.09	1
Intrapartum and Neonatal Death <28 days			
Parous home	—	0.59	1.16 (0.87–1.55)
Parous hospital (ref)	—	0.58	1
Apgar 5 Min <7			
Nulliparous home	—	8.85	0.95 (0.87–1.02)
Nulliparous hospital (ref)	—	7.90	1
Apgar 5 Min <7			
Parous home	—	4.57	0.77 (0.69–0.86)
Parous hospital (ref)	—	3.20	1
Severe Adverse Perinatal			
Nulliparous home	—	4.17	1.03 (0.92–1.15)
Nulliparous hospital (ref)	—	4.47	1
Severe Adverse Perinatal			
Parous home	—	1.82	0.87 (0.75–1.01)
Parous hospital (ref)	—	2.41	1
Neonatal Death			RR (95%) CI
Nulliparous	—	0.42	0.89 (0.34–2.33)
Multiparous (ref)	—	0.48	1
Perinatal Death			
Nulliparous	—	3.36	1.65 (1.11–2.45)
Multiparous (ref)	—	2.04	1

continued

TABLE 6-7 Continued

Study	Data Source/ Sample Size	Inclusion/Exclusion Criteria	Birth Setting
Hollowell et al., 2017 (ResQu: high, GRADE: fair) England	Birthplace in England national prospective cohort study data (Apr 2008–Apr 2010) 11,265 planned freestanding midwifery unit birth 16,673 alongside midwifery unit birth	Singleton, received prenatal care from an NHS midwife, no known risk factors. A composite defined as stillbirth after the start of care in labor, early neonatal death, neonatal encephalopathy, meconium aspiration syndrome, brachial plexus injury, fractured humerus or clavicle.	Nulliparous-freestanding midwifery unit Multiparous-freestanding midwifery unit Nulliparous-alongside midwifery unit Multiparous-alongside midwifery unit
Homer et al., 2014 (ResQu: high, GRADE: fair) Australia	Linked data from the New South Wales Perinatal Data Collection, Admitted Patient Data Collection, Register of Congenital Conditions, Registry of Birth Deaths and Marriages, and the Australian Bureau of Statistics (Jul 2000–Jun 2008) 242,936 hospital births 14,483 birth center births 742 home births Samples were restricted to women who were not missing any potential confounder data. Refer to article for sample sizes	Singleton, cephalic, spontaneous, >37 weeks	Hospital Birth center Home

Outcome	Morbidity/ Mortality %	Morbidity/ Mortality Rate per 1,000 Live Births	Risk
Birthplace Primary Perinatal			Adj. OR (95%) CI
Nulliparous-freestanding midwifery unit	4.5	—	0.96 (0.51–1.82)
Nulliparous-alongside midwifery unit (ref)	4.7	—	1
Birthplace Primary Perinatal			
Multiparous-freestanding midwifery unit	2.7	—	1.14 (0.52–2.50)
Multiparous-alongside midwifery unit (ref)	2.4	—	1
Neonatal Mortality			Adj. OR (95%) CI
Hospital	—	1.05	1
Birth center	—	0.69	0.66 (0.35–1.24)
Home	—	1.44	1.29 (0.18–9.23)

continued

TABLE 6-7 Continued

Study	Data Source/ Sample Size	Inclusion/Exclusion Criteria	Birth Setting
Hutton et al., 2009 (ResQu: high, GRADE: poor) Canada	Ontario Ministry of Health (Apr 2003–Mar 2006) 6,692 planned home 6,692 planned hospital	Low-risk planned home birth and planned hospital birth at the outset of labor. Groups matched by parity and previous lower-segment cesarean delivery. Death (stillbirth or neonatal death 0–27 days, excluding lethal anomalies and fetal demise before the onset of labor); Apgar 5 min <4; neonatal resuscitation requiring both positive pressure ventilations and cardiac compressions; admission to a neonatal or pediatric intensive care unit with a length of stay greater than 4 days; or birthweight less than 2,500 g.	Matched planned home Matched planned hospital
Janssen et al., 2009 (ResQu: high, GRADE: poor) Canada	Perinatal Database Registry and Department of Vital Statistics (2000–2004) 2,899 planned home births with midwife 4,752 planned hospital births with midwife 5,331 planned hospital births with physician	Home birth-singleton, cephalic, >36 and <41 weeks, no more than 1 previous cesarean delivery, spontaneous or induced. Labor on an outpatient basis, absence of significant preexisting disease, not transferred to hospital. Hospital midwife-planned hospital birth eligible for home birth. Hospital MD-matched births that met eligibility criteria for home birth on a 2:1 ratio.	Home midwife Hospital midwife Hospital MD

Outcome	Morbidity/ Mortality %	Morbidity/ Mortality Rate per 1,000 Live Births	Risk
Composite Outcome			RR (95%) CI
Home	2.4	—	0.84 (0.68–1.03)
Hospital	2.8	—	1
Perinatal Death			RR (95%) CI
Hospital midwife	—	0.35	1
Home midwife	—	0.57	0.61 (0.06–5.88)
Hospital MD	—	0.64	1
Home midwife	—	—	0.55 (0.06–5.25)
Apgar 5 Min <7			
Hospital midwife	—	—	1
Home midwife	—	—	0.92 (0.58–1.47)
Hospital MD	—	—	1
Home midwife	—	—	0.99 (0.61–1.61)

continued

TABLE 6-7 Continued

Study	Data Source/ Sample Size	Inclusion/Exclusion Criteria	Birth Setting
Kennare et al., 2010 (ResQu: moderate, GRADE: poor) Australia	South Australian perinatal birth and death data (1991–2006) N = 298,333	Live births and stillbirths, ≥400 g or 20 weeks' gestation.	Planned hospital Planned home born at home Planned home at hospital
Sprague et al., 2018 (ResQu: moderate, GRADE: poor) Canada	Better Outcomes Registry & Network (BORN) Information System (BIS), Canadian Institute for Health Information (CIHI) Discharge Abstract Database, the Statistics Canada Census Data for Ontario, birth center records, and birth center logs (Jan 2014–Feb 2015) 495 birth center admissions 1,980 matched midwifery hospital birth cohort	Birth center births matched on 1:4 basis to singleton, spontaneous labor in hospital midwifery care, gestational age (within 2 weeks), parity and maternal age, location of residence, and pregnancy complications (gestational diabetes and hypertension).	Birth center Hospital

Outcome	Morbidity/ Mortality %	Morbidity/ Mortality Rate per 1,000 Live Births	Risk
Perinatal Deaths			Adj. OR (95%) CI
Hospital	—	8.2	1
Home-home	—	2.5	0.48 (0.06–3.61)
Home-hospital	—	20.1	2.50 (0.82–7.35)
Apgar 5 Min <7			
Hospital	1.4	—	1
Home-home	0.5	—	0.62 (0.15–2.49)
Home-hospital	2.3	—	3.20 (1.24–8.26)
NICU Admission			Adj. RR (95%) CI
Birth center	5.5	—	1
Hospital	7.1	—	1.3 (0.9–2.0)

continued

TABLE 6-7 Continued

Study	Data Source/ Sample Size	Inclusion/Exclusion Criteria	Birth Setting
van der Kooy et al., 2011 (ResQu: high, GRADE: fair) Netherlands	Netherlands Perinatal Registry (2000–2007) 679,952 natural prospective approach 602,331 perfect guideline approach	Singleton, under the supervision of a community midwife at the onset of labor.	Home-NPA Home-PGA Hospital-NPA Hospital-PGA Planned place unknown-PGA Planned place unknown-NPA
Wiegerinck et al., 2018 (ResQu: high, GRADE: poor) Netherlands	National Perinatal Register (2005–2008) 46,764 midwife-led care 10,632 obstetrician-led care	Term (>37 to <42 weeks), in the Amsterdam region	Matched midwife-led care Matched obstetrician-led care

NOTE: CI = confidence interval; GRADE = Grading of Recommendations, Assessment, Development, and Evaluation; NICU = neonatal intensive care unit; NPA = natural prospective approach; OR = odds ratio; PGA = perfect guideline approach; ResQu = Birth Place Research Quality; RR = relative risk.

Outcome	Morbidity/ Mortality %	Morbidity/ Mortality Rate per 1,000 Live Births	Risk
Low Apgar Score			Adj. OR (95%) CI
Home-NPA	0.42	—	—
Home-PGA	0.41	—	—
Hospital-NPA	0.54	—	—
Hospital-PGA	0.50	—	—
Planned place unknown-PGA	0.50	—	—
Planned place unknown-NPA	0.47	—	—
Intrapartum and Neonatal Death 0–7 Days			
Home-NPA	0.15	—	1.05 (0.91–1.21)
Hospital-NPA (ref)	0.18	—	1
Unknown-NPA	0.18	—	0.77 (0.61–0.97)
Intrapartum and Neonatal Death 0–7 Days			
Home-PGA	0.09	—	1.11 (0.93–1.34)
Hospital-PGA (ref)	0.10	—	1
Unknown-PGA	0.05	—	0.57 (0.37–0.86)
Intrapartum and Neonatal Mortality			OR (95%) CI
Midwife-led care	—	0.08	4 (0.85–18.85)
Obstetrician-led care	—	0.02	1
Apgar 5 Min <7			
Midwife-led care	0.7	—	0.79 (0.58–1.07)
Obstetrician-led care	0.88	—	1

TABLE 6-8 Rate, Percentage, and Risk of Maternal Morbidity and Mortality in Australia, Canada, the Netherlands, and the United Kingdom

Study	Data Source/ Sample Size	Inclusion/Exclusion Criteria	Birth Setting
Birthplace in England Collaborative Group, 2011 (ResQu: high, GRADE: good) England	National Health Service (Apr 2008–Apr 2010) N = 64,538 16,840 planned home 11,282 planned freestanding midwifery unit 19,706 planned obstetrics unit 16,719 planned alongside midwifery unit Samples were restricted to women who were not missing any potential confounder data. Refer to article for sample sizes.	Women attended by a National Health Service (NHS) midwife during any phase of labor at ≥37 weeks gestation in spontaneous labor.	Obstetric unit Home Freestanding midwifery unit Alongside midwifery unit
Catling-Paul et al., 2013 (ResQu: low, GRADE: poor) Australia	12 publicly funded home birth programs (2005–2010) 1,807 home	Planned home birth at the onset of labor. Hospital transfers excluded.	Home

Outcome	Morbidity/ Mortality %	Morbidity/ Mortality Rate per 1,000 Live Births	Risk
Intrapartum Cesarean Section (per 100 births)			Adj. OR (99%) CI
Obstetric unit (ref)	—	11.1	1
Home	—	2.8	0.31 (0.23–0.41)
Freestanding midwifery unit	—	3.5	0.32 (0.24–0.42)
Alongside midwifery unit	—	4.4	0.39 (0.29–0.53)
3rd- or 4th-Degree Perineal Trauma (per 100 births)			
Obstetric unit (ref)	—	3.2	1
Home	—	1.9	0.77 (0.57–1.05)
Freestanding midwifery unit	—	2.3	0.78 (0.58–1.05)
Alongside midwifery unit	—	3.2	1.04 (0.79–1.38)
Syntocinon Augmentation (per 100 births)			
Obstetric unit (ref)	—	23.5	1
Home	—	5.4	0.25 (0.21–0.31)
Freestanding midwifery unit	—	7.1	0.26 (0.20–0.33)
Alongside midwifery unit	—	10.3	0.37 (0.30–0.46)
Cesarean Section	5.4	—	—
1st- or 2nd-degree tear	34.2	—	—
3rd-degree or more tear	1.1	—	—
Postpartum hemorrhage (>500 mL)	1.8	—	—
Maternal mortality	0	—	—

continued

TABLE 6-8 Continued

Study	Data Source/ Sample Size	Inclusion/Exclusion Criteria	Birth Setting
de Jonge et al., 2013 (ResQu: high, GRADE: fair) Netherlands	LEMMoN study merged with Netherlands Perinatal Registry (2004–2006) 92,333 planned home 54,419 planned hospital	Singleton birth, term (37–42 weeks), no risk factors prior to labor. We included cases in the LEMMoN study only if severe acute maternal morbidity occurred after the onset of labor.	Nulliparous-home Nulliparous-hospital Parous-home Parous-hospital
Hermus et al., 2017 Netherlands	Netherlands Perinatal Registry and case report form (Jul 2013–Dec 2013) 1,668 planned birth center 701 planned hospital 1,086 planned home	Data were collected for all term (≥37 weeks gestational age) women at the start of labor under care of a community midwife, regardless of their planned place of birth. A current version of the Dutch Optimality Index (OI-NL2015) was developed to measure differences between groups of low-risk women by comparing a sum score of optimal process and outcome items in perinatal care.	Birth center Midwife-led hospital Home

Outcome	Morbidity/ Mortality %	Morbidity/ Mortality Rate per 1,000 Live Births	Risk
Severe Acute Maternal Morbidity			Adj. OR (95%) CI
Nulliparous-home	—	2.3	0.77 (0.56–1.06)
Nulliparous-hospital (ref)	—	3.1	1
Parous-home	—	1.0	0.43 (0.29–0.63)
Parous-hospital (ref)	—	2.3	1
Postpartum Hemorrhage (>1,000 mL)			
Nulliparous-home	—	43.1	0.92 (0.85–1.00)
Nulliparous-hospital (ref)	—	43.3	1
Parous-home	—	19.6	0.50 (0.46–0.55)
Parous-hospital (ref)	—	37.6	1
OI-NL 2015 (mean)			
Nulli-birth center (ref)	25.8	—	—
Nulli-hospital midwife-led	26.0	—	—
Nulli-home	26.3	—	—

continued

TABLE 6-8 Continued

Study	Data Source/ Sample Size	Inclusion/Exclusion Criteria	Birth Setting
Hollowell et al., 2017 (ResQu: high, GRADE: fair) England	Birthplace in England national prospective cohort study data (Apr 2008–Apr 2010) 11,265 planned freestanding midwifery unit births 16,673 alongside midwifery unit births	Singleton, received prenatal care from an NHS midwife, no known risk factors. A composite defined as any of: stillbirth after the start of care in labor, early neonatal death, neonatal encephalopathy, meconium aspiration syndrome, brachial plexus injury, fractured humerus or clavicle.	Nulliparous-freestanding midwifery unit Multiparous-freestanding midwifery unit Nulliparous-alongside midwifery unit Multiparous-alongside midwifery unit

Outcome	Morbidity/ Mortality %	Morbidity/ Mortality Rate per 1,000 Live Births	Risk
Cesarean Section			Adj. OR (99%) CI
Nulliparous-freestanding midwifery unit	—	6.7	—
Nulliparous-alongside midwifery unit	—	7.7	—
Multiparous-freestanding midwifery unit	—	0.7	—
Multiparous-alongside midwifery unit	—	1.0	—
3rd- or 4th-Degree Perineal Trauma			
Nulliparous-freestanding midwifery unit	—	4.0	—
Nulliparous-alongside midwifery unit	—	4.9	—
Multiparous-freestanding midwifery unit	—	0.9	—
Multiparous-alongside midwifery unit	—	1.6	—
Cesarean Section			
Nulliparous-freestanding midwifery unit	—	—	0.84 (0.63–1.14)
Nulliparous-alongside midwifery unit	—	—	1
Cesarean Section			
Multiparous-freestanding midwifery unit	—	—	0.75 (0.41–1.38)
Multiparous-alongside midwifery unit	—	—	1
3rd- or 4th-Degree Perineal Trauma			
Nulliparous-freestanding midwifery unit	—	—	0.82 (0.59–1.15)
Nulliparous-alongside midwifery unit	—	—	1

continued

TABLE 6-8 Continued

Study	Data Source/ Sample Size	Inclusion/Exclusion Criteria	Birth Setting
Hollowell et al., 2017 (ResQu: high, GRADE: fair) England [continued]			
Homer et al., 2014 (ResQu: high, GRADE: fair) Australia	Linked data from the New South Wales Perinatal Data Collection, Admitted Patient Data Collection, Register of Congenital Conditions, Registry of Birth Deaths and Marriages, and Australian Bureau of Statistics (Jul 2000–Jun 2008) 242,936 hospital 14,483 birth center 742 home Samples were restricted to women who were not missing any potential confounder data. Refer to article for sample sizes	Singleton, cephalic, spontaneous, >37 weeks	Hospital Birth center Home

Outcome	Morbidity/ Mortality %	Morbidity/ Mortality Rate per 1,000 Live Births	Risk
3rd- or 4th-Degree Perineal Trauma			
Multiparous-freestanding midwifery unit	—	—	0.60 (0.36–1.00)
Multiparous-alongside midwifery unit	—	—	1
Caesarean Section (per 100 births)			Adj. OR (95%) CI
Hospital	—	10.6	1
Birth center	—	4.8	0.36 (0.34–0.39)
Home	—	3.3	0.27 (0.17–0.40)
3rd- or 4th-Degree Perineal Tear with Episiotomy Extensions (per 100 births)			
Hospital	—	3.3	1
Birth center	—	3.3	0.93 (0.84–1.02)
Home	—	2.0	0.66 (0.38–1.14)
Syntocinon Augmentation (per 100 births)			
Hospital	—	20.6	1
Birth center	—	11.1	0.43 (0.41–0.45)
Home	—	5.7	0.24 (0.17–0.33)

continued

TABLE 6-8 Continued

Study	Data Source/ Sample Size	Inclusion/Exclusion Criteria	Birth Setting
Hutton et al., 2009 (ResQu: high, GRADE: poor) Canada	Ontario Ministry of Health (Apr 2003–Mar 2006) 6,692 planned home 6,692 planned hospital	Low-risk planned home birth and planned hospital birth at the outset of labor. Groups matched by parity and previous lower-segment cesarean delivery. Death (stillbirth or neonatal death 0–27 days, excluding lethal anomalies and fetal demise before the onset of labor); Apgar 5 min <4; neonatal resuscitation requiring both positive pressure ventilations and cardiac compressions; admission to a neonatal or pediatric intensive care unit with a length of stay greater than 4 days; or birthweight less than 2,500 g.	Home Hospital

Outcome	Morbidity/ Mortality %	Morbidity/ Mortality Rate per 1,000 Live Births	Risk
Cesarean Section			RR (95%) CI
Home (ref)	5.2	—	0.64 (0.56–0.73)
Hospital	8.1	—	1
Any 2nd- to 4th-Degree Perineal, Labial, or Vaginal Tear, or Episiotomy			
Home (ref)	38.7	—	0.87 (0.83-0.90)
Hospital	44.5	—	1
Any Labor Augmentation			
Home (ref)	27.7	—	0.76 (0.72–0.80)
Hospital	36.3	—	1
Maternal Death			
Home	0	—	—
Hospital	0	—	—

continued

TABLE 6-8 Continued

Study	Data Source/ Sample Size	Inclusion/Exclusion Criteria	Birth Setting
Janssen et al., 2009 (ResQu: high, GRADE: poor) Canada	Perinatal Database Registry and Department of Vital Statistics (2000–2004) 2,899 planned home with midwife 4,752 planned hospital with midwife 5,331 planned hospital with physician	Home birth-singleton, cephalic, >36 and <41 weeks, no more than 1 previous cesarean delivery, spontaneous or induced labor on an outpatient basis, absence of significant preexisting disease, not transferred to hospital. Hospital midwife-planned hospital birth eligible for home birth. Hospital MD-matched births that met eligibility criteria for home birth on a 2:1 ratio (parameters were year of birth, parity, single parent, maternal age, and hospital where the midwife conducting the index home birth had hospital privileges), did not require oxytocin for induction of labor.	Home midwife Hospital midwife Hospital MD

Outcome	Morbidity/ Mortality %	Morbidity/ Mortality Rate per 1,000 Live Births	Risk
Augmentation			RR (95%) CI
Hospital midwife	39.9	—	1
Home midwife	23.7	—	0.59 (0.55–0.69)
Hospital MD	50.4	—	1
Home midwife	—	—	0.47 (0.44–0.51)
Cesarean			
Hospital midwife	10.5	—	1
Home midwife	7.2	—	0.76 (0.64–0.91)
Hospital MD	11.0	—	1
Home midwife	—	—	0.65 (0.56–0.76)
Postpartum Hemorrhage			
Hospital midwife	6.0	—	1
Home midwife	3.8	—	0.62 (0.45–0.70)
Hospital MD	6.7	—	1
Home midwife	—	—	0.57 (0.49–0.77)
Maternal Death			
Hospital midwife	0	—	—
Home midwife	0	—	—
Hospital MD	0	—	—
Home midwife	—	—	—
1st- or 2nd-Degree Perineal Tear			
Hospital midwife	50.2	—	—
Home midwife	43.5	—	—
Hospital MD	53.2	—	—
Home midwife	—	—	—
3rd- or 4th-Degree Perineal Tear			
Hospital midwife	1.2	—	1
Home midwife	2.9	—	0.34 (0.24–0.49)
Hospital MD	3.4	—	1
Home midwife	—	—	0.43 (0.29–0.63)

continued

TABLE 6-8 Continued

Study	Data Source/ Sample Size	Inclusion/Exclusion Criteria	Birth Setting
Kennare et al., 2010 (ResQu: moderate, GRADE: poor) Australia	South Australian perinatal birth and death data (1991–2006) 1,136 planned home (790 occurred at home, 346 transferred to hospital) 292,469 planned hospital	Live births and stillbirths, ≥400 g or 20 weeks' gestation.	Planned hospital Planned home, born at home Planned home, at hospital
Laws et al., 2014 (ResQu: high, GRADE: poor) Australia	New South Wales Midwives Data Collection; New South Wales Admitted Patient Data Collection; Registrar of the New South Wales Registry of Births, Deaths and Marriages; Australian Bureau of Statistics Mortality Data (2001–2009) 66,190 intended hospital 15,742 intended birth center	Singleton, ≥37 weeks, spontaneous labor, women intending to give birth in the collocated hospitals during the same period	Intended hospital Intended birth center

Outcome	Morbidity/ Mortality %	Morbidity/ Mortality Rate per 1,000 Live Births	Risk
Caesarean Section			Adj. OR (95%) CI
Hospital	27.1	—	1
Home (combined)	9.2	—	0.27 (0.22–0.34)
3rd- or 4th-Degree Perineal Tear			
Hospital	1.8	—	1
Home-home	0.4	—	0.37 (0.09–1.49)
Home-hospital	3.3	—	1.74 (0.62–4.89)
Postpartum Hemorrhage			
Hospital	5.5	—	1
Home-home	3.04	—	0.67 (0.39–1.14)
Home-hospital	7.5	—	0.84 (0.42–1.69)
Cesarean Section (emergency)			Adj. OR (95%) CI
Hospital (ref)	12.6	—	1
Birth center	3.9	—	0.23 (0.20–0.25)
3rd- or 4th-Degree Tear			
Hospital (ref)	3.0	—	1
Birth center	2.5	—	0.85 (0.74–0.99)
Postpartum Hemorrhage			
Hospital (ref)	10.6	—	1
Birth center	8.6	—	0.79 (0.73–0.86)
Postpartum Infection			
Hospital (ref)	1.4	—	1
Birth center	1.0	—	0.74 (0.59–0.92)
Maternal Death (n)			
Hospital (ref)	1	—	—
Birth center	0	—	—

continued

TABLE 6-8 Continued

Study	Data Source/ Sample Size	Inclusion/Exclusion Criteria	Birth Setting
Sprague et al., 2018 (ResQu: moderate, GRADE: poor) Canada	Better Outcomes Registry & Network (BORN) Information System (BIS), Canadian Institute for Health Information (CIHI) Discharge Abstract Database, Statistics Canada Census Data for Ontario, birth center records, and birth center logs (Jan 2014– Feb 2015) 495 birth center admissions 1,980 matched midwifery hospital birth cohort	Birth center births matched on 1:4 basis to singleton, spontaneous labor in hospital midwifery care Also matched on gestational age (within 2 weeks), parity and maternal age, location of residence, and pregnancy complications (gestational diabetes and hypertension) 50 cases of birth center births received a secondary review	Birth center Hospital
Wiegerinck et al., 2018 (ResQu: high, GRADE: poor) Netherlands	National Perinatal Register (2005–2008) 46,764 midwife-led care 10,632 obstetrician-led care	Term (>37 to <42 weeks), in the Amsterdam region	Matched midwife-led care Matched obstetrician-led care

NOTE: GRADE = Grading of Recommendations, Assessment, Development, and Evaluation; NPA = natural prospective approach; OR = odds ratio; PGA = perfect guideline approach; ResQu = Birth Place Research Quality; RR = relative risk.

Outcome	Morbidity/ Mortality %	Morbidity/ Mortality Rate per 1,000 Live Births	Risk
Augmentation			Adj. RR (95%) CI
Birth center (ref)	12.5	—	1
Hospital	24.5	—	2.0 (1.6–2.5)
Cesarean			
Birth center (ref)	7.7	—	1
Hospital	12.1	—	1.5 (1.1–2.1)
Maternal Mortality			
Birth center (ref)	0	—	—
Hospital	0	—	—
Secondary Review			
Postpartum hemorrhage (%)	2.4	—	—
4th-degree laceration (n)	1	—	—
Potential sepsis (n)	6	—	—
Caesarean Section			OR (95%) CI
Midwife-led care	2.5	—	0.26 (0.22–0.29)
Obstetrician-led care (ref)	8.9	—	1
Postpartum Hemorrhage (≥1,000 mL)			
Midwife-led care	4.3	—	0.68 (0.60–0.77)
Obstetrician-led care (ref)	6.2	—	1
3rd- or 4th-Degree Tear			
Midwife-led care	2.4	—	0.96 (0.80–1.14)
Obstetrician-led care (ref)	2.6	—	1

GRADE: fair]). They found no significant differences in composite perinatal and neonatal mortality/morbidity index score (7.1/1,000 for planned home births vs. 5.8/1,000 for planned hospital births), and a significant difference in cesarean delivery rates (3.3% vs. 10.6% for home and hospital births, respectively), but the authors also note they were unable to test the reliability of the differences because they did not have the statistical power.

In Canada, Janssen and colleagues (2009 [ResQu: high, GRADE: poor]) conducted a prospective cohort study and found no significant differences in perinatal mortality among three groups—midwife-attended home births (0.35/1,000), midwife-attended hospital births (0.57/1,000), and physician-attended hospital births (0.64/1,000). Maternal outcomes were significantly better in the home birth group than in the midwife-attended and physician-attended hospital groups, with the following specific outcomes, respectively: cesarean delivery rate: 7.2 percent vs. 10.5 percent vs. 11 percent, intact perineum rate: 54.4 percent vs. 46.1 percent vs. 43 percent, and postpartum hemorrhage rate: 3.8 percent vs. 6.0 percent vs. 6.7 percent. A second Canadian study (Hutton et al., 2009 [ResQu: high, GRADE: poor]) with a retrospective cohort design (N = 6,692 planned home births matched to 6,692 planned hospital births for comparable low-risk women) found no differences in combined perinatal/neonatal mortality rates (1/1,000 in both samples) or in composite perinatal and neonatal mortality/morbidity scores (2.4% for home vs. 2.8% for hospital). Cesarean delivery rates were significantly lower in the home group (5.2% vs. 8.1%), as was postpartum hemorrhage with more than 1,000 mL of blood loss.

The Birthplace in England Collaborative Group (2011 [ResQu: high, GRADE: good]) conducted a prospective cohort study comparing outcomes for births occurring in home, birth center, and midwifery and obstetric hospital units for 64,538 low-risk women at term. A composite outcome was created that combined stillbirth, early neonatal death, meconium aspiration, birth-related injuries, and encephalopathy. Overall, no significant differences in the composite outcome for the entire sample were found. When the sample was stratified by nulliparity, rates for the composite outcome were higher for home than for hospital for nulliparous women (9.3/1,000 vs. 5.3/1,000). A follow-up study focused on costs concluded that home birth was a cost-effective option for all low-risk women, including nulliparas (Schroeder et al., 2012).

Studies from Japan, New Zealand, Norway, and Sweden also found outcomes similar to those of the studies discussed above (see, e.g., Kataoka et al., 2013; Davis et al., 2011; Blix et al., 2012; Lindgren et al., 2008).

International Studies of Birth Center Outcomes

In other countries, including the United Kingdom, Australia, Canada, and the Netherlands, integration of birth center care into maternity care systems is much better than in the United States (Bailey, 2017; Birthplace in England Collaborative Group, 2011; Davis et al., 2012; Grigg et al., 2017; Hollowell et al., 2017; Sprague et al., 2018). In the United Kingdom, women have the option of choosing from multiple birth settings, including home, freestanding midwifery unit (FMU), a model similar to the U.S. birth center alongside midwifery unit (AMU) (a midwifery unit located in or collocated with a hospital), and obstetric hospital unit.

The Birthplace in England Collaborative Group (2011) was a prospective cohort study with a total sample size of 64,538, including 11,282 women planning births in an FMU. Researchers found no increased odds of poor outcomes for neonates born in FMUs versus obstetric units. Using the obstetric unit as the reference point, percentages and aORs for outcomes in the FMUs were spontaneous vaginal birth, 90.7 percent (aOR 3.38); cesarean birth, 3.5 percent (aOR 0.32); blood transfusion, 0.5 percent (aOR 0.48); and pitocin augmentation, 7.1 percent (aOR 0.26). Despite these outcomes, as of 2016, only about 2 percent of births in the United Kingdom occurred in FMUs (Walsh et al., 2018).[24]

A secondary analysis of the Birthplace in England Collaborative data (Hollowell et al., 2017 [ResQu: high, GRADE: fair]) compared outcomes in FMUs (n = 11,265) and AMUs (n = 16,673) and found no significant differences in adverse perinatal outcomes. Odds of "straightforward vaginal birth" were higher for planned FMU compared with planned AMU births (Hollowell et al., 2017). Compared with women with planned AMU births, women with planned FMU births had significantly lower odds of instrumental delivery and significantly lower rates of epistomy, epidurals, and augmentation of labor with syntocinon (Hollowell et al., 2017). In addition, one micro-costing study found a 40 percent reduction in costs for FMU care compared with hospital care for low-risk women, even when the cost of transfers was included (Schroeder et al., 2017).

A birth center study from Canada evaluated outcomes for all birth center admissions (n = 495) for the first year of operation in two Toronto-area facilities and compared them with outcomes among a low-risk group with midwife-led hospital births. No maternal deaths occurred; one fetal death was discovered at triage at the birth center, with immediate transfer to the hospital. Outcomes favored the birth center group, which evidenced lower rates of cesarean (7.7% vs. 12.1%) and synthetic oxytocin augmenta-

---

[24]Some confusion results from the fact that FMUs and AMUs are often reported together as "midwifery units," and in places where midwifery units exist, the percentage of women choosing them as their birth setting varies from 4 percent to 31 percent across England.

tion (12.5% vs. 24.5%) (Sprague et al., 2018 [ResQu: moderate, GRADE: poor]).

Appropriate maternity care in the Netherlands is determined based on risk level within an integrated system in which women have a choice of birth setting (Hermus et al., 2017; Schuit et al., 2016). All low-risk women have the option of being admitted when in labor for either home birth or primary labor care in a hospital with an independent midwife or a general practitioner. Birth center birth is also a primary care option for low-risk women in the Netherlands, though access to birth centers is limited in some regions. During the time period of the Schuit study, from 2000 to 2007, 52 percent of all women were admitted to primary hospital maternity care, and 32 percent of this group were transferred to secondary care during labor (Schuit et al., 2016; n = 746,642). During this time period, only 1 percent of women in the Netherlands planned to give birth in a birth center. For those women, odds of transfer from the birth center to a hospital were similar to the odds of transfer from primary to secondary care in the hospital, and greater than the odds of transfer from a planned home birth to a hospital (Schuitt et al., 2016).

In 2013, a national study of birth center care was conducted in the Netherlands, in which 21 of all 23 birth centers in the country participated (Hermus et al., 2017). Some of these birth centers were freestanding (3), but a majority were alongside a hospital (14). Outcomes were assessed using an optimality index, which focuses on processes and outcomes rather than adverse outcomes (Hermus et al., 2017). Of a total sample of 3,455 women, those in birth center care experienced optimality scores similar to those of women in midwife-led care in hospitals, but lower scores than those having home birth. Care in freestanding birth centers led to higher rates of spontaneous vaginal birth and fewer transfers relative to care in alongside hospital birth centers (Hermus et al., 2017).

A secondary analysis of matched cohort data in Denmark included 839 women each in birth center and hospital groups (Christensen and Overgaard, 2017 [ResQu: high, GRADE: poor]). Caesarean birth was lower in the birth center group, with odds ratios of 0.4 for nulliparous and 0.8 for multiparous women. For uncomplicated birth center births, the odds ratio was 2.2 for nulliparous and 2.9 for multiparous women (Christensen and Overgaard, 2017).

In Australia, the midwife-led units called "birth centers" are more similar to AMUs in the United Kingdom than to freestanding birth centers in the United States and New Zealand, usually being located within hospitals instead of being freestanding (Homer et al., 2014; Laws et al., 2014). Two cohort studies in Australia compared outcomes for women having planned births in midwife-led versus obstetric units. A study by Homer and colleagues (2014 [ResQu: high, GRADE: fair]) included 14,483 planning midwife unit care and 242,936 planning obstetric unit care, while a study by Laws and colleagues (2014 [ResQu: high, GRADE: poor]) included 15,742 participants in planned midwife unit care and 66,190 in obstetric unit care. In the midwife-led units, women were statistically more likely than those in the obstetric units to experience a normal vaginal birth, with cesarean rates of 4.8 percent versus 10.6 percent (aOR 0.36, 95% CI 0.34–0.39) in the Homer and colleagues study and 3.9 percent versus 12.6 percent (aOR 0.23, 95% CI 0.20–0.25) in the Laws and colleagues study. There were no statistically significant differences in stillbirth and early neonatal deaths among the three groups (Homer et al., 2014).

Studies from Japan, New Zealand, Norway, and Sweden also found outcomes similar to those of the studies discussed above (see, e.g., Kataoka et al., 2013; Suto et al., 2015; Christensen and Overgaard, 2017; Øian et al., 2018; Grigg et al., 2017; Davis et al., 2012; Bailey, 2017).

Summary

Two international studies suggest a small increase in adverse outcomes for the neonate in home versus hospital births for low-risk individuals (Caughey and Cheyney, 2019). The vast majority of international evidence, however, when limited to high-quality studies, particularly those from countries with well-integrated maternity care systems and clear collaboration guidelines, generally show no increase in neonatal morbidity or mortality for low-risk, planned home or birth center births versus low-risk hospital births, though notable exceptions exist. Taken together, U.S. and international studies suggest that for infants, home births for low-risk individuals may be as safe as hospital or birth center births when certain system-level features are in place, including collaboration and integration across birth settings, eligibility criteria for community birth, well-trained providers, appropriate risk selection, ability to manage first-line complications, interdisciplinary collaboration, choice among multiple birth settings that are covered through universal coverage policies, and low barriers to transfer. System-level features and the availability of institutional supports for physiologic childbearing and respectful care appear to play important roles in determining perinatal risk (Vedam et al., 2018). Conversely, in maternity care systems that lack these features, higher rates of infant morbidity and mortality are found. In the United States, integration of midwifery into maternity care delivery systems is fragmented, coverage is not available for all women or for all birth providers, and care is poorly coordinated, contributing to adverse perinatal outcomes.

Finding 6-5: International studies suggest that home and birth center births may be as safe as hospital births for low-risk women and infants when (1) they are part of an integrated, regulated system; (2) multiple provider options across the continuum of care are covered; (3) providers are well qualified and have the knowledge and training to manage first-line complications; (4) transfer is seamless across settings; and (5) appropriate risk assessment and risk selection occur across settings and throughout pregnancy. Such systems are currently not widespread in the United States.

As demonstrated by the international literature, risks in home and birth center settings may be mitigated by various strategies, including selection of low-risk mothers, referral to an obstetric or maternal fetal medicine provider for pregnancy complications, low thresholds for transfer, timely (20–30 minutes) transport when complications arise, barrier-free and mutually respectful transfers of care when needed, collaborative professional models of care, formal training of skilled practitioners (including in neonatal resuscitation), professional regulation, and oversight and accountability. Professional regulation may be particularly important. In the United States today, certified professional midwives, who attend a majority of U.S. home births, are regulated in only 33 states. In states where they are not regulated, there are no minimum standards for practice; regulated access to lifesaving, first-line medications, including anti-hemorrhagics; or access to continuing education, quality improvement opportunities, or professional development. In all international settings, where home and freestanding birth center births are better integrated into the maternity care system, these strategies have been widely implemented, and as a result, outcomes for both women and newborns tend to be better in these settings than in the United States, where health systems do not employ these strategies.

Finding 6-6: Lack of integration and coordination and unreliable collaboration across birth settings and maternity care providers are associated with poor birth outcomes for women and infants in the United States.

INTERPROFESSIONAL COLLABORATION ACROSS THE MATERNITY CARE TEAM AND BETWEEN BIRTH SETTINGS

Interprofessional teamwork is essential to the provision of high-quality maternity care (Guise and Segel, 2008). Previous research has shown that when professionals collaborate on decision making and coordination of care is seamless, fewer preventable intrapartum neonatal and maternal deaths occur during critical obstetric events (Cornthwaite et al., 2013). Poor communication, disagreement, and lack of clarity around provider roles are identified as primary determinant of these adverse outcomes (Guise and

Segel, 2008; The Joint Commission, 2004; Cornthwaite et al., 2013). When differences around defining risk and responsibility exist among providers, interprofessional cooperation and access to options for care are reduced (Barclay et al., 2016; Coxon et al., 2016; Healy et al., 2016).

Conversely, collaboration among health professionals can improve safety and quality, particularly as different members of the health care team contribute differing perspectives and areas of expertise. Two studies used data from the National Institutes of Health's (NIH's) Consortium on Safe Labor to compare outcomes from obstetric units having physician-only care with those from units in which midwives and physicians practiced together (Carlson et al., 2019; Neal et al., 2019). They both found that women receiving care in the latter units were less likely than women at physician-only centers to experience induction, oxytocin augmentation, and cesarean birth. Collaboration among health professionals can also greatly improve safety when care must be transferred across birth settings as interprofessional teamwork has been shown to be central to providing safe, effective, and efficient obstetric care (Guise and Segel, 2008).

In the United States, access to maternity care that is coordinated among homes, birth centers, and hospitals is unreliable, uncommon (Shah, 2015), highly variable, and generally shaped by physician perspectives (Leone et al., 2016; Rainey et al., 2017). U.S. obstetricians lack clear protocols for determining when and how to transfer patients to hospitals offering a higher level of care and risk-appropriate providers. Moreover, U.S. hospitals and birth centers often lack formal referral relationships and may face financial disincentives to transfer patients (Cheyney et al., 2014c; Shah, 2015; Vedam et al., 2014a).

Cheyney and colleagues (2014c) examined the views of hospital- and home-based clinicians in the context of 50 home-to-hospital transfers through open-ended, semistructured interviews (n = 40), and engaged in a process of reciprocal ethnography whereby results were returned to participants for comment and critique. Six key themes (three from receiving providers and three from referring midwives) that emerged from the interviews highlighted differences in referring and receiving providers' perspectives and experiences of transfer and interprofessional collaboration.

Hospital-based providers in this study described (1) the belief that home birth is substantially more dangerous than published studies suggest; (2) the experiences of fear and frustration generated when physicians or CNMs are forced to assume the risk of caring for another provider's patient; and (3) challenges related to unfamiliar charting and strained interprofessional communication during the heightened emotions of a transfer (Cheyney et al., 2014c, p. 446). Further, the perception that out-of-hosptial midwives, regardless of credential (i.e., certified professional midwives [CPMs], CNMs, or licensed midwives [LMs]), had mismanaged the needs of the woman and infant made hospital practitioners question the quality of data and publications that conclude that home birth is safe under certain conditions. The physicians in this study expressed fear and vulnerability over having to take over the care of a woman in labor who was transferred, even with the knowledge that few transfers are emergent.

Out-of-hospital midwives' transfer narratives focused on three key themes that differed from those of hospital-based colleagues: (1) midwives' tendency to defend the midwifery model of care; (2) physicians' tendency to judge midwives by "the exception, rather than the rule"; and (3) physicians' failure to take responsibility for their roles in poor state and national maternal–child health outcomes (Cheyney et al., 2014c, p. 449), instead blaming midwives. Clients worried about "punitive" cesarean sections and humiliating "blaming and shaming" for attempting a home birth, and this often led to a refusal of transfer until minor complications (i.e., a slow, nonprogressive labor) developed into something more severe (i.e., fetal distress). Fear on the part of clients and the lack of collaboration between community midwives and hospitals/providers sometimes led to a delay in transfer that could be detrimental (Cheyney et al., 2014c).

Following their analysis of common themes, Cheyney and colleagues (2014c) outlined a larger set of sociopolitical mechanisms that restrict collaboration between community midwives and receiving physicians. The first is the ethical conflict of interest providers face because professional associations ignore the reality that in some instances, care must be shared. The second is restrictive legislation that prevents CPMs in many states from gaining the legal status that is a precursor to the training and regulation that are likely to improve the quality of care and facilitate integration. The third is the cycle of liability concerns and fear of adverse outcomes that lead to delays in care and fractured communication, which in turn contribute to the actualization of the feared increased liability and bad outcomes. These mechanisms impede efficient and mutually respectful interactions and can result in costly delays (Cheyney et al., 2014c).

The authors also argue, however, that these mechanisms could lead to possible solutions. Midwives requested that, if a transfer is required, the receiving hospital staff show respect for them and the woman and include them in dialogues regarding the best course of treatment, while the hospital-based providers hoped the midwives would provide them with timely and clear charting. Hospital-based providers requested that midwives prepare their clients for the possibility of a transfer prior to labor, and the midwives encouraged the hospital staff to not assume that someone who has attempted a home birth will necessarily decline hospital procedures. These solutions can assist in creating an integrated maternity system premised on mutual accommodation and smooth articulations across birth settings and provider types (Cheyney et al., 2014c).

Fox and colleagues (2014) published a metasynthesis aimed at developing a more nuanced understanding of women's experiences of home-to-hospital transfer by synthesizing and interpreting the then existing body of qualitative research. Three categories emerged from their synthesis: (1) communication, connection, and continuity; (2) making the transition; and (3) making sense of events. Their review of four studies (n = 45) identified three factors that make transfers as seamless as possible from the perspective of the laboring woman: (1) quality and clarity of communication, (2) feeling connected to the backup hospital, and (3) continuity of midwifery care. Initial arrival at the hospital is a time of vulnerability and fear for clients who have spent their pregnancy planning for a community birth. Retaining the care of a known midwife is the core coping technique those women use to make the move—physically and ideologically—to a higher level of care. Receiving providers who are sensitive to women's needs to be reassured and accepted greatly reduce the tension, fear, and stress that mark the transfer experience for the patient. In addition, the reasons for transfer must be clearly communicated, both at the time of transfer and then again in more detail following the birth whenever possible. Fox and colleagues argue that women need to talk through their experiences of transfer, and that they need to have their feelings of disappointment acknowledged in order to move forward to the next phase of parenting. Focusing on the fact of a healthy baby is not sufficient and can be counterproductive if it omits the process of grieving the lost experience. Continuity of care provider was found to be essential to this process because it enables understanding and coping alongside a known caregiver. Several additional studies on the experiences of transfer have also been published as part of the Australian Birthplace Study (see Fox et al., 2018a, 2018b), as well as in other high-resource countries that are currently experiencing a rise in planned home births (Rowe et al., 2012; Ball et al., 2016; Blix et al., 2016; Patterson et al., 2017).

Following the 2011 Home Birth Consensus Summit in the United States, scholars from family medicine, midwifery, nursing, health administration, obstetrics, public health, pediatrics, and ethics, as well as consumers and childbirth educators, formed a collaborative work group with the goal of translating the existing body of literature on transfers from home or birth center to hospital into an applied set of best-practice guidelines for all professionals involved when a transfer is necessary (Vedam et al., 2014a).

Members of the work group reviewed national and international exemplars of best-practice protocols and standards for effective communication and documentation during transfer, examined the literature on strategies for promoting interprofessional coordination and collaboration, and developed a rating system to assess the relevance and clarity of each resource. Findings highlighted the need for "increased commitment to shared deci-

sion making, mutually respectful communication between maternity care
providers and health system staff, quality improvement processes and policies to ensure ongoing evaluation of outcomes of transfers, and expanded
interprofessional education opportunities" (Vedam et al., 2014a, p. 631).
The work group collated key components into Best Practice Guidelines for
Transfer from Home to Hospital (Home Birth Summit, n.d.).

After describing the methods used in the development of these transfer guidelines, Vedam and colleagues (2014a, p. 632) make the following statement: "Regardless of one's opinion of planned home birth, all
clinicians and researchers can agree on the importance of improving
interprofessional collaboration. Progress will require stakeholders with
historically opposing views to find common ground within the contested
space of home birth, especially when all share responsibility for care." As
Caughey and Cheyney (2019, p. 1042) have recently argued, "everyone
involved shares the responsibility for reducing the chasms between community and hospital care and between obstetricians and midwives where
these exist; a shorter distance to traverse literally, metaphorically, and
ideologically could mean improved outcomes for all." In fact, research
suggests that integration of midwives into regional health systems is a key
determinant of optimal maternal–newborn outcomes. A recent study of
midwifery integration in the United States (Vedam et al., 2018) showed
that states with midwifery-inclusive laws and regulations were correlated
with better maternal and neonatal health outcomes and had higher rates of
physiologic birth, breastfeeding, and vaginal birth after cesarean (VBAC).
Conversely, poor coordination of care across providers and birth settings
has been associated with adverse maternal–newborn outcomes. Yet prior
to this study, the characteristics of an integrated system had not been
described or linked to health disparities.

The study by Vedam and colleagues (2018) consisted of a multidisciplinary team of scholars who examined published regulatory data
that described the regulations around the practice of midwifery and interprofessional collaboration across each state in the United States. The team
used a modified Delphi process and selected 50 key items to create a
weighted, composite Midwifery Integration Scoring system (MISS). These
items measured the differences across jurisdictions in scope of practice,
autonomy, governance, and prescriptive authority for midwives, as well as
restrictions that can affect safety, quality, and access to providers across
birth settings. States were ranked by MISS scores, and using reliable indicators in the Centers for Disease Control and Prevention's (CDC's) Vital
Statistics Database, correlation coefficients were calculated between MISS
scores and maternal–newborn outcomes by state. Hierarchical linear regression analyses were used to control for confounding effects of race and
other factors.

MISS scores ranged from lowest at 17 (North Carolina) to highest at 61 (Washington) out of 100 points, indicating a wide range of integration across the United States, as well as generally low levels, as 61/100 was the highest score achieved. MISS scores correlated with the density of midwives and access to care across birth settings. States with higher MISS scores had significantly higher rates of spontaneous vaginal delivery, VBAC, and breastfeeding and significantly lower rates of cesarean, preterm birth, low-birthweight infants, and neonatal death. Significant differences in newborn outcomes, including preterm birth, low birthweight, and neonatal death, were accounted for by MISS scores and persisted after controlling for proportion of African American births in each state. Higher MISS scores were associated with significantly higher rates of physiologic birth, fewer obstetric interventions, and fewer adverse neonatal outcomes.

Overall, findings from this study suggest that states with higher levels of midwifery integration have improved outcomes for pregnant people and newborns, and states with lower levels of midwifery integration have poorer outcomes. Previous studies have also demonstrated similar relationships among midwifery care, systems integration, and improved maternity care outcomes (Cornthwaite et al., 2013; Manojlovich, 2014; Comeau et al., 2018; Reszel et al., 2018). The midwifery integration project is an ecological study, and as such, its main weaknesses is that it does not also assess patient-level data. Important individual-level confounders, moderators, and mediating factors could have affected the findings. In addition, as Vedam and colleagues (2018) are careful to note, the midwifery integration study has identified important correlations, but not necessarily causal relationships. Further research is needed to help clarify relationships among the policy environment, midwifery care across settings, individual-level risk factors, and birth outcomes in the United States.

CONCLUSION

There has yet to be a national, prospective, cohort study in the United States that utilizes an intention-to-treat model to compare outcomes by planned birth location and provider type, pays adequate attention to statistical power for rare outcomes, and controls for maternal risk factors and other confounders. Certainly, a better understanding of the true effect size of choice of birth setting with respect to fetal and neonatal outcomes would be achievable with a nationally validated, granular data registry (Caughey and Cheyney, 2019). With the rising rate of home and birth center births in the United States over the past several decades, it has become increasingly imperative to have a system that allows the tracking of outcomes by intended place of birth, provider type at the onset of labor, transfers over the course of care, and pregnancy characteristics.

Given both the acute and downstream risks of unnecessary interventions and the risks associated with potentially delayed access to lifesaving obstetric and neonatal interventions, birth setting decisions trade off some risks for others (Tilden et al., 2017), meaning there is no clear, risk-free option for giving birth (Caughey and Cheyney, 2019). In the United States, women and clinicians who desire access to medical intervetions generally prefer birth in a hospital (Tilden et al., 2017), while women and providers who do not want unneccesary interventions and who are focused on maternal autonomy and physiologic birth may consider home or birth center births. These distinctions are neither universal nor dichotomous: many hospital-based providers are committed to preventing unnecessary cesarean births and supporting physiologic birth, while some home birth and birth center midwives may overintervene (Caughey and Cheyney, 2019).

Taken together, the literature reviewed in this chapter makes clear that there are risks and benefits for pregnant women and newborns in each of the three birth settings in the United States. However, the literature (particularly from the international experience) also suggests that these risks are modifiable by systems through processes, policies, providers, and regulation.

CONCLUSION 6-1: In the United States, home, birth center, and hospital birth settings each offer risks and benefits to the childbearing woman and the newborn. While no setting is risk free, these risks may be modifiable within each setting and across settings.

The committee's review of the relevant literature on health outcomes by birth setting revealed a dearth of evidence related to the possible connection between maternal mortality and severe maternal morbidity and birth settings, likely because these events are so rare. Indeed, only one case of either of these outcomes following a planned home or birth center birth (see Cheyney et al., 2014a) has been reported in the literature on safety by birth setting.

CONCLUSION 6-2: A lack of data and the relatively small number of home and birth center births prevent exploration of the relationship between birth settings and maternal mortality and severe maternal morbidity.

In the next chapter, we turn to the question: How can each birth setting work to improve outcomes and make birth safer, where safety encompasses both clinical and psychosocial outcomes?

7

Framework for Improving
Birth Outcomes Across Birth Settings

The conceptual model presented in Chapter 1 (refer to Figure 1-7) identifies key areas for improving the knowledge base around birth settings and levers for improving policy and practice across settings. This model recognizes that three elements—access to care, quality of care, and informed choice and risk assessment among care options—contribute to the ultimate goal of positive outcomes in maternity care, and that the maternity care team, the systems and settings in which those personnel care for pregnant people and newborns, and collaboration and integration among providers and systems influence the presence and expression of those elements. It also shows that structural inequities and biases; social determinants of health; and the structure, policies, and financing of the health system itself influence quality, access, choice, and risk across birth settings. Each level of the model presents an opportunity to affect outcomes.

The system-level factors that influence outcomes across settings are responsive to intervention, yet these interventions are largely outside the scope of the health care system. Housing instability, transportation challenges, and intimate partner violence (i.e., social determinants of health) fall into this category. While Chapter 4 reviews these factors in detail and highlights some promising approaches to intervening in the context of maternal health care, given the committee's charge, we focus in this chapter on factors that can be influenced within the health care system, through changes to either service delivery or the services themselves. Of course, we acknowledge and emphasize that while many disparities in outcomes accrue within the health care system, drivers of inequities in these outcomes begin outside the health care system. This reality undergirds our framework for maternal and newborn care in the United States, described below, but there is a critical need for more research on how these factors affect birth outcomes (see, e.g., Krieger et al., 2014).

Given our charge to focus on health outcomes by birth setting, we focus our attention in this chapter on the question: How can each setting work to improve outcomes and make birth safer, where safety encompasses both clinical and psychosocial outcomes?

After first reviewing our framework for maternal and newborn care, we discuss opportunities for improving quality and outcomes in hospital births, the setting where the vast majority of pregnant people give birth in the United States. Next, we consider opportunities for improving quality and outcomes in home and birth center births, focusing on improving coordination, collaboration, integration, and regulation of these settings within the health care system. We then discuss efforts to improve informed choice and risk selection as well as access across settings. Finally, the chapter concludes with our assessment of priorities for future research. In each section, we highlight opportunities that prioritize respect for the woman and her infant and family, regardless of their circumstances (including race, ethnic origin or immigration status, gender identity, sexual orientation, family composition and marital status, religion, income, or education) or birth or health choices.

FRAMEWORK FOR MATERNAL AND NEWBORN CARE IN THE UNITED STATES

Culture of Health Equity

As described in Chapter 1, maternal and newborn care is embedded within the broader social context in which a person lives. As stated in Chapter 4 (Conclusion 4-1), **system-level factors and social determinants of health such as structural racism, lack of financial resources, availability of transportation, housing instability, lack of social support, stress, limited availability of healthy and nutritious foods, lower level of education, and lack of access to health care (including mental health care) are correlated with higher risk for poor pregnancy outcomes and inequity in care and outcomes.** That is, wherever a woman gives birth, the effects of the longitudinal, multifaceted, socially shaped health inputs she brings to her pregnancy and continuing through and beyond maternal and pediatric care influence her birth outcomes. These system-level factors, however, are modifiable, and improving maternal and newborn care in the United States will require interventions outside of the health care system.

Part of addressing these system-level factors is establishing a culture of health that ensures equitable access to quality care for all. As discussed in Chapter 4, a foundational driver of poor outcomes in maternity care is racism and biased attitudes toward women. The experiences of women of color, especially Black and Native American women, and those of women generally, create risk factors that bear on pregnancy and childbirth. These experiences include intergenerational trauma; marginalization, intolerance, and hostility; and continuing economic disadvantage.

A culture of health delivers on economic, social, environmental, restorative, and birthing justice. Such a culture ensures, for example, that families have clean air and water; fresh, healthy food; safe neighborhoods; freedom from violence; paid family and medical leave and paid sick days; respectful treatment; and other essential social supports. In a culture of health, pregnant people and their partners are able to bring their good health to bear on determining whether and when to have children and, when pregnant, on actively engaging in a high-quality maternity care system that leads to robust pregnancy outcomes and the lifelong health of their children, ultimately contributing to the health of the next generation (Koblinsky et al., 2016; National Academies of Sciences, Engineering, and Medicine, 2019).

"Right Amount at the Right Time"

As described in Chapter 6, "too little, too late (TLTL)" and "too much, too soon (TMTS)" patterns in the provision of maternity care contribute to excesses of morbidity and mortality, and in the context of inequality, these extremes often coexist within a single health care system. This means that **in the United States, home, birth center, and hospital birth settings each offer risks and benefits to the childbearing woman and the newborn. While no setting is risk free, these risks may be modifiable within each setting and across settings** (Conclusion 6-1). We assert that a goal for the nation is to move beyond both TLTL and TMTS to the "right amount at the right time." Moreover, this care should be delivered "in the right way," that is, in a way that respects the autonomy and dignity of all birthing people, given that, as reported in Chapter 6, Finding 6-4: *Some women experience a gap between the care they expect and want and the care they receive. Women want safety, freedom of choice in birth setting and provider, choice among care practices, and respectful treatment. Individual expectations, the amount of support received from caregivers, the quality of the caregiver–patient relationship, and involvement in decision making appear to be the greatest influences on women's satisfaction with the experience of childbirth.* The committee sees potential for providers with experience across settings to collaborate on strategies for reducing intervention-related morbidity and to find a more beneficial balance between TMTS and TLTL.

Therefore, the committee envisions a transformed maternal and newborn care system that places women and their infants at the center. In such a system, policies and structures are based on the best interests of these service users. Available care is matched to the physical, emotional, and social goals, preferences, needs, and life circumstances of the woman and her fetus/ infant. The woman and infant are matched to appropriate care, including type and intensity of services, with vigilance being exercised to determine whether a change in status calls for a different level of care, which might be of either greater or lesser intensity. Rigorous attention to the best available evidence limits overuse of unneeded care and underuse of beneficial care.

Respectful Treatment

In order to facilitate equitable access to maternity care services, the maternity care system must provide respectful treatment to all women in its care. The objective of respectful maternity care is to support pregnant and birthing women and remove barriers to receiving health care services before, during, and after birth. Across cultures and contexts, the components of respectful care are largely consistent. In a review of 67 qualitative studies on women's and health care providers' perspectives, Shakibazadeh and colleagues (2018) identify 12 components of respectful maternity care:

1. being free from harm and mistreatment;
2. maintaining privacy and confidentiality;
3. preserving women's dignity;
4. sharing information and seeking informed consent;
5. ensuring continuous access to family and community support;
6. enhancing the quality of the physical labor and birth environment and resources;
7. treating all women equally, regardless of age, race, ethnicity, religion, ability, or other subgroups;
8. using effective communication, including the use of interpreters when needed;
9. respecting women's choices that strengthen their capabilities to give birth;
10. having competent and motivated maternity care providers available;
11. providing effective and efficient care; and
12. ensuring continuity of care.

Based on our review of the literature and of public testimony before the committee, *listening to women* should be added to this list, as women may describe important symptoms not obvious to caregivers. Respectful maternity care is not a given for all women and pregnant individuals. Recent studies from the United States, the United Kingdom, Canada, and Australia document women's experiences of disrespect and mistreatment across lines of race/ethnicity (McLemore et al., 2018; Vedam et al., 2018), ability (Hall, 2018), and nativity (Hennegan et al., 2014). Black and American Indian/Alaska Native women, immigrant women, and other women and individuals from marginalized groups face both structural racism and interpersonal bias within the health system, which likely contributes to disparities in pregnancy outcomes. To rectify these inequities, the maternity care system needs to strive to provide respectful care to all women by listening to them and responding appropriately, providing risk information in understandable terminology, providing culturally and linguistically appropriate care, providing informed choices around care and interventions, and providing clear and supportive communication for women who seek delivery care in hospitals before labor onset or too early in labor to admit.

HOSPITAL SETTINGS

Quality Improvement

The committee recognizes that many interventions are overused in U.S. hospital settings today. As discussed in Chapter 6, Finding 6-3: *In the United States, low-risk women choosing home or birth center birth compared with women choosing hospital birth have lower rates of intervention, including cesarean birth, operative vaginal delivery, induction of labor, augmentation of labor, and episiotomy, and lower rates of intervention-related maternal morbidity, such as infection, postpartum hemorrhage, and genital tract tearing. These findings are consistent across studies. The fact that women choosing home and birth center births tend to select these settings because of their desire for fewer interventions contributes to these lower rates.* There are promising strategies and approaches for lowering the rates of nonmedically indicated morbidity-related interventions, for example, the primary cesarean rate in hospital settings (American College of Obstetricians and Gynecologists, 2019a; Gams et al., 2019).

Such initiatives take a variety of forms and can be implemented at the regional or state level, in a particular health care system, or by an individual hospital or group of hospitals. Perinatal quality collaboratives (PQCs)—"networks of perinatal care providers and public health professionals working to improve health outcomes for women and newborns through continuous quality improvement" (Centers for Disease Control and Prevention, 2016, p. 6)—are a major mechanism for large-scale quality improvement. Within these networks, members from different stakeholder groups (health system administrators, physicians, midwives, state departments of health, childbearing women and their advocates, and others) work together to identify and address deficiencies in perinatal care processes as quickly as possible (Centers for Disease Control and Prevention, 2019a). These state—and occasionally regional—networks contribute to important improvements in health care and outcomes for childbearing women and infants, as well as cost savings for hospitals and systems (Horbar et al., 2017). The National Network for Perinatal Quality Collaboratives is a driving force for communication across PQCs and shared learning and teaching.

For example, the California Maternal Quality Care Collaborative (CMQCC), founded by the California Department of Public Health (Maternal, Child and Adolescent Health Division) and the California Perinatal Quality Care Collaborative and headquartered at Stanford University, now includes more than 40 partner organizations and 200 participating hospitals. Since its inception in 2006, the CMQCC has developed a number of evidence-based quality improvement (QI) toolkits, which are combined with outreach efforts to help hospitals implement the initiatives. It uses data-driven approaches to understand the root causes of maternal mortality, including conducting mock emergencies, making quality improvements in hospital settings, and training staff to work more collaboratively. Its efforts have resulted in measurable improvements in maternal and infant outcomes:

- Among 56 participating hospitals, low-risk first-birth cesarean rates were reduced from 29.1 percent in 2015 to 24.6 percent in 2017, with no worsening of maternal and infant outcomes (Main et al., 2019).
- In contrast to the rise in maternal mortality in the United States as a whole, California's maternal mortality rate was cut in half by 2013, down to 7.0 deaths per 100,000 live births (Main et al., 2018).
- Among 99 hospitals that used a collaborative mentorship approach to implement a hemorrhage safety bundle, severe maternal morbidity was reduced by 20.8 percent between 2014 and 2016 (Main et al., 2017).
- After the release of a toolkit designed to reduce elective early induction, along with an implementation playbook by the National Quality Forum, an additional 8 percent of California births were full term (California Maternal Quality Care Collaborative, n.d.).

While these results are encouraging, ethnic group differences in improvements show that significant racial disparities persist (Main et al., 2018; McLemore, 2019). To address these persistent racial disparities, the CMQCC has initiated a new hospital-based racial equity pilot throughout several communities to redesign obstetric practices. Results from the pilot initiative are expected in 2020 (McLemore, 2019).

Other states have also seen striking results from PQCs. Participating hospitals in Ohio saw their nonmedically indicated early-term birth rate decrease by 68 percent between 2008 and 2015. Participating hospitals in New York experienced a 92 percent decrease in the proportion of early-term scheduled births that were not medically indicated between 2012 and 2013 (Centers for Disease Control and Prevention, 2014, 2016). In terms of maternal outcomes, PQCs have also contributed to reductions in primary cesarean births and maternal morbidity in some states. For example, the New York PQC saw a decrease of 91 percent in scheduled early-term primary cesarean births without medical indication among participating hospitals (Centers for Disease Control and Prevention, 2014). Additionally, the Health Resources and Services Administration (HRSA) supports QI through its infant mortality Collaborative Improvement and Innovation Networks (CoIINs). Through infant mortality CoIINs, multidisciplinary teams of local, state, and federal leaders work together to reduce infant mortality and related perinatal outcomes. These teams use real-time data to determine effective strategies and support distribution of best practices across states. Currently, there are four infant mortality CoIIN teams covering 25 states (Health Resources and Services Administration, 2018).

In an assessment of the CMQCC, Markow and Main (2019) attribute improvement through the QI initiatives to four key components: engagement of many disciplines and partner organizations, mobilization of low-burden data to create a rapid-cycle data center to support QI efforts, provision of up-to-date guidance for implementation using safety bundles and toolkits, and availability of coaching and peer learning to support implementation through multihospital quality collaboratives. While PQCs have shown promising results, currently they include primarily hospital settings in their initiatives. To promote improvement across settings and better outcomes for all women and infants, it is essential for all birth settings to participate in sentinel event reporting and root-cause analyses as part of PQC efforts.

Moreover, 13 states either do not yet have a PQC or their status in this regard is unknown (see Figure 7-1). As noted above, while QI initiatives can lead to cost savings, many such initiatives are currently underfunded and receive no federal funding support. At present, the Centers for Disease Control and Prevention (CDC) provides support for state-based PQCs in Colorado, Delaware, Florida, Georgia, Illinois, Louisiana, Massachusetts, Minnesota, Mississippi, New Jersey, New York, Oregon, and Wisconsin. Sufficient and sustainable financing of QI initiatives by both government and private entities is needed if QI is to be implemented effectively at all levels of health care.

At the national level, the Alliance for Innovation on Maternal Health (AIM) is another example of a QI initiative. AIM—a collaboration among numerous associations, including the American College of Nurse-Midwives (ACNM), the American College of Obstetricians and Gynecologists (ACOG), and the American Hospital Association (AHA), funded through a cooperative agreement with HRSA's Maternal and Child Health Bureau—produces patient safety bundles and provides implementation and data sup-

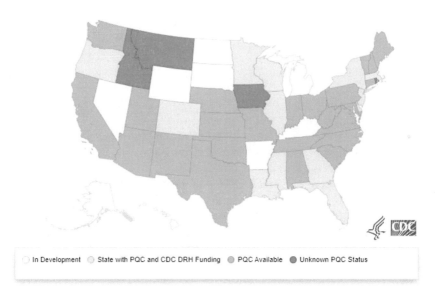

FIGURE 7-1 Status of perinatal quality collaboratives in the United States.
SOURCE: Centers for Disease Control and Prevention (2019b).

port for states or health systems that wish to implement these care practices. There are currently eight AIM patient safety bundles, on issues that include opioid use disorder and reduction of racial/ethnic disparities. Preliminary evaluation of the initiative showed promising results, with reductions in the maternal morbidity rate in states that implemented the hemorrhage and hypertension bundles (American College of Obstetricians and Gynecologists, 2018b). Federal and state government support for and implementation of national data-driven maternal and newborn safety and QI initiatives such as AIM and the National Network of Perinatal Quality Collaboratives would enhance the use of maternal safety and rescue protocols and best practices.

Specific national practice guidelines and adoption of those guidelines could also improve outcomes in hospital settings. For example, professional organizations such as the Association of Women's Health, Obstetrics and Neonatal Nurses (AWHONN) (2018), ACNM (2015), ACOG (2019a), the Society for Maternal-Fetal Medicine (SMFM) (American College of Obstetricians and Gynecologists and Society for Maternal-Fetal Medicine, 2014), and AIM (Lagrew et al., 2018) have published recommendations and clinical guidelines outlining the importance of supportive nursing care during labor and birth, such as nurse staffing. These guidelines are informed by research on the content of care and practice. For instance, researchers in several studies evaluated nursing care during labor as part of an overall approach to decreasing cesarean birth. One study showed that labor care that included such nursing interventions as repositioning and use of a peanut ball was associated with lower cesarean birth rates when incorporated in a comprehensive program that implemented the ACOG-SMFM (2014) labor management guidelines proposed to prevent the first cesarean (Bell et al., 2017). Likewise, a unit culture in which nurses were encouraged to be at the bedside of women in labor as part of a program designed to reduce cesarean births and incorporating the ACOG-SMFM guidelines was found to be associated with lower cesarean birth rates (White VanGompel et al., 2019). The California Maternal Quality Care Collaborative project (56 hospitals with more than 119,000 births) saw similar results in decreasing the cesarean birth rate among nulliparous term singleton vertex (NTSV) women by using the ACOG-SMFM guidelines regarding supportive nursing care, such as increased ambulation, upright positioning, peanut balls, and interpersonal coaching (Main et al., 2019). Finally, two randomized controlled trials of nursing care involving use of a peanut ball during labor had favorable results: Roth and colleagues (2016) found that nurses' use of a peanut ball for nulliparous women shortened first-stage labor, while Tussey and colleagues (2015) found that this practice both shortened labor and deceased the risk of cesarean birth.

The quality of maternity care would also be improved if hospitals and hospital systems universally adopted national standards and guidelines promulgated by ACOG, SMFM, AWHONN, the Society for Obstetric Anesthesia and Perinatology, the American Academy of Pediatrics (AAP), and ACNM for care in hospital settings—in particular, the ACOG-SMFM guidelines on levels of maternal care and the AAP guidelines on neonatal levels of care.

> **CONCLUSION 7-1:** Quality improvement initiatives—such as the Alliance on Innovation in Maternal Health and the National Network of Perinatal Quality Collaboratives—and adoption of national standards and guidelines—such as the Maternal Levels of Care of the American College of Obstetricians and Gynecologists and Society for Maternal-Fetal Medicine; the American Academy of Pediatrics' Neonatal Levels of Care; and guidelines for care in hospital settings developed by the Association of Women's Health, Obstetric, and Neonatal Nurses, the Society for Obstetric Anesthesia and Perinatology, and the American College of Nurse-Midwives—have been shown to improve outcomes for pregnant people and newborns in hospital settings.

QI initiatives may also lead to cost savings. For hospitals, such initiatives provide timely performance feedback (Henderson et al., 2018), training measures, and toolkits for quality improvement, all of which can lead to better individual outcomes and greater efficiency, as well as cost savings. For example, hospitals that participated in neonatal infection prevention initiatives saved an estimated $2.2 million (Centers for Disease Control and Prevention, 2017a). Similarly, in Ohio, participating hospitals saw an estimated savings of $28 million over 7 years by reducing the number of early-term births without a medical indication (Centers for Disease Control and Prevention, 2016). States also see benefits when PQCs work to improve birth certificate data; for example, a 10 percent increase in the accuracy of birth certificates in Illinois resulted from a PQC-led QI initiative (Centers for Disease Control and Prevention, 2017b). However, QI initiatives can sometimes lead to financial losses for hospitals, depending on the revenue streams and mix of payers involved. For this reason, financial support from federal and state sources is critical to the successful implementation of such initiatives at all levels of health care. For example, in California, the state provides an incentive for hospitals to participate in the Perinatal Quality Care Collaborative. Hospitals that participate and provide a quality report to the state for ongoing evaluation and certification purposes receive extra reimbursement. This way, the hospital benefits, the Collaborative receives stable member funding to run its operations, and the state benefits from better care and lower cost.

Additionally, key to improving outcomes for pregnant women and infants in the United States is the ability to measure and report performance on meaningful aspects of care and priority outcomes. Box 7-1 addresses performance measures for quality improvement.

BOX 7-1
Performance Measures

A more comprehensive set of nationally endorsed maternal and newborn performance measures would provide timely feedback to the entities being measured about their own and peer performance, and to purchasers, payers, and policy makers. Public reporting using well-publicized, evidence-based, and user-friendly online interfaces would also enable childbearing women to make informed choices among health plans, maternity care providers, and birth settings.

Currently, National Quality Forum–endorsed measures include Cesarean Birth, Unexpected Complications of the Term Newborn, Exclusive Breast Milk Feeding, and Contraceptive Care-Postpartum, among others. However, the present portfolio of nationally endorsed measures has major gaps. To fill these gaps, the Agency for Healthcare Research and Quality (AHRQ) could develop and submit for national endorsement performance measures for maternity and newborn care for all providers in all settings. Implementation of such measures will require a performance measurement and improvement infrastructure for maternity and newborn care, including mechanisms for public reporting, accountability, quality improvement, and funding.

BOX 7-1 Continued

Additional performance measures to be considered could include the following:

- Access to choice of type of provider and type of setting
- Patient engagement and respect for choices throughout pregnancy, childbirth, and postpartum care
- Composite woman-reported measure of maternal outcomes of maternity care
- Woman-reported measures of the experience of maternal and newborn care, adapting for this clinical area generic Consumer Assessment of Healthcare Providers and Systems (CAHPS) provider and group, facility, and health plan surveys
- Physiologic childbearing, aligned with the definition in reVITALize Obstetric Data Definitions,[a] which has been endorsed by leading professional societies
- Access to a choice of labor pain relief and comfort measures
- Severe maternal morbidity, risk-adjusted
- Composite measure of routine newborn health checks
- Access to and/or rate of vaginal birth after cesarean in hospitals with 24/7 access to surgical teams
- Prenatal and postpartum anxiety screening and follow-up
- Prenatal and postpartum depression screening and follow-up
- Exclusive breast milk feeding to 6 months and any breast milk feeding to 12 months, reflecting the consensus professional standard (Chantry et al., 2015)
- Care coordination in maternity care
- Use of shared decision making in maternity care
- Use of health information technology to engage, inform, and support childbearing women
- Measures of key concepts at the clinician/group and health plan levels, including those aligned with priority currently endorsed facility-level measures
- Measures of peripartum nursing care of women and newborns
- Facility engagement in maternal and newborn quality improvement activities

To promote optimal integration, safety, and accountability, consideration is needed of facility-level measures that apply to birth centers as well as hospitals, and clinician-level measures that apply to all midwives with nationally recognized credentials, whenever feasible and appropriate. To promote equity, measures would need to be stratified to make it possible to determine whether care differs by the race and ethnicity, ability, knowledge, and language of childbearing women, whenever appropriate. Providing these measures in eMeasure format, whenever appropriate, would also promote efficiency.

---

[a] See https://www.acog.org/About-ACOG/ACOG-Departments/Patient-Safety-and-Quality-Improvement/reVITALize-Obstetric-Data-Definitions.

Access to Care Options

While some women desire vaginal birth, and births for high-risk pregnancies require well-equipped hospital settings (Bovbjerg et al., 2017), some
women cannot find hospitals and physicians offering such care. This includes such maternity care services as planned vaginal birth after cesarean,
external cephalic version, vaginal breech birth, and planned vaginal twin
birth. Further, some women face challenges in finding hospitals that support
intermittent auscultation, nonpharmacologic measures for labor comfort
and progress, freedom to drink fluids and eat solids, freedom of movement
in labor, and freedom of choice of birth positions, as well as the related
essential care option of the choice between midwifery- or medical-led care
(National Partnership for Women & Families, 2018).

Women's ability to exercise choice with regard to birth setting is limited
by this lack of access to care options. To promote safety, it is essential for
informed choice of care that fosters physiologic childbearing to be readily
available in all settings for women who desire such care. Moreover, access
to such options is important for improving outcomes, as care that supports
physiologic birth offers benefits for both childbearing women and their
fetuses/newborns. These include onset of labor when the woman is ready
to give birth and the fetus is ready to be born; comfort, progress, and safety
in labor; healthy transitions of the woman and newborn after birth; and
readiness and support for mother–infant attachment and establishment of
breastfeeding (Buckley, 2015).

To promote better outcomes for pregnant woman and newborns, the
majority of whom receive care in hospital settings in the United States,
hospitals—individually and within geographic areas—have a clear and
urgent responsibility to make available forms of care that appear to be
safest in the hospital setting (e.g., planned vaginal breech birth), recognizing that comparative safety may change with greater integration within
maternity care (Bovbjerg et al., 2017). Hospitals could meet this responsibility by developing in-hospital, low-risk, midwifery-led units; adopting
these services in existing maternity units; and enabling greater collaboration among maternity care providers (including midwives, physicians, and
nurses) at all levels of education and practice, as well as ensuring cultivation
of these skills in obstetric residency and maternal–fetal medicine fellowship
programs.

Evidence from the international literature also shows that alongside midwifery units (AMUs) (a midwifery unit located in or collocated
with a hospital) have been successful in reducing the number of non–
medically indicated interventions as compared with traditional obstetric
units (Schroeder et al., 2017; Homer et al., 2014; Laws et al., 2014). The
Vanderbilt University Medical Center (VUMC) model provides an illustra-

tive case study in the U.S. context. Certified nurse midwives manage care for both low- and moderate-risk patients, collaborating with physician colleagues to co-manage the care of women with high-risk pregnancies (e.g., gestational diabetes requiring medication, hypertensive disorders, chronic disease). Most recently, the obstetrical unit committed to the ACOG/ACNM Reducing Primary Cesareans Project initiative and has seen a decline in these rates (American College of Nurse-Midwives, 2017b). As part of that initiative, measures to support physiologic birth are routinely employed. These include use of birth and peanut balls, intermittent auscultation as the standard of care for all low-risk women, an in-house volunteer doula program, and use of hydrotherapy in labor. Mercy Hospital in St. Louis offers an additional example of a hospital setting providing access to midwifery care within the context of a minimal- to low-intervention model and a more conventional maternity care unit (see Box 7-2).

> **CONCLUSION 7-2: Providing currently underutilized nonsurgical maternity care services that some women have difficulty obtaining, including vaginal birth after cesarean, external cephalic version, planned vaginal breech, and planned vaginal twin birth, according to the best evidence available, can help hospitals and hospital systems ensure that all pregnant people receive care that is respectful, appropriate for their condition, timely, and responsive to individual choices. Developing in-hospital, low-risk, midwifery-led units or adopting these practices within existing maternity units, enabling greater collaboration among maternity care providers (including midwives, physicians, and nurses), and ensuring cultivation of skills in obstetric residency and maternal-fetal medicine fellowship programs can help support such care.**

Moreover, there is evidence to suggest that socially and financially disadvantaged women may thrive in midwifery models of care across all birth settings. (Raisler and Kennedy, 2005; Huynh, 2014; Hill et al., 2018; Hardeman et al., 2019). The woman-centered philosophy of care that characterizes these models affirms agency among women of color, and group prenatal care models offer needed social support. Thus these models likely mitigate the harmful impact of medical models that have historically failed to trust the competence and capabilities of women, particularly Black women, including the experiences of disregard and disrespect described by many Black women in traditional care (Huynh, 2014; Vedam et al., 2019; Yoder and Hardy, 2018; Davis, 2018).

The available evidence is inadequate to determine health outcomes among women of color associated with hospital births that follow the midwifery model of care. Until more data are available to guide policy, there may be important opportunities to integrate midwifery models of care

BOX 7-2
Mercy Birthing Center, St. Louis, Missouri

The Birthing Center at Mercy Hospital, St. Louis, opened in 2014 in response to the growing interest of childbearing women in physiologic childbirth. In its first year, the center employed two midwives and had 136 births. Today, the center employs seven midwives (6.7 full-time equivalents) and sees more than 550 births annually, and a second clinic has opened in St Charles, Missouri, for prenatal visits.

The birthing center is located on the first floor of the medical center adjacent to the Maternity Welcome Center and obstetric triage unit. There are four rooms for prenatal visits, four homelike labor–birth–recovery–postpartum rooms, a living room and kitchen, and a classroom for various childbirth and infant care classes. The center offers women the option of a low-risk nonintervention birth with midwifery care in the context of a safety net if complications should arise or conditions change. Routine care includes intermittent auscultation for monitoring the fetal heart status, nitrous oxide and drug-free measures for comfort, freedom to eat and drink according to the woman's interest, freedom of movement in labor, and the woman's birth position of choice.

The birthing center is connected to the labor and birth unit, located on the sixth and seventh floors of the medical center, by a dedicated elevator. Approximately 12 percent of women who are initially admitted to the center in labor are transferred to the labor and birth unit. Reasons for transfer include a desire for epidural analgesia or the need for continuous electronic fetal monitoring, which are unavailable in the center. When a transfer occurs, the attending midwife is able to care for the woman on the labor and birth unit, where rooms are allocated for care of low-risk women in this situation. Medical coverage for women who develop complications is provided by the obstetrician hospitalists who are inhouse on a 24/7 basis. Co-management occurs when appropriate. Maternal–fetal medicine specialists are available for consultation as needed.

The average length of stay in the birthing center is about 13 hours. The midwives provide the initial newborn care until discharge. Parents are encouraged to make an appointment with their pediatric care provider within 3 days postpartum.

The clinic and the midwives have received multiple awards for their patient satisfaction surveys, which hover at the 97th–99th percentile. Over the past 4 years, 100 percent of patients indicated they would recommend the birthing center to friends. Clinical outcomes include a cesarean birth rate of 9.5 percent, a vaginal birth after cesarean success rate of 84 percent, an episiotomy rate of 0.4 percent, an epidural rate of 6.4 percent, and an induction of labor rate of 8.7 percent. Based on existing 2019 data, approximately 600 births and 9,000 clinic visits were anticipated for the year.[a]

---

[a]Personal Communication, Elizabeth Cook, Director, Mercy Birthing Center.

and doulas (dedicated support persons for laboring women) for labor support into hospital-based delivery settings. Doing so would enable women of color, particularly those with elevated medical, social, or obstetric risk factors, to still garner the benefits of woman-centered midwifery models of care and labor support.

Incentivizing High-Value Care

High-value payment models with measures, performance targets, and value-based payment are a mechanism for accountability. In the current system, 23 percent of persons discharged from hospitals are childbearing women and newborns (Agency for Healthcare Research and Quality, 2016), and giving birth and being born have together been the most costly hospital conditions for commercial insurance, Medicaid, and all payers (Wier and Andrews, 2011). While costs have risen through fee-for-service models, performance has routinely fallen short and is worsening for some indicators. Payment tied to value, rather than reimbursement for providing services whether or not optimal care occurred or an optimal outcome was achieved, can incentivize quality, create conditions for innovative systems and leaders to lead delivery system reform, improve care and outcomes, reduce costs, allocate resources to most effective services, and foster emulation and competition, among other improvements. While a number of high-value payment models exist, efforts are needed to pilot, evaluate, and refine these models more extensively and across state Medicaid agencies, Medicaid managed-care organizations, and commercial payers.

CONCLUSION 7-3: Efforts are needed to pilot and evaluate high-value payment models in maternity care and identify and develop effective strategies for value-based care.

Two high-value payment models in particular provide promising approaches for fostering care transformation, curbing overuse and underuse, encouraging members of the care team to work toward shared aims, and meeting the individualized needs of women and newborns: episode payment and the maternity care home (Avery et al., 2018). These models are described in detail below. They may be used in tandem and can include other important but less transformative payment reforms, such as increased payments for sustainability of maternity services in low-volume rural settings and blended case rates. See Box 7-3 for an example of implementation of a blended case rates model.

When implementing episode and maternity care home high-value care models, continuous evaluation, refinement, and learning from initial models and pioneer programs are important for accelerating care

---

BOX 7-3
Rapidly Reduced Cesarean Rate with
Blended Case Rate Payment Reform Pilot

In response to the broad consensus that cesarean rates in the United States are too high (American College of Obstetricians and Gynecologists and Society for Maternal Fetal Medicine, 2014), a pilot project sponsored by the Pacific Business Group on Health aimed to reduce the cesarean rate among nulliparous women laboring at term with a single baby in a head-first position (i.e., the nationally endorsed Cesarean Birth measure), in three participating California hospitals.

The hospitals negotiated a blended case rate designed to be a disincentive for unnecessary cesarean births with multiple health plans. The facility and professional fees for vaginal and cesarean birth were made equal. In addition, the California Maternal Quality Care Collaborative provided the facilities with data management, rapid-cycle performance feedback, and customized technical support to enable each to pursue approaches to cesarean reduction tailored to its local culture (Pacific Business Group on Health, 2015).

Whereas the national cesarean rate has plateaued for about a decade, participating hospitals reduced low-risk cesarean rates by more than 20 percent overall across just five quarters, averting nearly 400 cesareans and saving an estimated $4 million after factoring in repeat cesareans for subsequent births. Cesarean rates dropped for women both covered and not covered under the negotiated contracts. While not a part of the pilot, rates of vaginal birth after cesarean increased during the pilot by 40 percent in the two sites that had had relatively low rates. (See also Kozhimannil et al., 2018b.)

---

transformation and achieving gains in quality, experience, outcomes, and resource use.

Maternity Care Episode Payment

Episode payment encourages collaboration of members of the care team across the three phases of care toward shared goals, and allocation of resources where they are likely to be most effective among a flexible array of services. The timing and types of services included in the episode and the price of the episode are defined. Quality measures are also defined to ensure that mechanisms to decrease costs within the episode foster and do not harm the quality of care. Appropriate adjustments are made for the level of risk involved.

A maternity episode payment program provides a single payment for all services across the episode and encourages members of the team to work together toward shared aims. When designed well, this model offers benefits:

> The biggest beneficiary of bundled payments will be the patients, who will receive better care and have access to more choice. The best providers will also prosper. Many already recognize that bundled payments enable them to compete on value, transform care, and put the health care system on a sustainable path for the long run (Porter and Kaplan, 2016).

Innovative developers of episode payment models that drive toward high-value care will recognize that high-performing forms of care such as midwives, doulas, and birth centers are keys to success, including by reducing cesarean birth and increasing breastfeeding rates, improving performance on quality measures, minimizing overuse/waste and underuse/forgoing valuable care, and fostering women's satisfaction. Proposals for episode payment of birth center care explore this potential (Center for Healthcare Quality and Payment Reform, 2018; Nijagal et al., 2018; Calvin, 2019).

While some bundling of services occurs in conventional codes for paying maternity care providers and in some hospital payments, these do not constitute an episode model. For example, the fee-for-service model involves separate billing from multiple entities (including maternity care provider, newborn provider, anesthesia services, facility maternal services, and facility newborn services), with payments not tied to quality and outcomes, as well as reliable periodic payment increases, providing little or no pressure for more judicious use of appropriate services.

Core elements of optimal, mature maternity care episode payment programs include the following (Health Care Payment Learning and Action Network, 2016, n.d.; Avery et al., 2018):

- inclusion of the woman and the baby;
- inclusion of the vast majority of women and newborns of varied levels of risk who benefit from greater accountability for quality and outcomes;
- limited exclusion of selected high-cost health conditions and further adjustments to limit service provider risk (e.g., risk adjustment, stop loss);
- duration from the initial entry into prenatal care through the postpartum and newborn periods;
- single payment for all services across the episode;
- a willing person who assumes role of coordinator;
- meaningful performance indicators that impact a large segment of the population (e.g., the nationally endorsed Cesarean Birth, Unexpected Complications of the Term Newborn, Exclusive Breast Milk Feeding, and Contraceptive Care-Postpartum measures, as well as woman-reported measures of the experience of maternal and newborn care and the outcomes of maternal care), and targets

for each measure that progressively raise the bar over time as systems develop ways to improve;

- performance impact on the revenue of all service providers, which begins with "upside" gainsharing and with experience over time moves to include downside potential for risk/revenue reduction;
- inclusion of high-performing care elements such as midwives, doulas, and birth centers, including services that may lack conventional billing codes;
- integration into practice, e.g., to foster communication across the care team, monitor performance, and manage payments;
- meaningful engagement of women and families (e.g., in informed choice of care provider and birth setting, shared care planning, shared decision making, access to health records, and completion of woman-reported measures of experience and outcomes), adding great value; and
- QI initiatives to support continuous improvement and success with high levels of accountability.

Maternity Care Home

The second high-value payment model with potential for reducing costs is maternity care homes. Four of five dollars paid on behalf of the woman and newborn across the entire episode from pregnancy through the postpartum and newborn periods cover the relatively brief hospital phase of maternity care (Truven Health Analytics, 2013). In that context, prenatal and postpartum office visits are limited to about 15 minutes, and a dearth of resources is available to meet the individualized needs of women and families that arise during office visits. As this inability to provide meaningful help for women's identified needs likely contributes to disparities that could readily be averted or reduced, the maternity care home, modeled on the primary care patient-centered medical home (PCMH), can make a major contribution. The PCMH model has been shown to help reduce disparities (National Committee for Quality Assurance, 2019).

By linking with social and community services, maternity care homes address social determinants of health, for example, by helping with smoking cessation, maternal mood disorders, or intimate partner violence. Similarly, they help coordinate clinical care across the episode, such as by helping the woman make care plans that include shared decision-making processes—for example, carefully weighing birth options after prior cesarean or postpartum contraception options. The care setting could be a birth center, OB/GYN practice, community health center, or health plan. The key attribute would be responsibility across the episode of care for meeting the individualized needs of the woman and newborn.

Core elements of optimal, mature maternity-care home programs include the following (Rakover, 2016; Avery et al., 2018; Hill et al., 2018; Milliman, 2019):

- payment mechanism, such as a fixed amount per member per month (PMPM);
- personnel ("care coordinators," "care navigators") who are tasked with and prepared, resourced, and accountable for helping meet the individualized needs of pregnant and postpartum women (e.g., nurses, community health workers, or social workers);
- performance indicators (e.g., relating to care coordination, engagement, activation, shared decision making, care planning, access to convenience services such as support during evenings and weekends and prescription refills) and performance targets for each indicator;
- program incentives, including health plan support for infrastructure development and a recognition program demonstrating that the entity has developed capacities and meets standards of a maternity care home;
- performance incentives, for example, a health plan bonus or increased PMPM associated with performance;
- dual focus both to connect women and families with community and social services as needed and to plan and coordinate clinical care across episode settings and providers;
- commitment to addressing individualized needs of any woman in the practice, versus risk screening and premature, often faulty, case management segmentation, with potentially undermining "high-risk" labels and exclusion of some who may need services;
- support for women during the prenatal and postpartum periods, extending to 12 months after birth, reflecting the growing awareness that women's postpartum needs and vulnerabilities are considerable and extend beyond the traditional care trajectory of about 2 months after birth; and
- integration into practice, for example, to foster communication between care navigators and maternity care providers, develop knowledge of/relationships with community and online resources, acquire and develop care coordination tools (e.g., patient portal, decision aids), and keep records.

HOME AND BIRTH CENTER SETTINGS

In reviewing the literature on outcomes in home birth settings, the committee found that statistically significant increases in the relative risk of neonatal death in the home compared with the hospital setting have been reported in most U.S. studies of low-risk births using vital statistics data (see Finding 6-1 in Chapter 6). With regard to birth center settings, we similarly found that, as reported in Chapter 6, Finding 6-2: *Vital statistics studies of low-risk births in freestanding birth centers show a slightly increased risk of poor neonatal outcomes, while studies conducted in the United States using models indicating intended setting of birth have demonstrated that low-risk births in birth centers and hospitals have similar to slightly elevated rates of neonatal and perinatal mortality. Studies of the comparative risk of neonatal morbidity between low-risk birth center and hospital births were mixed, with variation across studies by outcome and provider type.* Conversely, low-risk pregnant women showed lower rates of interventions and reductions in intervention-related morbidities in home and birth center settings as compared with hospital births (see Finding 6-3).

Because of the committee's consensus on a woman's right to choose where and with whom she gives birth, because we recognize that no birth setting is risk-free, because the data are imperfect, and because births are in fact already occurring in homes, birth centers, and hospitals in the United States, we focus in this section on how to improve outcomes and make birth safer in home and birth center settings in the United States.

International studies suggest that home and birth center births may be as safe as hospital births for low-risk women and that neonatal risk can be substantially reduced when (1) they are part of an integrated, regulated system; (2) providers are well qualified and have the knowledge and training to manage first-line complications; (3) transfer is seamless across settings; and (4) appropriate risk assessment and risk selection occur across settings and throughout pregnancy. Such systems are currently not widespread in the United States (see Finding 6-5 in Chapter 6). Thus, we focus on improved collaboration, integration, licensure, and regulation of these settings within the health care system—each representing key levers for improving birth outcomes in home and birth center settings. An integrated and regulated maternity care system aims to promote communication, collaboration, and coordination among health services providers and across care settings, and includes shared care and ready access to safe and timely consultation, collaborative care agreements that ensure seamless transfer across settings, appropriate risk assessment and risk selection across settings and throughout the episode of care, and well-qualified maternity care providers with the knowledge and training to manage first-line complications. Importantly, systems integration appears to influence safety and outcomes, as does patient selection and matching of risk to setting.

Integration and Collaboration

To support equitable, high-quality maternity care, effective structures that shape care settings, providers, and practices need to be in place (Berwick, 2002). In fact, as observed in Chapter 6, Finding 6-6: *Lack of integration and coordination and unreliable collaboration across birth settings and maternity care providers are associated with poor birth outcomes for women and infants in the United States.*

Integration creates a single, coordinated, high-functioning system and is an important driver of safety. Moreover, as discussed in Chapter 6, a recent U.S. study suggests that integration of midwifery professionals within a state's maternal care system may be related to improved maternal and newborn health outcomes (Vedam et al., 2018). Greater midwifery integration was found to be associated with significantly higher rates of spontaneous vaginal birth, vaginal birth after cesarean, and breastfeeding and significantly lower rates of cesarean birth, preterm birth, low-birthweight infants, and neonatal mortality. In the United States, midwifery integration varies from very low in North Carolina to moderate in Washington State (Comeau et al., 2018; Vedam et al., 2018).

A highly integrated maternity and newborn care system also requires the existence of respectful, collaborative relationships across settings and types of providers. The development and maintenance of respectful, collaborative relationships among providers of birth center and home birth care and providers of care in hospitals would foster seamless transfer to hospital care when needed. However, in the current fragmented system, collaboration is often hampered by systems or policies, such as those whereby physicians are not allowed to create these relationships on their own, or legal liability coverage does not permit collaboration with other providers, such as midwives (Sakala et al., 2013a).[1] An integrated system offers women planning home and birth center births the safety of ready access to safe and timely consultation, shared care, and transfer of care and seamless transport when additional risk-appropriate care is needed. Such a system recognizes that all maternity care providers need places to turn when circumstances exceed their scope of practice and areas of competence.

---

[1] Collaboration among providers may be hampered by professional liability concerns. Currently, professional liability restrictions may prevent professionals from providing appropriate care and negatively impact women's access to maternity care choices. Some policies, for instance, impose surcharges for care, such as vaginal birth after cesarean, obstetricians' collaborative practice with midwives, and family physicians' provision of maternity care (Benedetti et al., 2006; Hale, 2006).

CONCLUSION 7-4: Integrating home and birth center settings into a regulated maternity and newborn care system that provides shared care and access to safe and timely consultation; written plans for discussion, consultation, and referral that ensure seamless transfer across settings; appropriate risk assessment and risk selection across settings and throughout the episode of care; and well-qualified maternity care providers with the knowledge and training to manage first-line complications may improve maternal and neonatal outcomes in these settings.

Multidisciplinary guidelines for transport from home and birth center settings are an essential tool for fostering safe, responsible integration of maternity services. As discussed in Chapter 6, the manner in which transfers are conducted, including the level of collaboration between the hospital and the community midwife, impacts birth outcomes (Vedam et al., 2014a). Model consensus guidelines for such transfers were developed through a multidisciplinary process that emerged from the 2011 Home Birth Consensus Summit (see Chapter 6).

The collaborative care model at Cheshire Medical Center (CMC) within the Dartmouth-Hitchcock Health System in New Hampshire is one example of a hospital system collaborating with home and birth center providers. In 2010, the Northern New England Perinatal Quality Improvement Network began work to improve communication and interprofessional collaboration between community midwives and the hospital system. Early products included a Situation, Background, Assessment, Recommendation (SBAR) report form to be used by the midwife calling in to the hospital, resources for hospital personnel about scope of practice, and transfer guidelines. CMC also adopted protocols for the ambulatory setting and for in-labor transfers related to unaffiliated providers. Out-of-hospital midwives coordinate with the obstetrics and gynecology practice at CMC if their clients need particular tests or consultations. In the case of intrapartum transfer, the relationship is already established, and the transfer is smooth. Midwives retain primary responsibility for their patients, and hospital obstetricians complement their care. Postpartum women are released back into the care of the out-of-hospital midwife unless further collaborative follow-up is needed. Providers can quickly share information and work together effectively when care plans need to change. Postpartum follow-up and communication have improved as a result of home birth and birth center midwives having access to their clients' electronic health records (Cheshire Medical Center, 2019).

The U.S. Military Health System also offers cross-cutting lessons for implementing a coordinated and integrated maternal and newborn care system, as described in Box 7-4.

BOX 7-4
Comprehensive Direct Care Maternity Services in the
Military Health System, a Universal Health Care Model

The Military Health System (MHS), which provides care to military members and their families, is one of the largest health care systems in the United States (Smith et al., 2017), providing care for 9.4 million military beneficiaries in hospitals, clinics, and dental clinics across the globe (Defense Health Agency, 2019). All military members and their families are entitled to medical care that is free of cost through the TRICARE program. Military families receive care through military treatment facilities (MTFs) or through contracts with private-sector providers.

In 2017, the Department of Home Affairs (DHA) provided direct care for 41,164 births in MTFs. Direct maternity care providers are educated, board certified, licensed, and credentialed according to national standards. Evidence-based prenatal care is guided by the Department of Veterans Affairs (VA)/Department of Defense (DoD) *Clinical Practice Guideline for the Management of Pregnancy*, a peer-reviewed document that identifies sound relationships among various care options and health outcomes (Veterans Affairs/Department of Defense Management of Pregnancy Work Group, 2018).

Intrapartum care is provided in accordance with national professional recommendations (e.g., American College of Obstetricians and Gynecologists [ACOG], American College of Nurse-Midwives [ACNM], Association of Women's Health, Obstetric and Neonatal Nurses [AWHONN], American Academy of Pediatrics [AAP]). A range of care options, from intermittent auscultation, to continuous electronic fetal monitoring, to physiologic labor support (e.g., hydrotherapy), to epidural pain management, to noninterventional vaginal birth, to emergent cesarean section, are available, depending on location. Many MTFs offer labor, birth, and recovery in the same room. Medical providers and nurses involved in the care of the laboring woman include registered nurses, certified nurse midwives, and MDs/DOs (including obstetricians and family medicine physicians). Certified nurse midwives have full practice authority in DHA. Further, women are able to choose birth center or home births.

Women have the option of receiving care outside of the MTFs. However, outcomes outside of MTFs, considered "purchased care," differ from those in the military system. From 2006 to 2010, direct care was associated with higher vaginal birth rates relative to purchased care, and women with low comorbidity and low cesarean risks had greater odds of having a cesarean birth in purchased care (Ranjit et al., 2017). Overall, purchased care had higher rates and adjusted odds of cesarean birth and severe acute maternal morbidity (Ranjit et al., 2017). About one-quarter of active duty women had a cesarean birth from 2012 to 2016 (Stahlman et al., 2017), which is lower than the national average for cesarean birth.

Maternal and infant mortality is also lower in the MHS relative to rates reported nationally through the National Perinatal Information Center (NPIC). The MHS rate of infant mortality was 2.51 deaths per 1,000 live births from January 2009 through June 2018, and the NPIC rate was statistically significantly greater

continued

BOX 7-4 Continued

than that at 4.76 deaths per 1,000 live births. Maternal mortality rates were also lower in the MHS, with pregnancy-related maternal mortality at 7.40 deaths per 100,000, compared with 11.3 deaths per 100,000 in the NPIC database for the same time period. Both maternal and infant mortality rates were even lower for women who chose to give birth in the MTF instead of going outside the system to use purchased care (Office of the Secretary of Defense, 2019).

Direct care in MTFs is analogous to universal health care coverage in that it allows for unlimited access without payment. TRICARE coverage includes well-woman, prenatal, postpartum, newborn, pediatric, and gynecologic care, all within the same system, and often at the same location. This system provides multiple opportunities for women to optimize their health prior to pregnancy, seek preconception counseling, and access contraceptive care when pregnancy is not desired. Additionally, with decreased concern about insurance coverage of procedures, providers are free to recommend and perform all clinically indicated procedures, and similarly, to avoid procedures that are not clinically indicated. Another unique feature of the MHS is that the threat of malpractice is minimized by statutory limits on military members filing malpractice suits against the United States.

Safety and accountability in MTFs are enhanced at multiple levels through federal statutes, DoD specifications, and service-specific requirements for training and reporting of quality metrics. With national transparency, TRICARE is federally mandated to report to Congress on metrics of access, quality, and outcomes of maternity care (National Defense Authorization Act for Fiscal Year 2016,). There are standardized training requirements for all providers (including MDs/DOs, certified nurse midwives, advanced practice nurses, licensed practical nurses/licensed vocational nurses, registered nurses, and licensed and unlicensed personnel who care for pregnant women and babies). To enforce accountability, the MTF and military services are required to report training status biannually. MTF and service-level reports plus an annual summary are submitted to service leadership and MHS governance (Defense Health Agency, 2019).

Teamwork has been a hallmark of the MHS for years, from TeamSTEPPS© to simulation training in obstetric emergencies (Deering, 2009; Agency for Healthcare Research and Quality, 2011). Collaborative practice in the MHS is carried out in accordance with the recommendations of the joint consensus of ACOG/ACNM. Further enhancing collaborative practice through interprofessional education, certified nurse midwives in the MHS train residents in maternity care practices, including prenatal, intrapartum, and postpartum care.

In summary, the MHS provides a unique model of maternity care that combines a universal payment model, a diminished malpractice threat, safety and accountability of care, and collaborative practice.

Licensure and Regulation

Currently, nine states do not license birth centers (American Association of Birth Centers, 2016d). Licensure of birth centers in all states and territories would support safety. Licensing statutes, generally written with great specificity, ensure that planned births in birth centers are limited, to the extent feasible, to healthy, low-risk women, and that midwives provide care that keeps their clients healthy and continually assess and identify problems early so they can be properly and rapidly addressed. The American Public Health Association (APHA) has adopted model guidelines for writing state regulations licensing birth centers.[2] These regulations cover such topics as definitions, staffing, the facility, fire and building codes, and the services that can and cannot be provided. For example, no states allow cesarean births in birthing centers.

The American Association of Birth Centers (AABC) establishes national standards to enable quality measurement of services provided in freestanding birth centers (American Association of Birth Centers, 2017). Components of external quality evaluation of birth centers include federal and state regulation, licensure, and national accreditation. The standards also encompass a strong internal quality improvement program, as well as criteria for appropriate clinical risk status for birth center admission. The committee supports the accreditation of freestanding birth centers, which provides an additional layer of assurance for women and families. The AABC standards provide the basis for accreditation and the indicators used by the Commission for Accrediting Birth Centers (American Association of Birth Centers, 2017). The standards cover seven areas: philosophy and scope of service; planning, governance, and administration; human resources; facility, equipment, and supplies; the health record; research; and quality evaluation and improvement. Accreditation of a birth center indicates that a high standard of evidence-based and widely recognized benchmarks has been met for clinical care and safety (American Association of Birth Centers, 2016a). The AABC regularly reviews the standards

---

[2] APHA recommends the following: increasing legislative funding support to strengthen the public health workforce infrastructure, including public health nurses, with a focus on prevention, health promotion, and population-focused practice; developing academic–practice partnerships to prepare public health nurses for changes in the public health delivery system; developing the capacity for public health nurses to function at their highest levels of education, competence, and licensure; developing opportunities for public health nurses to build their capacity for health system and health policy leadership; developing effective strategies to recruit and retain qualified public health nurses; and increasing funding to support a research agenda that measures the effectiveness of public health nurse–sensitive interventions with respect to population health outcomes. See https://www.apha.org/policies-and-advocacy/public-health-policy-statements/policy-database/2014/07/10/13/29/guidelines-for-licensing-and-regulating-birth-centers.

to ensure that they remain consistent with current evidence-based maternity care. No research has been conducted specifically on variation in outcomes for birth centers that follow these standards and those that do not (Illuzzi et al., 2015).

> CONCLUSION 7-5: The availability of mechanisms for all freestanding birth centers to access licensure at the state level and requirements for obtaining and maintaining accreditation could improve access to and quality of care in these settings. Additional research is needed to understand variation in outcomes for birth centers that follow accreditation standards and those that do not.

As discussed in Chapter 4, Finding 4:3: *Access to midwifery care is limited in some settings because some types of midwives are not licensed in some states and do not have admitting privileges in some medical facilities, but this varies across the country. The wide variation in regulation, certification, and licensing of maternity care professionals across the United States is an impediment to access across all birth settings.* Much of the discussion related to the education, training, and licensure of maternity and newborn care providers in the United States has focused on the midwifery profession. The U.S. Midwifery Education, Regulation, and Association (U.S. MERA), a coalition of representatives from seven national midwifery associations, credentialing bodies, and accreditation agencies, was formed in 2013 with the goal of creating a more cohesive midwifery workforce in the United States.[3] The global midwifery standards and competencies of the International Confederation of Midwives (ICM) (adopted in 2011) were used to underpin the group's recommendations. Organizations participated in U.S. MERA signed on to support legislative language that includes the following: "by 2020 any new states adding midwifery licensure use language stating that all new applicants for midwifery licensure in that state *must* have completed an educational program *or* pathway accredited by an organization recognized by the U.S. Department of Education *or* have obtained the Midwifery Bridge Certificate. All applicants for licensure must pass a national certification exam, as well as hold CPM, CNM, or CM [certified professional midwife, certified nurse midwife, or certified midwife] credentials" (U.S. Midwifery Education, Regulation, and Association Professional Regulation Committee, 2015b).

---

[3] The U.S. MERA participating organizations include the Accreditation Commission for Midwifery Education, American Midwifery Certification Board, Midwifery Education Accreditation Council, Midwives Alliance of North America, National Association of Certified Professional Midwives, North American Registry of Midwives, and American College of Nurse-Midwives. The International Center for Traditional Childbearing (ICTC) became a member of the U.S. MERA coalition in 2016.

The committee supports the certification and licensure of midwives who complete midwifery education at an accredited organization recognized by the U.S. Department of Education and who pass a national certification exam. We also discussed the evidence around the efficacy of endorsing licensure for the approximately two-thirds of current certified professional midwives who were trained in apprenticeship and self-study programs that lack accreditation. Under the U.S. MERA model language, the bridge certificate program is a pathway for these certified professional midwives credentialed through nonaccredited apprenticeship programs to meet the higher educational and training standards specified by the ICM. Bridge certificate applicants must complete 50 continuing education units of accredited coursework within 5 years of application.[4] The committee did not reach consensus on the evidence for licensing credentialed midwives who use the bridge pathway. We recognize that in 2016, ACOG issued a statement supporting the ICM educational standards as the minimum education and licensure requirement for all midwives practicing in the United States and endorsed the Midwifery Bridge Certificate.[5] However, the committee calls on professional organizations, such as those participating in the U.S. MERA process, to continue to study the appropriate level of education and training needed to offer high-quality, safe care to all women and infants.

CONCLUSION 7-6: The inability of all certified nurse midwives, certified midwives, and certified professional midwives whose education meets International Confederation of Midwives Global Standards, who have completed an accredited midwifery education program, and who are nationally certified to access licensure and practice to the full extent of their scope and areas of competence in all jurisdictions in the United States is an impediment to access across all birth settings.

INFORMED CHOICE AND RISK SELECTION

As discussed in Chapters 3 and 4, informed choice requires a set of real options, accurate information about the risks and benefits of those options, appropriate and ongoing medical/obstetrical risk assessment, respect for women's informed decisions, and recognition that those choices may change over the course of care. True choice occurs when

---

[4] See https://www.acog.org/-/media/Departments/State-Legislative-Activities/2017CPMLicensureLaws-EducationStandards.pdf.

[5] See https://www.acog.org/About-ACOG/News-Room/Statements/2016/ACOG-Statement-on-the-US-MERA-Bridge-Certificate and https://www.acog.org/About-ACOG/News-Room/Statements/2016/ACOG-Statement-on-the-US-MERA-Bridge-Certificate?IsMobileSet=false.

- choice among care providers and birth settings is available;
- choice among care options is available across the episode of care in all birth settings, including safe low-tech alternatives to common practices;
- women have access to high-quality information provided at appropriate literacy levels in culturally and linguistically concordant ways about the experience of birth across the variety of settings and types of providers and possible benefits and harms of the various care options, ideally through shared decision making and quality up-to-date decision aids and with support from a care navigator as needed;
- women receive professional guidance about the suitability of those options given the woman's specific risk level and circumstances;
- the care team genuinely supports women's informed choice and recognizes that perceptions of risk may differ among women and between a woman and her care provider; and
- women and their care team recognize that circumstances may change, and women's choices may change.

However, women's knowledge of their options and ability to exercise choice with regard to birth setting is limited by systemic barriers to knowledge, including a lack of systematic, objective information on the various options provided in plain lay English or an appropriate language.

A key component of informed choice is risk assessment, which accounts for a woman's unique physical, social, financial, and emotional needs. In light of this assessment, women are then informed about all choices that align with their unique risk profile and circumstances. To enable this process, high-quality, evidence-based online decision aids and risk assessment tools incorporating medical, obstetric, and social factors that influence outcomes and facilitating clinical risk assessment and a culturally appropriate assessment of the woman's risk preferences and tolerance are needed. A key feature of such tools would be helping women make decisions related to risk, including settings, providers, and specific care practices, leading to an overall birth plan for use in concert with their providers and care navigators. These tools need to be widely available, and their availability needs to be publicized.

CONCLUSION 7-7: Ongoing risk assessment to ensure that a pregnant person is an appropriate candidate for home or birth center birth is integral to safety and optimal outcomes. Mechanisms for monitoring adherence to best-practice guidelines for risk assessment and associated birth outcomes by provider type and settings is needed to improve birth outcomes and inform policy.

CONCLUSION 7-8: To foster informed decision making in choice of birth settings, high-quality, evidence-based online decision aids and risk-assessment tools that incorporate medical, obstetrical, and social factors that influence birth outcomes are needed. Effective aids and tools incorporate clinical risk assessment, as well as a culturally appropriate assessment of risk preferences and tolerance, and enable pregnant people, in concert with their providers, to make decisions related to risk, settings, providers, and specific care practices.

The committee notes a special challenge with respect to a woman's ability to exercise informed choice regarding care provider and birth setting. In important respects, these choices are best made before entry into maternity care, a time when such discussions could be awkward, could involve conflicts of interest, and could inhibit women from acting on their informed preferences if doing so involved leaving a provider with whom they had initiated care. Thus, it is ideal to provide high-quality sources of information about these options and access to decision aids when women are planning pregnancy or have just become pregnant and have not yet entered care. Further support for these decisions can be provided by independent care navigators. If a woman pursues care that is not appropriate for her situation, her prospective maternity care provider has the responsibility to facilitate a more suitable match, whether to a higher or lower level of care (see Chapter 3).

In addition, it is important for women with low-risk pregnancies who present for physician-led care to be counseled about options for midwife-led care in the home, freestanding birth center, or hospital. For women who desire home or birth center births, midwives working in those settings need to apply protocols in assessing their eligibility. These protocols need to be aligned with state statutes and developed in concert with midwives, physicians, and policy makers, and to include guidance on physician consultation and facilitation of transfer aligned with model guidelines.

ACCESS

Ability to Pay

As discussed in Chapter 4, Finding 4-4: *Access to all types of birth settings and providers is limited because of the lack of universal coverage for all women, for all types of providers, and at levels that cover the cost of care.* Currently, only a limited number of insurance providers offer coverage for care in home or birth center settings. Models for increasing access to birth settings for low-risk women that have been implemented at the state level include expanding Medicaid, Medicare, and commercial payer coverage to cover care provided in home and birth center settings within their accreditation and licensure guidelines and to cover care provided by certified nurse midwives, certified midwives, and certified professional midwives whose education meets ICM Global Standards, who have completed an accredited midwifery education program, and who are nationally certified.

As an example, the Oregon Health Plan, the state's Medicaid program, covers home birth for low-risk women in a limited set of circumstances. Out-of-hospital birth is covered if women meet low-risk criteria based on appropriate risk assessment (both initially and throughout pregnancy, labor, and delivery), no exclusion criteria are present, and criteria for consultation and transfer are met. Only pregnancies that meet the Oregon Health Authority's (OHA's) criteria for low-risk pregnancy, which include criteria for maternal, fetal, and placental complications for the current and any previous pregnancies, can be covered, and OHA delineates which conditions are allowable for out-of-hospital birth (Oregon Health Authority, 2015). Some risk criteria, such as multiple gestation and placenta previa, must be ruled out by ultrasound, while others, such as gestational hypertension, require continuous assessment over the course of the pregnancy. Out-of-hospital providers must perform clinical and diagnostic assessment for each risk criterion. If a woman refuses a required risk assessment, she is ineligible for an out-of-hospital birth because her risk status cannot be ascertained. The presence of high-risk complications, such as breech presentation, previous preeclampsia or eclampsia, or preexisting hypertension, renders the woman ineligible for a covered out-of-hospital birth (Oregon Health Authority, 2015). In addition to the requirements for risk selection, the Oregon Health Plan delineates situations in which an out-of-hospital midwife is required to consult with a hospital-based maternity care provider (Oregon Health Authority, 2015). When caring for women with high-risk conditions, such as more than one previous preterm birth, consultation between out-of-hospital and hospital-based providers is required to meet coverage criteria. Finally, coverage of out-of-hospital births under the Oregon Health Plan requires out-of-hospital providers to initiate transfer to a hospital during the intrapartum or postpartum period under certain conditions (Oregon Health Authority, 2015). These conditions include maternal infection or fever, hemorrhage, laceration requiring hospital repair, and failure to progress, among others. In the case of out-of-hospital deliveries, certain neonatal complications, such as very low birthweight (weight less than 3 lb 4 oz at birth), low Apgar scores (less than 5 at 5 minutes, and less than 7 at 10 minutes), and unexpected significant or life-threatening congenital anomalies, require transfer to a hospital for the midwife's pretransfer services to be covered by the Oregon Health Plan (Oregon Health Authority, 2015).

The committee discussed the efficacy of national, universal adoption of Medicaid, Medicare, and commercial payer reimbursement for home birth. In addition to Oregon, Washington State outlines administrative certification/licensure guidelines for midwives and home births that designate scope of practice standards in that state. Based on those guidelines, payers then designate reimbursable services. As detailed above, Oregon and Washington, for instance, have such licensure requirements for midwives (certified professional midwives, certified nurse midwives, and certified midwives), and Medicaid reimburses providers only for the care they provide within the scope of their licensure.[6] These state-based models that include extensive licensure and certification guidelines are consistent with best practices. Unlike these leading states, however, the majority of U.S. states lack widely available integrated health care systems or requirements for collaborative care, as well as high-quality monitoring systems. In addition to these concerns, the committee is aware that disproportionate rates of such risk factors as obesity, hypertension, diabetes, depression and other mental illness, substance use, and smoking are present among the Medicaid population. Therefore, the committee did not reach consensus as to whether national expansion of Medicaid and Medicare for home births would be efficacious or cost-effective, but rather points to the need for additional research, demonstration, and evaluation of these state-level models.

An additional model for increasing access to birth settings for low-risk women and improving outcomes is to cover care provided by community-based doulas. As discussed in Chapter 5, the support of labor doulas offers many benefits for childbearing women (Bohren et al., 2017, 2019). In addition, the extended model of doula support (beginning during pregnancy, supporting childbirth, and continuing into the postpartum period), although less rigorously studied, appears to have benefits beyond those provided by labor doulas, such as reduced preterm birth and low birthweight and increased breastfeeding (Gruber et al., 2013). Overall, providing financing to support women's use of doulas has been shown to be associated with both better outcomes for women and infants and cost savings (Kozhimannil et al., 2016; Greiner et al., 2019). New York, Minnesota, and Oregon have extended coverage for the services of doulas through Medicaid. Evaluation of such efforts to determine the potential impact of these state-level models is needed, particularly with regard to effects on reduction of racial/ethnic disparities in access, quality, and outcomes of care (Meyerson, 2019).

The rise of community-based perinatal health worker groups, which may include or focus exclusively on doula services, also holds promise. Such groups provide respectful, culturally concordant care and may fill a void in the availability of affirming, supportive, salutogenic services within the health care system (Karbeah et al., 2019; Davis, 2018; National Partner-

---

[6] See http://www.gencourt.state.nh.us/rules/state_agencies/mid500.html for an example of licensure/certification regulations for midwives in New Hampshire.

ship for Women & Families, 2019a). Thus, they may serve as a major part of the solution to addressing disparities in access to maternity care, as well as a key to community development (Hardeman and Kozhimannil, 2016; Kozhimannil et al., 2016; Ireland et al., 2019; National Partnership for Women & Families, 2019a). These groups often include training components, and have various models for financial support and various degrees of financial sustainability. While initial evaluations of their services are favorable, further evaluations are needed.

When considering expansion of coverage for care, it is important that reimbursement levels be adequate to support quality and allow providers across settings to sustain the services they offer. Currently, payment to providers through Medicaid and Medicare does not always cover the full cost of care and prevents some providers from accepting more women with Medicaid coverage. To address this issue, the Medicaid and CHIP Payment and Access Commission (MACPAC) could analyze levels of payment for maternity and newborn care across birth settings to ensure that payment is adequate to support access to maternity care options nationwide. Just as Congress relies on the payment expertise of the Medicare Payment Advisory Commission (MedPAC) and the Centers for Medicare & Medicaid Services (CMS) to determine the adequacy of payment, the Medicaid program needs similar analysis to ensure access to quality, affordable maternity care for Medicaid beneficiaries. This analysis would also ensure that guidelines for billing under the various fee schedules are appropriate to all types of maternity providers—a point of particular importance to enable providers to care for a high proportion of uninsured or Medicaid patients.

Moreover, as noted throughout this report, evidence demonstrates that the postpartum period is critical for the adjustment and development of the woman and her infant and continues to set the stage for their long-term health and well-being (see, e.g., National Academies of Sciences, Engineering, and Medicine, 2019). It is a period of exceptional change and transition for families, and there is increasing awareness of their considerable needs at this time. For example, ACOG terms this period the "fourth trimester," and calls for postpartum care that is continuous throughout the postpartum period rather than a single encounter, as well as coordination between a woman's maternity care providers and the rest of her health care team (American College of Obstetricians and Gynecologists, 2018a). In addition, awareness is increasing of the extent of adverse pregnancy-related outcomes that occur throughout the first year after birth, including maternal mortality and many types of new-onset and often persistent morbidity (Declercq et al., 2013; Petersen et al., 2019). This awareness is leading to a reconceptualizing of postpartum care needs, including growing calls for extending pregnancy-related Medicaid coverage to 1 year postpartum (American College of Obstetricians and Gynecologists, 2019b).

CONCLUSION 7-9: Access to choice in birth settings is curtailed by a pregnant person's ability to pay. Models for increasing access to birth settings for low-risk women that have been implemented at the state level include expanding Medicaid, Medicare, and commercial payer coverage to cover care provided at home and birth centers within their accreditation and licensure guidelines; cover care provided by certified nurse midwives, certified midwives, and certified professional midwives whose education meets International Confederation of Midwives Global Standards, who have completed an accredited midwifery education program, and who are nationally certified; and cover care provided by community-based doulas. Additional research, demonstration, and evaluation to determine the potential impact of these state-level models is needed to inform consideration of nationwide expansion, particularly with regard to effects on reduction of racial/ethnic disparities in access, quality, and outcomes of care.

CONCLUSION 7-10: Ensuring that levels of payment for maternity and newborn care across birth settings are adequate to support maternity care options across the nation is critical to improving access.

Underserved Rural and Urban Areas

While the above section focuses on improving access to maternity care services for women lacking access as a result of their socioeconomic status, additional efforts are needed to improve access to services for women in underserved geographic areas. As described in Chapter 4, Finding 4-2: *Women living in rural communities and underserved urban areas have greater risks of poor outcomes, such as preterm birth and maternal and infant mortality, in part because of lack of access to maternity and prenatal care in their local areas.* Rural and urban maternity care deserts present a challenge to improving maternal and newborn care in the United States, and research is needed to develop sustainable models for safe, effective, and adequately resourced maternity care in underserved areas to resolve disparities in outcomes by geographic location. One approach to making quality maternity care more widely accessible is to build on the concept of community mental health centers, rural health centers, and federally qualified health centers. These centers were established to fulfill a need for services that might not be offered absent some public subsidies. HRSA could establish demonstration model birth centers and hospital services in underserved rural and urban areas and evaluate their impact on birth outcomes and access to care. Such models could focus, for example, on ensuring access by improving health equity. Use of telemedicine may also be appropriate as part of these centers, particularly in rural areas. The Strong Start initiative's findings with respect to the results of midwife-led care for Medicaid beneficiaries in birth centers also suggest that such policies could make inroads in lowering rates of preterm birth, low birthweight, and cesarean birth and increasing rates of breastfeeding while reducing costs (see the discussion of Strong Start in Chapter 4). Any intervention effective in reducing preterm birth and low birthweight—two of the most costly and intractable areas of inequality in maternity care in the United States—is worth pursuing (Petrou, 2019; Petrou et al., 2019).

Improving access to underserved rural and urban areas will also require increasing the pipeline of maternal and newborn care providers in these areas. Beyond specific efforts to rightsize and match the distribution of the maternity care workforce described below, research could explore the potential for using a variety of providers, including community health workers, public health nurses, certified nurse midwives, certified professional midwives, and certified midwives. These providers could be used in underserved communities to increase access to maternal and newborn care, including prenatal and postpartum care, while maintaining seamless transfer of information and continuity of care during the intrapartum period. Commonsense Childbirth's Easy Access Clinic provides a model for extending such care to underserved areas through use of midwives. The clinic provides prenatal services for low-income and racial minority women who are at risk for not receiving prenatal care. Prenatal care is provided by midwives, and women may then choose to give birth in a birth center or an affiliated hospital setting. Designed to address higher-than-average rates of preterm birth, the clinic has succeeded in reducing disparities in the rate of preterm birth and greatly reducing cesarean births in the women served (National Partnership for Women & Families, 2019a). The Family Health and Birth Center (FHBC) in Washington, DC, offers another example of this type of care (see Box 7-5). These models demonstrate the promise of wraparound support for women of color and other underserved communities.

CONCLUSION 7-11: Research is needed to study and develop sustainable models for safe, effective, and adequately resourced maternity care in underserved rural and urban areas, including establishment of sustainably financed demonstration model birth centers and hospital services. Such research could explore options for using a variety of maternity care professionals—including nurse practitioners, certified nurse midwives, certified professional midwives, certified midwives, public health nurses, home visiting nurses, and community health workers—in underserved communities to increase access to maternal and newborn care, including prenatal and postpartum care. These programs would need to be adequately funded for evaluation, particularly with regard to effects on reduction of racial/ethnic and geographic disparities in access, quality, and outcomes of care.

BOX 7-5
Family Health and Birth Center

The Family Health and Birth Center (FHBC) in Washington, DC, is one of the only freestanding birth centers in the district. Midwives at the FHBC have been serving the city for more than 20 years and provide assistance to those who choose to give birth at their birth center and local hospitals. The FHBC serves mostly low-income, Black women and provides additional services beyond health care, such as inhouse childcare. Women utilizing the FHBC for prenatal care receive an individualized prenatal care plan in which social and medical risks are identified, and services are afforded to meet those needs. In this way, the FHBC model recognizes that not only is it meeting the medical needs of the people it serves critical to improving outcomes, but also providing for social needs, particularly for historically disadvantaged populations (Benatar et al., 2013).

Benatar and colleagues (2013) examined a 3-year period of birth certificate data to measure maternal and infant outcomes for women who gave birth with an FHBC midwife, either in the hospital or at the birthing center; women who initiated prenatal care at the FHBC but transferred care prior to birth; and those who received usual care. Characteristics of women who received prenatal care were matched with those of women who received usual care, and a logistic regression model was used to compute a propensity score; an instrumental variable analysis was also conducted.

The results from the propensity score analysis showed that women who received prenatal care at the FHBC were less likely to have a cesarean section, an instrumental birth, and a preterm birth and were more likely to have a vaginal birth after cesarean section compared with those who received usual care. The rates of low birthweight and a 5-minute Apgar score of less than 7 were not significantly different between women receiving FHBC care and usual care. However, those who received FHBC care were significantly more likely to have an infant with an average birthweight (3,245 grams vs. 3,166 grams) compared with the usual care group. The instrumental variable analysis showed results similar to those of the propensity score model.

The researchers also performed an analysis on a subgroup of Black women using the same methods described above. Black women who received FHBC care were less likely to have a cesarean section, an instrumental birth, or a preterm birth and were more likely to have a vaginal birth after cesarean compared with Black women who received usual care. There were no statistically significant differences in low birthweight and 5-minute Apgar score of less than 7 between the two subgroups. Women who received FHBC care had infants with a higher average birthweight compared with those in usual care (3,198 grams vs. 3,130 grams).

Maternity Care Workforce Pipeline

The evidence reviewed in Chapter 4 documents forms of disrespect and abuse in maternity care, including blatant and intentional acts of racism and discrimination. In addition, quality of care may be affected through implicit bias or poor cross-cultural communication. To address racial/ethnic inequities in quality of care, attention is needed to ensure that the workforce resembles the ethnic composition of the population of childbearing women, as well as its linguistic, geographic, and socioeconomic diversity. Such efforts are important to providing culturally concordant care, fostering trust in providers, and achieving optimal birth outcomes. To strengthen the diversity of the workforce, investments are needed to enable and support prospective maternity care providers from historically underrepresented groups to enroll in qualified education programs. Some additional strategies for achieving workforce diversity include

- creating pipeline recruitment programs beginning in high school and establishing professional and career pathways through such ancillary roles as community health workers;
- casting a wider net for recruitment and reducing both barriers to application and biases in selection criteria;
- increasing opportunities for mentoring and peer support;
- fostering inclusive professional organization practices;
- requiring training in implicit bias for faculty and students; and
- providing preferential selection for applicants with the potential to address unmet population needs (Avery et al., 2018; Institute of Medicine, 2004).

In addition, access to choice in birth settings is limited by the availability and distribution of the maternity care workforce. As discussed in Chapter 4, Finding 4-1: *Birthing facilities and maternity care providers are unevenly distributed across the United States, leaving many women without access to prenatal, birthing, and postpartum care and choices among options near home.* While the current U.S. maternity care system relies primarily on a surgical specialty to provide front-line care, most childbearing women in the United States are largely healthy and do not need that level of care in first-line providers. The reliance on surgical specialties in the United States contrasts sharply with the situation in most other countries. The ratio of midwives to obstetricians, for example, is much higher in Australia, the Netherlands, and the United Kingdom than in Canada or the United States (see Table 7-1). Thus, in addition to greater diversity, the maternity care workforce needs to develop so that a larger portion focuses on healthy pregnancy and childbirth and optimal care for lower-risk women.

TABLE 7-1 Ratio of Obstetricians and Midwives in Australia, Canada, the Netherlands, the United Kingdom, and the United States

	Australia	Canada	Netherlands	UK	U.S.
Live births/year	305,000	376,600	163,800	754,000	3,885,500
Obstetricians	1,742	2,213	931	2,600	36,915
Midwives[a]	15,000	1,740	3,221	21,500	12,436[b]
Total providers	16,742	3,953[c]	3,752	24,100	49,351
Midwife/obstetrician ratio	8.61/1	0.79/1	3.46/1	8.27/1	0.34/1

[a]Midwives in active practice.

[b]There are three types of midwifery certification in the United States. Certified nurse midwives (n = 12,331) and certified midwives (n = 105) are certified by the American Midwifery Certification Board (American Midwifery Certification Board, 2019). Certified professional midwives are certified by the North American Registry of Midwives. Their numbers are not publicly available and are not included in the total of U.S. midwives shown.

[c]This number does not reflect general practitioners/family physicians, who were not included because of a lack of data. In 2018 there were 43,500 family practitioners in Canada (CMA, 2018). It is estimated that approximately 11 percent of family practitioners in Canada attend births and are responsible for 30 percent of all births. Family practitioners provide approximately 50 percent of prenatal care, but not all attend births (personal communication, Professor Michael Klein, University of British Columbia, July 21, 2019). It is also important to note that in Canada, as in the United States, the majority of women giving birth in a hospital will have an obstetric nurse. Thus, the number of providers for Canada appears skewed when compared with the numbers for Australia, the Netherlands, and the United Kingdom, which do not have a model of obstetric nursing and in which midwives are the primary attendant during labor and birth.

As discussed in Chapter 4, the growing shortage of obstetricians offers an opportunity to rectify this situation by focusing finite resources on growing the cadre of midwives with nationally recognized credentials, who are especially prepared to provide care to healthy lower-risk women or to higher-risk women in collaboration with physicians and can be educated more quickly and at lower cost than physicians (Fagerlund and Germano, 2009). Moreover, supporting the education of midwives yields a favorable return on investment (Bushman, 2015; Avery et al., 2018). The Strong Start study, discussed above and in Chapter 4, further demonstrates the contributions of the midwifery model of care and the value added of expanding this segment of the maternity care workforce (Hill et al., 2018).

The most significant challenges to expanding the certified nurse midwife, certified midwife, and certified professional midwife workforce are the current limited number of accredited schools or midwifery programs and the limited availability of preceptors. Currently, only 37 programs for midwifery education in the United States that are accredited by the Accreditation Commission for Midwifery Education and just 12 midwifery schools are accredited by the Midwifery Education Accreditation Council.[7] Certified nurse midwife and certified midwife education programs consistently report that obtaining sufficient preceptors is the primary barrier to educating more certified nurse midwives and certified midwives (Germano et al., 2014). To eliminate these barriers and increase the pipeline of midwives for the maternity and newborn care workforce, funds under Title 7 and Title 8 of the Public Health Service Act could be used to support midwifery students in accredited schools or programs, establish or expand such schools or programs, and support qualified preceptors for such students.

The geographic maldistribution of the maternity care workforce is also a concern, as geography is a risk factor for poor birth outcomes and limits women's access and choice. To foster optimal geographic distribution of providers by region of the country and to avoid rural and urban maternity care deserts, strategies are needed to retain and reverse the losses of maternity care services in rural areas (March of Dimes, 2018a). Specifically, HRSA could expand the National Health Service Corps (NHSC) for maternity care providers so that maternity care could be provided in areas with shortages of these professionals. NHSC awards scholarships and loan repayment to primary care providers in eligible disciplines, including physicians, nurse practitioners, physician assistants, and certified nurse midwives, who commit to providing services for at least 2 years in sites with shortages of health professionals.[8] HRSA could also expand the Maternity Provider Shortage designation to include freestanding birth centers located in shortage areas as NHSC loan repayment sites.

Efforts to retain obstetricians currently in the workforce are also needed. In 2009, obstetricians were retiring from the obstetrical portion of their practice on average at age 44 (women) or age 52 (men). Avery and colleagues (2018) suggest, as one possible strategy for retention, experimentation with collaborative practice arrangements, including flexible work schedules, to increase the relatively low professional satisfaction of obstetricians. Laborist (also referred to as obstetrician hospitalist) models may also be fruitful, and additional research to assess the benefits of laborist models in increasing professional satisfaction and improving patient outcomes is needed (Avery et al., 2018).

Interprofessional health professions education is also needed to prepare various members of the maternity care workforce to work together as one high-functioning team. As noted in Chapter 6, interdisciplinary team collaboration and communication can improve the quality of maternity care and increase favorable maternal and infant birth outcomes among childbearing

---

[7] See http://meacschools.org/member-school-directory/ and https://portal.midwife.org/education/accredited-programs?reload=timezone.

[8] See https://nhsc.hrsa.gov.

women (Guise and Segel, 2008; The Joint Commission, 2004; Cornthwaite et al., 2013; Barclay et al., 2016; Coxon et al., 2016; Healy et al., 2016). To promote greater interdisciplinary collaboration, professional associations, academic medical centers, educational programs, philanthropies, the National Institutes of Health (NIH), the CDC, and HRSA could increase opportunities for interprofessional education, collaboration, and research across all birth settings. Interprofessional education and collaboration can be fostered through shared learning and teaching that impart understanding and respect for the roles and competencies of the various team members and provide opportunities for trainees to work with and learn about the roles and expertise of other members of the care team, including community health workers, doulas, lactation personnel, childbirth educators, and diabetes educators. Supporting interprofessional research would also require substantial resources and effort in several areas (including schools of medicine, nursing, public health, and midwifery). More important, truly encouraging interdisciplinary research would require incentivizing conducting research across disciplinary silos, which is currently disincentivized.

Additional steps to promote interprofessional collaboration could be taken by professional organizations themselves. For instance, AABC, ACNM, ACOG, AWHONN, SMFM, the National Association of Certified Professional Midwives (NACPM), and other professional organizations could work together on initiatives to build trust and collaboration across professions and settings of care. Such initiatives could be undertaken during undergraduate and graduate education and continue through continuing education programs and various quality improvement efforts to increase relationship building across provider types. OB/GYN residencies could require observation of at least one birth at a home or birth center birth, and midwifery schools could incorporate experience working with OB/GYNs as well. VUMC offers one example of collaborative practice and integration of nurse midwives into the education of medical students and OB/GYN residents (see Box 7-6).

CONCLUSION 7-12: To improve access and reduce racial/ethnic disparities in quality of care and treatment, investments are needed to grow the pipeline for the maternity and newborn care workforce—including community health workers, doulas, maternity nurses, nurse practitioners and physicians' assistants, public health nurses, family medicine physicians, pediatricians, midwives, and obstetricians—with the goal of increasing its diversity, distribution, and size. Greater opportunities for interprofessional education, collaboration, and research across all birth settings are also critical to improving quality of care.

BOX 7-6
Interprofessional Education:
Vanderbilt University Medical Center

Vanderbilt University Medical Center (VUMC) is home to two nurse midwifery practices—one within Vanderbilt University School of Medicine (VUSOM) and the other within Vanderbilt University School of Nursing (VUSON)—as well as an OB/GYN residency program. The nurse midwifery practice owned by VUSON was formed more than 20 years ago and functions largely as a private practice, with the primary charge of educating nurse midwifery students (Vanderbilt University School of Nursing, 2019). Nurse midwifery students are also incorporated in the outpatient clinical environment to work with the VUSOM certified nurse midwives (CNMs). The VUSOM nurse midwifery practice was formed within the past 10 years and has a primary charge of working with medical students and OB/GYN residents (Vanderbilt University Medical Center, 2019). Both services have outpatient sites off of the main hospital campus, with all births occurring at VUMC.

At VUMC, nurse midwives are fully integrated into the education of medical students and resident training (Vanderbilt University Medical Center, 2019). For example, medical students may attend births at the midwifery practice under the supervision of CNMs, and VUSON CNMs regularly give postpartum and lactation lectures to the medical students. On the labor deck, if an attending CNM or physician of VUSOM is unavailable to attend a birth, the VUSON CNM will step in as attending.

Under this model, nurse midwives are fully integrated into the education and work of medical students and residents. Medical students are given gradually advancing responsibility from the beginning to the end of residency (Vanderbilt University Medical Center, 2019). As interns, they manage the least complex patients initially, under the direction of the nurse midwives. As they advance through residency, they become more knowledgeable and capable of caring for higher-risk and more complex patients (Vanderbilt University Medical Center, 2019).

PRIORITY AREAS FOR FUTURE RESEARCH

Despite decades of advancement in medical science and technology, much remains unknown about perinatal health. Research gaps remain at the levels of human biology, clinical epidemiology, and implementation science. The scientific challenge is to better understand the science of childbirth—from biology to policy—to improve outcomes for mothers, infants, and society as a whole.

While the literature examining outcomes by birth setting has increased since the 2013 National Academies workshop on this topic, a key priority for future research is continued efforts to understand safety, quality, and outcomes of each birth setting by type of provider and the profiles of pregnant people, such as race/ethnicity, socioeconomic status, gender identity and sexual orientation, and immigrant status, as well as risk factors. Just as it is now acknowledged that racial/ethnic disparities in birth outcomes are unacceptable and require remediation, it is likely that other dimensions of identity and social systems affect outcomes (e.g., immigrant status, sexual orientation). However, research is very limited in this area, with some suggestion that there are disparities between sexual and gender minority people and heterosexuals.

The committee also emphasizes that any policy and practice changes need to be evaluated based on whether they affect racial/ethnic inequities, in addition to overall population health. It is possible for general population policies to exacerbate disparities even if they improve overall health. This has occurred in the past when policies have reached or been taken up only by the most advantaged members of populations (i.e., leaving marginalized people at the same prepolicy level with a wider disparity) (Frohlich and Potvin, 2008; Kozhimannil et al., 2018c).

Additional future research efforts are needed in the following areas:

- Understanding the impact of home and birth center births on disparities in outcomes by race and ethnicity, as well as socioeconomic status.
- Understanding variation in outcomes by setting and by provider type, including outcomes for midwives with accredited education compared with those without such education.
- Improving the source data and data collection mechanisms for research on maternal and newborn outcomes. Outcomes need to be measured from the prenatal period through at least 1 year postpartum, and beyond when feasible. Data collection mechanisms need to be designed such that data are collected and available to be used for multiple purposes, including research and performance improvement.
- Using the best available methods, investigating practices—regardless of setting—that show promise for being both safe and effective. This includes practices that support physiologic childbearing, one-to-one labor support practices by nurses, and doula care.
- Understanding the impact of widely used intrapartum interventions on maternal and infant health in the weeks and months after birth, including on maternal behaviors, maternal anxiety and depression, maternal–infant attachment, and establishment and continuation of breastfeeding; and developing a research program to assess longer-term, potentially lifelong effects given growing knowledge of the microbiome, epigenetics, life-course health development, and hormonal physiology.

- Evaluating the impact and return on investment of community-based perinatal health worker groups providing clinical and non-clinical support across the full episode of care, and developing a systems science approach to evaluate, refine, and spread effective practices.
- Studying and developing sustainable models for culturally appropriate care that are safe, effective, and adequately resourced.
- Developing, peer reviewing, and publishing a consensus core set of outcomes for studying birth settings, aligned with the Core Outcomes in Women's and Newborns' Health Initiative.
- Developing and carrying out a biannual survey of childbearing women on childbearing experiences and maternity care, including questions specific to access to services, respectful care, utility of information, willingness to listen, patient engagement, and safety. The survey would need to oversample women of color, low socioeconomic status, and underserved health care areas.
- Through evaluation, identifying the most effective components of episode payment programs and maternity care homes that improve care and outcomes, foster wise spending, and avoid unintended consequences (e.g., stinting) to enable coalescence of support for these models.
- Assessing the return on investment of incorporating quality improvement through all levels of professional education and as a core component of professional practice.
- Multidisciplinary research on interprofessional communication and collaboration across all birth settings, as well as studies on models and best practices for transfer and integrated home-to-hospital care.

CONCLUSION

An international perspective and pockets of high-performing care in the United States suggest many opportunities for improving care, experiences, outcomes, and patterns of expenditure in the nation's maternity care system. Potential improvements include reversing rising rates of maternal mortality and severe maternal morbidity, making more judicious use of cesarean birth and other consequential interventions, providing better support for needs and preferences of childbearing women and newborns, and advancing equity in childbearing across all areas. Above all, all stakeholders need to join together (1) to use quality improvement and health professions education to better align maternal and newborn care in all settings with best evidence and the needs and preferences of women and newborns; (2) to move expeditiously toward a fully integrated system across settings and care providers; and (3) to increase access to informed choice of setting, care providers, and specific care practices. Growth of the midwifery profession can help address workforce shortages and women's care preferences in a timely, cost-effective manner.

While the committee acknowledges that change will not occur instantaneously, there is an urgent need for all stakeholders—pregnant people, policy makers, payers, health care systems, professional organizations, and providers—to come together to improve maternity care in the United States and build a high-functioning, integrated, regulated, and collaborative maternity care system, a system that fosters respect for all woman, newborns, and families, regardless of their circumstances or birth or health choices.

References

Abuya, T., Warren, C.E., Miller, N., Njuki, R., Ndwiga, C., Maranga, A., Mbehero, F., Njeru, A., and Bellows, B. (2015). Exploring the prevalence of disrespect and abuse during childbirth in Kenya. *PLOS One*, *10*(4), p. e0123606.

Acevedo-Garcia, D., Soobader, M.J., and Berkman, L.F. (2007). Low birthweight among US Hispanic/Latino subgroups: the effect of maternal foreign-born status and education. *Social Science and Medicine*, *65*(12), pp. 2503–2516.

Acevedo-Garcia, D., and Stone, L.C. (2008). State variation in health insurance coverage for U.S. citizen children of immigrants. *Health Affairs*, *27*(2), pp. 434–446.

Admon, L.K., Bart, G., Kozhimannil, K.B., Richardson, C.R., Dalton, V.K., and Winkelman, T.N. (2019). Amphetamine- and opioid-affected births: incidence, outcomes, and costs, United States, 2004–2015. *American Journal of Public Health*, *109*(1), pp. 148–154.

Aetna. (2019). *Home Births*. Available: http://www.aetna.com/cpb/medical/data/300_399/0329.html.

Agency for Healthcare Research and Quality. (2011). *TeamSTEPPS©: National Implementation*. Available: http://teamstepps.ahrq.gov.

Agency for Healthcare Research and Quality. (2016). *Healthcare Cost and Utilization Project*. Available: https://hcupnet.ahrq.gov/inpatient.

Agency for Healthcare Research and Quality. (2018). *National Healthcare Quality and Disparities Report*. Available: https://www.ahrq.gov/sites/default/files/wysiwyg/research/findings/nhqrdr/2018qdr-final.pdf.

Aiken, L.H., Sermeus, W., Van den Heede, K., Sloane, D.M., Busse, R., McKee, M., Bruyneel, L., Rafferty, A.M., Griffiths, P., Moreno-Casbas, M.T., and Tishelman, C. (2012). Patient safety, satisfaction, and quality of hospital care: Cross sectional surveys of nurses and patients in 12 countries in Europe and the United States. *The BMJ*, *344*, p. e1717.

Aizer, A. (2011). Poverty, violence, and health the impact of domestic violence during pregnancy on newborn health. *Journal of Human Resources*, *46*(3), pp. 518–538.

Aizer, A., and Currie, J. (2014). The intergenerational transmission of inequality: Maternal disadvantage and health at birth. *Science*, *344*(6186), pp. 856–861.

Alaska Department of Health and Social Services. (2019). *Annual Alaskan Births (2014–2018 Average*). Available: https://alaska-dhss.maps.arcgis.com/apps/MapSeries/index.html?appid=6b6e14aa8c764e21ae96e94b25d0adde.

Alcalay, R., Ghee, A., and Scrimshaw, S. (1993). Designing prenatal care messages for low-income Mexican women. *Public Health Reports*, 108(3), p. 354.

Alderdice, F., Henderson, J., Opondo, C., Lobel, M., Quigley, M., and Redshaw, M. (2019). Psychosocial factors that mediate the association between mode of birth and maternal postnatal adjustment: Findings from a population-based survey. *BMC Women's Health*, 19(1), p. 42.

Alhusen, J.L., Ray, E., Sharps, P., and Bullock, L. (2015). Intimate partner violence during pregnancy: Maternal and neonatal outcomes. *Journal of Women's Health*, 24(1), pp. 100–106.

Alhusen, J.L., Bower, K.M., Epstein, E., and Sharps, P. (2016). Racial discrimination and adverse birth outcomes: An integrative review. *Journal of Midwifery and Women's Health*, 61(6), pp. 707–720.

Alliman, J., and Phillippi, J.C. (2016). Maternal outcomes in birth centers: An integrative review of the literature. *Journal of Midwifery and Women's Health*, 61(1), pp. 21–51.

Alliman, J., Stapleton, S.R., Wright, J., Bauer, K., Slider, K., and Jolles, D. (2019). Strong Start in birth centers: Sociodemographic characteristics, care processes, and outcomes for mothers and newborns. *Birth*, 46(2), pp. 234–243.

Alston, C., Berger, Z., Bownlee, S., Elwyn, G, Fowler, F. Jr., Hall, L.K, Montori, V.M., Moulton, B., Paget, L., Haviland-Shebel, B., Singerman, R., Walker, J., Wynia, M.K., and Henderson, D. (2014). *Shared Decision-Making Strategies for Best Care: Patient Decision Aids*. Available: https://nam.edu/perspectives-2014-shared-decision-making-strategies-for-best-care-patient-decision-aids.

American Academy of Pediatrics and American College of Obstetricians and Gynecologists. (2017). *Guidelines for Perinatal Care (8th ed.)*. American Academy of Pediatrics: Elk Grove Village, IL.

American Academy of Physicians Assistants. (2019). *Become a PA*. Available: https://www.aapa.org/career-central/become-a-pa.

American Association of Birth Centers. (2016a). *Birth Center Definitions*. Available: https://cdn.ymaws.com/www.birthcenters.org/resource/resmgr/about_aabc_-_documents/Birth_Center_Definitions-12.pdf.

American Association of Birth Centers. (2016b). *The Birth Center Experience*. Available: https://www.birthcenters.org/page/bc_experience.

American Association of Birth Centers. (2016c). *What Is a Birth Center?* Available: https://cdn.ymaws.com/www.birthcenters.org/resource/resmgr/About_AABC_-_Documents/aabc_press_kit.pdf.

American Association of Birth Centers. (2016d). *Birth Center Regulations*. Available: https://www.birthcenters.org/page/bc_regulations.

American Association of Birth Centers. (2016e). *Will My Insurance Pay for Birth Center Care?* Available: https://www.birthcenters.org/page/insurance_coverage.

American Association of Birth Centers. (2017). *Standards for Birth Centers*. Available: https://cdn.ymaws.com/www.birthcenters.org/resource/resmgr/AABC-STANDARDS-RV2017.pdf.

American Association of Birth Centers. (2019). *What Does Accreditation Mean?* Available: https://www.birthcenteraccreditation.org/find-accredited-birth-centers/accreditation-is-the-mark-of-quality.

American Association of Nurse Practitioners. (2019). *Nurse Practitioners: Improving Patient Outcomes for Opioid Use Disorder*. Available: https://storage.aanp.org/www/documents/advocacy/NPs-Improving-Patient-Outcomes-for-OUD.pdf.

American College of Nurse-Midwives. (n.d.a). *Pathways to Midwifery Education*. Available: https://portal.midwife.org/education/education-pathway?reload=timezone.

American College of Nurse-Midwives. (n.d.b). *Midwives and Medicare after Health Care Reform*. Available: http://www.midwife.org/Midwives-and-Medicare-after-Health-Care-Reform.

American College of Nurse-Midwives. (n.d.c). *ACME Accredited Programs*. Available: https://portal.midwife.org/education/accredited-programs?reload=timezone.

American College of Nurse-Midwives. (2009). *ACOG Endorses Full Equity for CNM and CM Reimbursement under Medicare*. Available: https://www.midwife.org/acnm/files/ccLibraryFiles/Filename/000000006564/ACOG-SupportofACNM061209.pdf.

American College of Nurse-Midwives. (2011). *Definition of Midwifery and Scope of Practice of Certified Nurse-Midwives and Certified Midwives*. Available: https://www.midwife.org/acnm/files/ccLibraryFiles/Filename/000000007043/Definition-of-Midwifery-and-Scope-of-Practice-of-CNMs-and-CMs-Feb-2012.pdf.

American College of Nurse-Midwives. (2015). *ACNM Department of Advocacy and Government Affairs: Grassroots Advocacy Resources*. Available: http://www.midwife.org/acnm/files/cclibraryfiles/filename/000000005600/acnmstatefactsheets8-21-15.pdf.

American College of Nurse-Midwives. (2016). *Shared Decision Making in Midwifery Care*. Available: http://www.midwife.org/acnm/files/ACNMLibraryData/UPLOADFILENAME/000000000305/Shared-Decision-Making-in-Midwifery-Care-10-13-17.pdf.

American College of Nurse-Midwives. (2017a). *Comparison of Certified Nurse-Midwives, Certified Midwives, Certified Professional Midwives Clarifying the Distinctions Among Professional Midwifery Credentials in the U.S.* Available: https://www.midwife.org/acnm/files/ccLibraryFiles/FILENAME/000000006807/FINAL-ComparisonChart-Oct2017.pdf.

American College of Nurse Midwives. (2017b). *The American College of Nurse-Midwives Reducing Primary Cesareans Project Welcomes Three New Hospitals*. Available: https://www.midwife.org/RPC-welcomes-new-hospitals.

American College of Nurse-Midwives. (2018). *Quick Reference: Practice Environments for Certified Nurse-Midwives as of June 2018*. Available: https://campaignforaction.org/wp-content/uploads/2018/08/Quick-Reference-Practice-Environment-as-of-June-2018.jpg.

American College of Nurse-Midwives. (2019). *Essential Facts about Midwives*. Available: http://www.midwife.org/acnm/files/cclibraryfiles/filename/000000007486/EssentialFactsAboutMidwives-UPDATED.pdf.

American College of Obstetricians and Gynecologists. (n.d.). *How ACOG is Combating Maternal Mortality*. Available: https://www.acog.org/About-ACOG/News-Room/ACOG-on-the-Record/Eliminate-Preventable-Maternal-Mortality/How-ACOG-is-Combating-Maternal-Mortality?IsMobileSet=false.

American College of Obstetricians and Gynecologists. (2012). *Intimate Partner Violence*. ACOG Committee Opinion, 518. Available: https://www.acog.org/Clinical-Guidance-and-Publications/Committee-Opinions/Committee-on-Health-Care-for-Underserved-Women/Intimate-Partner-Violence.

American College of Obstetricians and Gynecologists. (2014). *Health Disparities in Rural Women*. ACOG Committee Opinion, 586. (Replaces Committee Opinion, 429, March 2009). Available: https://www.acog.org/Clinical-Guidance-and-Publications/Committee-Opinions/Committee-on-Health-Care-for-Underserved-Women/Health-Disparities-in-Rural-Women.

American College of Obstetricians and Gynecologists. (2016a). *Refusal of Medically Recommended Treatment During Pregnancy*. ACOG Committee Opinion, 664. Available: https://www.acog.org/Clinical-Guidance-and-Publications/Committee-Opinions/Committee-on-Ethics/Refusal-of-Medically-Recommended-Treatment-During-Pregnancy.

American College of Obstetricians and Gynecologists. (2016b). *ACOG Statement on the U.S. MERA Bridge Certificate.* Available: https://www.acog.org/About-ACOG/News-Room/Statements/2016/ACOG-Statement-on-the-US-MERA-Bridge-Certificate.

American College of Obstetricians and Gynecologists. (2017a). *Emergent Therapy for Acute-Onset, Severe Hypertension During Pregnancy and the Postpartum Period.* ACOG Committee Opinion, 692. *Obstetrics and Gynecology, 129*(4), pp. e90–e95.

American College of Obstetricians and Gynecologists. (2017b). Opioid use and opioid use disorder in pregnancy. *ACOG Committee Opinion, 711.* Available: https://www.acog.org/-/media/Committee-Opinions/Committee-on-Obstetric-Practice/co711.pdf?dmc=1.

American College of Obstetricians and Gynecologists. (2017c). *CPM Licensure Legislation: Education Standards.* Available: https://www.acog.org/-/media/Departments/State-Legislative-Activities/2017CPMLicensureLaws-EducationStandards.pdf.

American College of Obstetricians and Gynecologists. (2018a). *Presidential Task Force on Redefining the Postpartum Visit.* ACOG Committee Opinion, 736. (Replaces Committee Opinion, 666, June 2016). Available: https://www.acog.org/Clinical-Guidance-and-Publications/Committee-Opinions/Committee-on-Obstetric-Practice/Optimizing-Postpartum-Care.

American College of Obstetricians and Gynecologists. (2018b). *AIM Program Awarded Millions to Expand Efforts to Reduce Maternal Mortality and Morbidity.* Available: https://www.acog.org/About-ACOG/News-Room/News-Releases/2018/AIM-Program-Maternal-Mortality-and-Morbidity?IsMobileSet=false.

American College of Obstetricians and Gynecologists. (2018c). Gestational diabetes mellitus: ACOG practice bulletin, 190. *Obstetrics and Gynecology, 131*(2), pp. e49–e64.

American College of Obstetrics and Gynecology. (2018d). *Mode of Term Singleton Breech Delivery.* ACOG Committee Opinion, 745. (Replaces Committee Opinion, 340, July 2006). Available: https://www.acog.org/Clinical-Guidance-and-Publications/Committee-Opinions/Committee-on-Obstetric-Practice/Mode-of-Term-Singleton-Breech-Delivery?IsMobileSet=false.

American College of Obstetrics and Gynecology. (2018e). Gestational hypertension and preeclampsia: ACOG practice bulletin, 202. *Obstetrics and Gynecology, 133*(1), pp. e1–e25.

American College of Obstetricians and Gynecologists. (2019a). *Obstetric Care Consensus: Safe prevention of the primary cesarean delivery, reaffirmed 2019.* Available: https://www.acog.org/Clinical-Guidance-and-Publications/Obstetric-Care-Consensus-Series/Safe-Prevention-of-the-Primary-Cesarean-Delivery.

American College of Obstetricians and Gynecologists. (2019b). *Levels of Maternal Care.* Available: https://www.acog.org/Clinical-Guidance-and-Publications/Obstetric-Care-Consensus-Series/Levels-of-Maternal-Care?IsMobileSet=false.

American College of Obstetricians and Gynecologists. (2019c). *American College of Obstetricians and Gynecologists and Society for Maternal-Fetal Medicine Release Updated Guidance to Help Hospitals Provide Risk Appropriate Maternal Care.* Available: https://www.acog.org/About-ACOG/News-Room/News-Releases/2019/ACOG-and-SMFM-Release-Updated-Guidance-to-Help-Hospitals-Provide-Risk-Appropriate-Maternal-Care?IsMobileSet=false.

American College of Obstetricians and Gynecologists. (2019d). *Emergent Therapy for Acute- Onset, Severe Hypertension During Pregnancy and the Postpartum Period.* ACOG Committee Opinion, 767. (Replaces Committee Opinion, 692, September 2017). Available: https://www.acog.org/Clinical-Guidance-and-Publications/Committee-Opinions/Committee-on-Obstetric-Practice/Emergent-Therapy-for-Acute-Onset-Severe-Hypertension-During-Pregnancy-and-the-Postpartum-Period.

American College of Obstetricians and Gynecologists. (2019d). Emergent therapy for acute-onset, severe hypertension during pregnancy and the postpartum period: ACOG committee opinion, 767. *Obstetrics and Gynecology, 133*(2), pp. e174–80.

American College of Obstetricians and Gynecologists. (2019e). Vaginal birth after cesarean delivery: ACOG practice bulletin, 205. *Obstetrics and Gynecology, 133*(2), pp. e110–e127.

American College of Obstetricians and Gynecologists. (2019f). *Approaches to Limit Intervention During Labor and Birth: ACOG Committee Opinion, 766.* Available: https://www.acog. org/-/media/Committee-Opinions/Committee-on-Obstetric-Practice/co766.pdf?dmc= 1&ts=20190204T2356061672.

American College of Obstetricians and Gynecologists and Society for Maternal-Fetal Medicine. (2014). *Safe Prevention of the Primary Cesarean Delivery: Obstetric care consensus 1.* Available: https://www.acog.org/-/media/Obstetric-Care-Consensus-Series/oc001.pdf.

American Diabetes Association. (2019). Management of diabetes in pregnancy: Standards of medical care in diabetes—2019. *Diabetes Care, 42*(1), pp. S165–S172.

American Medical Association. (2017). *State law chart: Nurse practitioner prescriptive authority.* Available: https://www.ama-assn.org/media/14406/download.

American Public Health Association. (1982). *Guidelines for Licensing and Regulating Birth Centers.* Available: https://www.apha.org/policies-and-advocacy/public-health-policy-statements/policy-database/2014/07/10/13/29/guidelines-for-licensing-and-regulating-birth-centers.

American Public Health Association. (2019). *Community Health Workers.* Available: https:// www.apha.org/apha-communities/member-sections/community-health-workers.

Ananth, C.V. (2005). Perinatal epidemiologic research with vital statistics data: Validity is the essential quality. *American Journal of Obstetrics and Gynecology, 193*(1), pp. 5–6.

Anderson, L.M., Scrimshaw, S.C., Fullilove, M.T., and Fielding, J.E. (2003). The Community Guide's model for linking the social environment to health. *American Journal of Preventive Medicine, 24*(3), 12–20.

Andreyeva, T., Puhl, R.M., and Brownell, K.D. (2008). Changes in perceived weight discrimination among Americans, 1995–1996 through 2004–2006. *Obesity, 16*(5), pp. 1129–1134.

Angelini, D., and Howard, E. (2014). Obstetric triage: A systematic review of the past fifteen years 1998–2013. *The American Journal of Maternal/Child Nursing, 39*(5), pp. 284–297.

Arabin, B., and Baschat, A.A. (2017). Pregnancy: An underutilized window of opportunity to improve long-term maternal and infant health: An appeal for continuous family care and interdisciplinary communication. *Frontiers in Pediatrics, 5*, p. 69.

Artiga, S., and Diaz, M. (2019). *Health Coverage and Care of Undocumented Immigrants.* Available: https://www.kff.org/disparities-policy/issue-brief/health-coverage-and-care-of-undocumented-immigrants.

Association of State and Territorial Health Officials. (2015). *From the Bottom to the Top: How Alaska Became a Leader in Perinatal Regionalization.* Available: http://www. astho.org/Programs/Maternal-and-Child-Health/Documents/From-the-Bottom-to-the-Top--How-Alaska-Became-a-Leader-in-Perinatal-Regionalization.

Association of State and Territorial Health Officials. (2018). *State Policy Approaches to Incorporating Doula Services into Maternal Care.* Available: https://www.astho.org/ StatePublicHealth/State-Policy-Approaches-to-Incorporating-Doula-Services-into-Maternal-Care/08-09-18.

Association of Women's Health, Obstetric and Neonatal Nurses. (2010). Guidelines for professional registered nurse staffing for perinatal units. *Journal of Obstetric, Gynecologic & Neonatal Nursing, 40*(1), pp. 131–134. Available: https://doi.org/10.1111/j.1552-6909.2010.01214.x

Association of Women's Health, Obstetric and Neonatal Nurses. (2015). *Maternal Fetal Triage Index*. Available: https://www.awhonn.org/page/MFTI.

Association of Women's Health, Obstetric and Neonatal Nurses. (2018). Continuous labor support for every woman. *Journal of Obstetric, Gynecologic, and Neonatal Nursing*, 47(1), pp. 73–74.

Austin, A., Langer, A., Salam, R.A., Lassi, Z.S., Das, J.K., and Bhutta, Z.A. (2014). Approaches to improve the quality of maternal and newborn health care: An overview of the evidence. *Reproductive Health*, 11(2), p. S1.

Australian Institute of Health and Welfare. (2019). *Australia's Mothers and Babies*. Available: https://www.aihw.gov.au/getmedia/2a0c22a2-ba27-4ba0-ad47-ebbe51854cd6/aihw-per-100-in-brief.pdf.aspx?inline=true.

Avery, M.D., Bell, A.D., Bingham, D., Corry, M.P., Delbanco, S., Gullo, S.L., Ivory, C.H., Jennings, J.C., Kennedy, H.P., Kozhimannil, K.B., Leeman, L., Lothian, J.A., Miller, H.D., Ogburn, T., Romano, A., Sakala, C., and Shah, N.T. (2018). *Blueprint for Advancing High-Value Maternity Care Through Physiologic Childbearing*. Washington, DC: National Partnership for Women and Families. Available: http://www.nationalpartnership.org/blueprint.

Bachilova, S., Czuzoj-Shulman, N., and Abenhaim, H.A. (2018). Effect of maternal and pregnancy risk factors on early neonatal death in planned home births delivering at home. *Journal of Obstetrics and Gynaecology Canada*, 40(5), pp. 540–546.

Bailey, J. (2017). Birth outcomes for women using freestanding birth centers in Aukland, New Zealand. *Birth*, 44(3), pp. 246–251.

Ball, C., Hauck, Y., Kuliukas, L., Lewis, L., and Doherty, D. (2016). Under scrutiny: Midwives' experience of intrapartum transfer from home to hospital within the context of a planned homebirth in Western Australia. *Sexual and Reproductive Healthcare*, 8, pp. 88–93.

Ball, J.E., Bruyneel, L., Aiken, L.H., Sermeus, W., Sloane, D.M., Rafferty, A.M., Lindqvist, R., Tishelman, C., Griffiths, P. and RN4Cast Consortium. (2018). Post-operative mortality, missed care and nurse staffing in nine countries: A cross-sectional study. *International Journal of Nursing Studies*, 78, pp. 10–15.

Barclay, L., Kornelsen, J., Longman, J., Robin, S., Kruske, S., Kildea, S., Pilcher, J., Martin, T., Grzybowski, S., Donoghue, D. and Rolfe, M. (2016). Reconceptualising risk: Perceptions of risk in rural and remote maternity service planning. *Midwifery*, 38, pp. 63–70.

Bateman, B.T., Shaw, K.M., Kuklina, E.V., Callaghan, W.M., Seely, E.W., and Hernández-Díaz, S. (2012). Hypertension in women of reproductive age in the United States: NHANES 1999–2008. *PLOS One*, 7(4), p. e36171

Bauer, K., Bushman, J.S., and Lawlor, M. (n.d). *Letter to CMS on Birth Center Regulation*. Available: https://www.midwife.org/acnm/files/ccLibraryFiles/Filename/000000005105/AABC-ACNM-NACPM-LettertoCMSonBirthCenterRegulation.pdf.

Becker, M., Weinberger, T., Chandy, A., and Schmukler, S. (2016). Depression during pregnancy and postpartum. *Current Psychiatry Reports*, 18(3), p. 32.

Bell, A.F., and Andersson, E. (2016). The birth experience and women's postnatal depression: A systematic review. *Midwifery*, 39, pp. 112–123.

Bell, A.D., Joy, S., Gullo, S., Higgins, R., and Stevenson, E. (2017). Implementing a systematic approach to reduce cesarean birth rates in nulliparous women. *Obstetrics and Gynecology*, 130(5), pp. 1082–1089.

Benatar, S., Garrett, A.B., Howell, E., and Palmer, A. (2013). Midwifery care at a freestanding birth center: A safe and effective alternative to conventional maternity care. *Health Services Research*, 48(5), pp. 1750–1768.

Benedetti, T.J., Baldwin, L.M., Skillman, S.M., Andrilla, C.H.A., Bowditch, E., Carr, K.C., and Myers, S.J. (2006). Professional liability issues and practice patterns of obstetric providers in Washington State. *Obstetrics and Gynecology*, 107(6), pp. 1238–1246.

Bennett, H.A., Einarson, A., Taddio, A., Koren, G., and Einarson, T.R. (2004). Prevalence of depression during pregnancy: Systematic review. *Obstetrics and Gynecology*, *103*(4), pp. 698–709.

Berhan, Y., and Haileamlak, A. (2016). The risks of planned vaginal breech delivery versus planned caesarean section for term breech birth: A meta-analysis including observational studies. *British Journal of Obstetrics and Gynaecology*, *123*(1), pp. 49–57.

Berwick, D.M. (2002). A user's manual for the IOM's 'Quality Chasm' report. *Health Affairs*, *21*(3), pp. 80–90.

Birthplace in England Collaborative Group. (2011). Perinatal and maternal outcomes by planned place of birth for healthy women with low risk pregnancies: The Birthplace in England national prospective cohort study. *The BMJ*, *343*, p. d7400.

Blix, E., Huitfeldt, A. S., Øian, P., Straume, B., and Kumle, M. (2012). Outcomes of planned home births and planned hospital births in low-risk women in Norway between 1990 and 2007: A retrospective cohort study. *Sexual and Reproductive Healthcare*, *3*(4), pp. 147–153.

Blix, E., Kumle, M., Kjærgaard, H., Øian, P., and Lindgren, H.E. (2014). Transfer to hospital in planned home births: A systematic review. *BMC Pregnancy and Childbirth*, *14*(1), p. 179.

Blix, E., Kumle, M.H., Ingversen, K., Huitfeldt, A.S., Hegaard, H.K., Ólafsdóttir, Ó.Á., Øian, P., and Lindgren, H. (2016). Transfers to hospital in planned home birth in four Nordic countries: A prospective cohort study. *Acta Obstetricia et Gynecologica Scandinavica*, *95*(4), pp. 420–428.

Bloom, K.C., Bednarzyk, M.S., Devitt, D.L., Renault, R.A., Teaman, V., and Van Loock, D.M. (2004). Barriers to prenatal care for homeless pregnant women. *Journal of Obstetric, Gynecologic, and Neonatal Nursing*, *33*(4), pp. 428–435.

Blumenshine, P., Egerter, S., Barclay, C.J., Cubbin, C., and Braveman, P. (2010). Socio-economic disparities in adverse birth outcomes: A systematic review. *American Journal of Preventive Medicine*, *39*(3), pp. 263–272.

Bohren, M.A., Hofmeyr, G.J., Sakala, C., Fukuzawa, R.K., and Cuthbert, A. (2017). Continuous support for women during childbirth. *Cochrane Database of Systematic Reviews*, 7.

Bohren, M.A., Berger, B.O., Munthe-Kaas, H., and Tunçalp, Ö. (2019). Perceptions and experiences of labour companionship: A qualitative evidence synthesis. *Cochrane Database of Systematic Reviews*, 3.

Bolten, N., De Jonge, A., Zwagerman, E., Zwagerman, P., Klomp, T., Zwart, J.J., and Geerts, C.C. (2016). Effect of planned place of birth on obstetric interventions and maternal outcomes among low-risk women: A cohort study in the Netherlands. *BMC Pregnancy and Childbirth*, *16*(1), p. 329.

Bossano, C.M., Townsend, K.M., Walton, A.C., Blomquist, J.L., and Handa, V.L. (2017). The maternal childbirth experience more than a decade after delivery. *American Journal of Obstetrics and Gynecology*, *217*(3), p. 342e1.

Boucher, D., Bennett, C., McFarlin, B., and Freeze, R. (2009). Staying home to give birth: Why women in the United States choose home birth. *Journal of Midwifery and Women's Health*, *54*(2), pp. 119–126.

Bovbjerg, M.L., Cheyney, M., Brown, J., Cox, K.J., and Leeman, L. (2017). Perspectives on risk: Assessment of risk profiles and outcomes among women planning community birth in the United States. *Birth*, *44*(3), pp. 209–221.

Boyko, E. (2013). Observational research opportunities and limitations. *Journal of Diabetes and Its Complications*, *27*(6), pp. 642–648.

Braveman, P., and Gottlieb, L. (2014). The social determinants of health: It's time to consider the causes of the causes. *Public Health Reports*, *129*(1, suppl2), pp. 19–31.

Braveman, P.A., Cubbin, C., Egerter, S., Chideya, S., Marchi, K.S., Metzler, M., and Posner, S. (2005). Socioeconomic status in health research: One size does not fit all. *Journal of the American Medical Association, 294*(22), pp. 2879–2888.

Braveman, P., Marchi, K., Egerter, S., Kim, S., Metzler, M., Stancil, T., and Libet., M. (2010). Poverty, near-poverty, and hardship around the time of pregnancy. *Maternal and Child Health Journal, 14*(1), pp. 20–35.

Braveman, P.A., Egerter, S.A., Woolf, S.H., and Marks, J.S. (2011). When do we know enough to recommend action on the social determinants of health? *American Journal of Preventive Medicine, 40*(1), pp. S5–S66.

Brody, D.J., Pratt, L.A., and Hughes, J.P. (2018). *Prevalence of Depression among Adults Aged 20 and Over: United States, 2013–2016.* Available: https://www.cdc.gov/nchs/products/databriefs/db303.htm#ref1.

Brown, J.B., Beckhoff, C., Bickford, J., Stewart, M., Freeman, T.R., and Kasperski, M.J. (2009). Women and their partners' perceptions of the key roles of the labor and delivery nurse. *Clinical Nursing Research, 18*(4), pp. 323–335.

Brownridge, D.A., Taillieu, T.L., Tyler, K.A., Tiwari, A., Chan, K.L., and Santos, S.C. (2011). Pregnancy and intimate partner violence: Risk factors, severity, and health effects. *Violence Against Women, 17*(7), pp. 858–881.

Buckley, S.J. (2015). *Hormonal Physiology of Childbearing: Evidence and Implications for Women, Babies and Maternity Care.* Washington, DC: National Partnership for Women & Families. Available: http://www.nationalpartnership.org/our-work/resources/health-care/maternity/hormonal-physiology-of-childbearing.pdf.

Buerhaus, P. (2018). Nurse practitioners: A solution to America's primary care crisis. In *American Enterprise Institute.* Available: https://www.aei.org/research-products/report/nurse-practitioners-a-solution-to-americas-primary-care-crisis.

Burcher, P., Cheyney, M.J., Li, K.N., Hushmendy, S., and Kiley, K.C. (2016). Cesarean birth regret and dissatisfaction: A qualitative approach. *Birth, 43*(4), pp. 346–352.

Bureau of Labor Statistics. (2019). *Employee Benefits in the United States–March 2019.* Available: https://www.bls.gov/news.release/pdf/ebs2.pdf.

Bushman, J.S. (2015). *The Role of Certified Nurse-Midwives and Certified Midwives in Ensuring Women's Access to Skilled Maternity Care.* Available: https://www.midwife.org/acnm/files/ccLibraryFiles/Filename/000000005794/MaternityCareWorkforce-11-18-15.pptx.

Cahill, A.G., and Macones, G.A. (2006). Vital considerations for the use of vital statistics in obstetrical research. *American Journal of Obstetrics and Gynecology, 194*(4), pp. 909–910.

Cahill, H.A. (2001). Male appropriation and medicalization of childbirth: An historical analysis. *Journal of Advanced Nursing, 33*(3), pp. 334–342.

Cai, C., Vandermeer, B., Khurana, R., Nerenberg, K., Featherstone, R., Sebastianski, M., and Davenport, M.H. (2019). The impact of occupational shift work and working hours during pregnancy on health outcomes: A systematic review and meta-analysis. *American Journal of Obstetrics and Gynecology, 221*(6), pp. 563–576.

California Health Care Foundation. (2014). *A Tale of Two Births: High-and Low-Performing Hospitals on Maternity Measures in California.* Available: https://www.chcf.org/publication/a-tale-of-two-births-high-and-low-performing-hospitals-on-maternity-measures-in-california.

California Maternal Quality Care Collaborative. (n.d.). *Early Elective Deliveries.* Available: https://www.cmqcc.org/qi-initiatives/early-elective-deliveries.

Calvin, S. (2019). *The Minnesota Birth Center and the Birth Bundle.* Presentation to the Committee. April 9, 2019. Washington, DC: National Academies of Sciences, Engineering, and Medicine.

Canadian Association of Midwives. (2019). *Midwifery-Led Births Per Province and Territory.* Available: https://canadianmidwives.org/2018/08/08/midwifery-assisted-births.

Carlson, N.S., Neal, J.L., Tilden, E.L., Smith, D.C., Breman, R.B., Lowe, N.K., Dietrich, M.S., and Phillippi, J.C. (2019). Influence of midwifery presence in United States centers on labor care and outcomes of low-risk parous women: A Consortium on Safe Labor study. *Birth*, 46(3), pp. 487–499.

Carmichael, S.L., and Snowden, J.M. (2019). The ARRIVE Trial: Interpretation from an epidemiologic perspective. *Journal of Midwifery and Women's Health*, 64(5), pp. 657–663.

Carrion, B.V., Earnshaw, V.A., Kershaw, T., Lewis, J.B., Stasko, E.C., Tobin, J.N., and Ickovics, J.R. (2015). Housing instability and birth weight among young urban mothers. *Journal of Urban Health: Bulletin of the New York Academy of Medicine*, 92(1), pp. 1–9.

Catalano, P.M., and Shankar, K. (2017). Obesity and pregnancy: Mechanisms of short-term and long-term adverse consequences for mother and child. *The BMJ*, 356, p. j1.

Catling-Paull, C., Coddington, R.L., Foureur, M.J., and Homer, C.S. (2013). Publicly funded homebirth in Australia: A review of maternal and neonatal outcomes over 6 years. *Medical Journal of Australia*, 198(11), pp. 616–620.

Caughey, A.B., and Cheyney, M. (2019). Home and birth center birth in the United States: Time for greater collaboration across models of care. *Obstetrics and Gynecology*, 133(5), pp. 1033–1050.

Cavazos-Rehg, P.A., Krauss, M.J., Spitznagel, E.L., Bommarito, K., Madden, T., Olsen, M.A., Subramaniam, H., Peipert, J.F., and Bierut, L.J. (2015). Maternal age and risk of labor and delivery complications. *Maternal and Child Health Journal*, 19(6), pp. 1202–1211.

Centers for Disease Control and Prevention. (2014). *New York State Perinatal Quality Collaborative Increases the Proportion of Babies Born Full-Term*. Available: https://www.cdc.gov/reproductivehealth/maternalinfanthealth/pdf/New-York-Success-Story_508tagged.pdf.

Centers for Disease Control and Prevention. (2016). *Developing and Sustaining Perinatal Quality Collaboratives: A Resource Guide for States*. Available: https://www.cdc.gov/reproductivehealth/maternalinfanthealth/pdf/Best-Practices-for-Developing-and-Sustaining-Perinatal-Quality-Collaboratives_tagged508.pdf.

Centers for Disease Control and Prevention. (2017a). *Severe Maternal Morbidity in the United States*. Available: https://www.cdc.gov/reproductivehealth/maternalinfanthealth/severematernalmorbidity.html.

Centers for Disease Control and Prevention. (2017b). *User Guide to the 2017 Natality Public-Use File*. Available: http://ftp.cdc.gov/pub/Health_Statistics/NCHS/Dataset_Documentation/DVS/natality/UserGuide2017.pdf.

Centers for Disease Control and Prevention. (2017c). *Illinois Perinatal Quality Collaborative Improves the Accuracy of Birth Certificate Data*. Available: https://www.cdc.gov/reproductivehealth/maternalinfanthealth/pdf/Illinois-success-story_508tagged.pdf.

Centers for Disease Control and Prevention. (2017d). *North Carolina PQC Leads a National Project to Reduce Infections in the NICU*. Available: https://www.cdc.gov/reproductivehealth/maternalinfanthealth/pdf/North-Carolina-PQC_TAGGED508.pdf.

Centers for Disease Control and Prevention. (2018). *Type 1 or Type 2 Diabetes and Pregnancy*. Available: https://www.cdc.gov/pregnancy/diabetes-types.html.

Centers for Disease Control and Prevention. (2019a). *Pregnancy Mortality Surveillance System*. Available: https://www.cdc.gov/reproductivehealth/maternalinfanthealth/pregnancy-mortality-surveillance-system.htm.

Centers for Disease Control and Prevention. (2019b). *Pregnancy-Related Deaths*. Available: https://www.cdc.gov/reproductivehealth/maternalinfanthealth/pregnancy-relatedmortality.htm.

Centers for Disease Control and Prevention. (2019c). *Data on Selected Pregnancy Complications in the United States*. Available: https://www.cdc.gov/reproductivehealth/maternalinfanthealth/pregnancy-complications-data.htm#hyper.

Centers for Disease Control and Prevention. (2019d). *Fetal Alcohol Spectrum Disorders (FASDs): Data and Statistics*. Available: https://www.cdc.gov/ncbddd/fasd/data.html.

Centers for Disease Control and Prevention. (2019e). *Perinatal Quality Collaboratives*. Available: https://www.cdc.gov/reproductivehealth/maternalinfanthealth/pqc.htm.

Centers for Disease Control and Prevention. (2019f). *State Perinatal Quality Collaboratives*. Available: https://www.cdc.gov/reproductivehealth/maternalinfanthealth/pqc-states.html.

Centers for Disease Control and Prevention. (2019g). *Racial/Ethnic Disparities in Pregnancy-Related Deaths—United States, 2007-2016*. Available: https://www.cdc.gov/reproductivehealth/maternal-mortality/disparities-pregnancy-related-deaths/infographic.html.

Center for Healthcare Quality and Payment Reform. (2018). *An Alternative Payment Model for Maternity Care*. Available: http://www.chqpr.org/downloads/MaternityCare_APM.pdf.

Centers for Medicare & Medicaid Services. (n.d.). *Newborns' and Mothers' Health Protection Act (NMHPA)*. Available: https://www.cms.gov/CCIIO/Programs-and-Initiatives/Other-Insurance-Protections/nmhpa_factsheet.html.

Centers for Medicare & Medicaid Services. (2011). *Recent Developments in Medicaid and CHIP Policy*. Available: https://downloads.cms.gov/cmsgov/archived-downloads/CMCSBulletins/downloads/CMCS-Info-Bulletin-March-2011-Final.pdf.

Centers for Medicare & Medicaid Services. (2012). *Emergency Medical Treatment and Labor Act* (EMTLA). Available: https://www.cms.gov/regulations-and-guidance/legislation/emtala.

Centers for Medicare & Medicaid Services. (2013). *Improving Maternal and Infant Health Outcomes: Crosswalk Between Current and Planned CMCS Activities and Expert Panel Identified Strategies*. Available: https://www.medicaid.gov/Medicaid-CHIP-Program-Information/By-Topics/Quality-of-Care/Downloads/Crosswalk-of-Activities.pdf.

Centers for Medicare & Medicaid Services. (2016). *Beneficiary Engagement and Incentives Models: Direct Decision Support Model*. Available: https://www.cms.gov/newsroom/fact-sheets/beneficiary-engagement-and-incentives-models-direct-decision-support-model#_ftnref10 [May 2019].

Centers for Medicare & Medicaid Services. (2019). *Improving Access to Maternal Health Care in Rural Communities*. Available: https://www.cms.gov/About-CMS/Agency-Information/OMH/equity-initiatives/rural-health/09032019-Maternal-Health-Care-in-Rural-Communities.pdf.

Chamberlain, M., and Barclay, K. (2000). Psychosocial costs of transferring indigenous women from their community for birth. *Midwifery*, 16(2), pp. 116–122.

Chantry, C.J., Eglash, A., and Labbok, M. (2015). *ABM Position on Breastfeeding—Revised 2015*. Available: https://www.bfmed.org/assets/DOCUMENTS/abm-position-breastfeeding.pdf.

Chapple, W., Gilliland, A., Li, D., Shier, E., and Wright, E. (2013). An economic model of the benefits of professional doula labor support in Wisconsin births. *Wisconsin Medical Journal*, 112(2), pp. 58–64.

Charles, C., Gafni, A., and Whelan, T. (1997). Shared decision-making in the medical encounter: What does it mean? (Or it takes at least two to tango). *Social Science and Medicine*, 44(5), pp. 681–692.

Charles, C., Gafni, A., and Whelan, T. (1999). Decision-making in the physician–patient encounter: Revisiting the shared treatment decision-making model. *Social Science and Medicine*, 49(5), pp. 651–661.

Chawanpaiboon, S., Vogel, J.P., Moller, A.B., Lumbiganon, P., Petzold, M., Hogan, D., Landoulsi, S., Jampathong, N., Kongwattanakul, K., Laopaiboon, M., Lewis, C., Rattanakanokchai, S., Teng, D.N., Thinkhamrop, J., Watananirun, K., Zhang, J., Zhou, W., and Gülmezoglu, A.M. (2019). Global, regional, and national estimates of levels of preterm birth in 2014: A systematic review and modelling analysis. *The Lancet Global Health*, 7(1), pp. e37–e46.

Cheng, Y.W., Snowden, J.M., King, T.I., and Caughey, A.B. (2013). Selected perinatal outcomes associated with planned home births in the United States. *American Journal of Obstetrics and Gynecology*, 209(4), pp. 325.e1–e8.

Cheshire Medical Center. (2019). *Departments and Services: Midwifery.* Available: https://www.cheshire-med.com/pregnancy_birth/midwifery.html.

Cheyney, M. (2010). *Born at Home: The Biological, Cultural and Political Dimensions of Maternity Care in the United States.* Belmont, CA: Wadsworth, Cengage Learning.

Cheyney, M., Bovbjerg, M., Everson, C., Gordon, W., Hannibal, D., and Vedam, S. (2014a). Outcomes of care for 16,924 planned home births in the United States: The Midwives Alliance of North America Statistics Project, 2004 to 2009. *Journal of Midwifery and Women's Health*, 59(1), pp. 17–27.

Cheyney, M., Bovbjerg, M., Everson, C., Gordon, W., Hannibal, D., and Vedam, S. (2014b). Development and validation of a national data registry for midwife-led births: The Midwives Alliance of North America Statistics project 2.0 dataset. *Journal of Midwifery and Women's Health*, 59(1), pp. 8–16.

Cheyney, M., Everson, C., and Burcher, P. (2014c). Homebirth transfers in the United States: Narratives of risk, fear, and mutual accommodation. *Qualitative Health Research*, 24(4), pp. 443–456.

Cheyney, M., Olsen, C., Bovbjerg, M., Everson, C., Darragh, I., and Potter, B. (2015). Practitioner and practice characteristics of certified professional midwives in the United States: Results of the 2011 North American Registry of Midwives Survey. *Journal of Midwifery and Women's Health*, 60(5), pp. 534–545.

Cheyney, M.M., Bovbjerg, M.L., Leeman, L., and Vedam, S. (2019). Community versus out-of-hospital birth: What's in a name? *Journal of Midwifery and Women's Health*, 64(1).

Childbirth Connection. (2013). *How Do Childbearing Experiences Differ across Racial and Ethnic Groups in the United States? A Listening to Mothers III Data Brief.* Available: https://www.nationalpartnership.org/our-work/health/maternity.

Chisholm, C.A., Bullock, L., and Ferguson, J., 2nd. (2017). Intimate partner violence and pregnancy: Epidemiology and impact. *American Journal of Obstetrics and Gynecology*, 217(2), pp. 141–144.

Christensen, L.F., and Overgaard, C. (2017). Are freestanding midwifery units a safe alternative to obstetric units for low-risk, primiparous childbirth? An analysis of effect differences by parity in a matched cohort study. *BMC Pregnancy and Childbirth*, 17(1), p. 14.

Christiaens, W., and Bracke, P. (2009). Place of birth and satisfaction with childbirth in Belgium and the Netherlands. *Midwifery*, 25(2), pp. e11–e19.

Citizens for Midwifery. (2008). *The Midwives Model of Care.* Available: http://cfmidwifery.org/mmoc/define.aspx.

Collins, J.W., and Hammond, N.A. (1996). Relation of maternal race to the risk of preterm, non-low birth weight infants: A population study. *American Journal of Epidemiology*, 143(4), pp. 333–337.

Collins, J.W., Wu, S.Y., and David, R.J. (2002). Differing intergenerational birth weights among the descendants of U.S.-born and foreign-born Whites and African Americans in Illinois. *American Journal of Epidemiology*, 155(3), pp. 210–216.

Collins, N.L., Dunkel-Schetter, C., Lobel, M., and Scrimshaw, S.C. (1993). Social support in pregnancy: Psychosocial correlates of birth outcomes and postpartum depression. *Journal of Personality and Social Psychology, 65*(6), p. 1243.

Comeau, A., Hutton, E.K., Simioni, J., Anvari, E., Bowen, M., Kruegar, S., and Darling, E.K. (2018). Home birth integration into the health care systems of eleven international jurisdictions. *Birth, 45*(3), pp. 311–321.

Commission for the Accreditation of Birth Centers. (2019). *Find CABC Accredited Alongside Maternity Centers.* Available: https://www.birthcenteraccreditation.org/find-cabc-accredited-alongside-maternity-centers.

Commonwealth Fund. (2018). *A Community-Based Approach to Reducing Disparities in Maternal Health Outcomes.* Available: https://www.commonwealthfund.org/publications/newsletter-article/2018/sep/community-based-approach-reducing-disparities-maternal.

Cooper, L.A., Roter, D.L., Johnson, R.L., Ford, D.E., Steinwachs, D.M., and Powe, N.R. (2003). Patient-centered communication, ratings of care, and concordance of patient and physician race. *Annals of Internal Medicine, 139*(11), pp. 907–915.

Corbett, C.A., and Callister, L.C. (2000). Nursing support during labor. *Clinical Nursing Research, 9*(1), pp. 70–83.

Cornthwaite, K., Edwards, S., and Siassakos, D. (2013). Reducing risk in maternity by optimising teamwork and leadership: An evidence-based approach to save mothers and babies. *Best Practice and Research: Clinical Obstetrics and Gynaecology, 27*(4), pp. 571–581.

Council on Patient Safety in Women's Health Care. (2019). *Patient Safety Bundles.* Available: https://safehealthcareforeverywoman.org/patient-safety-bundles.

Cox, K.J., Bovbjerg, M.L., Cheyney, M., and Leeman, L.M. (2015). Planned home vaginal birth after cesarean in the United States, 2004–2009: Outcomes, maternity care practices, and implications for shared decision making. *Birth, 42*(4), pp. 299–308.

Coxon, K., Homer, C., Bisits, A., Sandall, J., and Bick, D. (2016). Reconceptualising risk in childbirth. *Midwifery, 38*, pp. 1–5.

Cuellar, A., Simmons, A., and Finegold, K. (2012). *The Affordable Care Act and Women.* Available: https://aspe.hhs.gov/report/affordable-care-act-and-women.

Dahlen, H.G., Kennedy, H.P., Anderson, C.M., Bell, A.F., Clark, A., Foureur, M., Ohm, J.E., Shearman, A.M., Taylor, J.Y., Wright, M.L., and Downe, S. (2013). The EPIIC hypothesis: Intrapartum effects on the neonatal epigenome and consequent health outcomes. *Medical Hypotheses, 80*(5), pp. 656–662.

David, R.J., and Collins, J.W. (1997). Differing birth weight among infants of U.S.-born blacks, African-born blacks, and U.S.-born whites. *The New England Journal of Medicine, 337*(17), pp. 1209–1214.

Davis, D.A. (2018). Obstetric racism: The racial politics of pregnancy, labor, and birthing. *Medical Anthropology*, pp. 1–14.

Davis, D., Baddock, S., Pairman, S., Hunter, M., Benn, C., Wilson, D., Dixon, L., and Herbison, P. (2011). Planned place of birth in New Zealand: Does it affect mode of birth and intervention rates among low-risk women? *Birth, 38*(2), pp. 111–119.

Davis, D., Baddock, S., Pairman, S., Hunter, M., Benn, C., Anderson, J., Dixon, L. and Herbison, P. (2012). Risk of severe postpartum hemorrhage in low-risk childbearing women in New Zealand: Exploring the effect of place of birth and comparing third stage management of labor. *Birth, 39*(2), pp. 98–105.

Davis-Floyd, R., and Johnson, C.B. (Eds.). (2006). *Mainstreaming Midwives: The Politics of Change.* Routledge: New York, NY.

Davis-Floyd, R. (2018). *Ways of Knowing About Birth: Mothers, Midwives, Medicine and Birth Activism.* Prospect Heights IL: Waveland Press.

Daw, J.R., Hatfield, L.A., Swartz, K., and Sommers, B.D. (2017). Women in the United States experience high rates of coverage 'churn' in months before and after childbirth. *Health Affairs*, 36(4), pp. 598–606.

Daysal, N.M., Trandafir, M., and Van Ewijk, R. (2015). Saving lives at birth: The impact of home births on infant outcomes. *American Economic Journal: Applied Economics*, 7(3), pp. 28–50.

de Jonge, A., van der Goes, B.Y., Ravelli, A.C., Amelink-Verburg, M.P., Mol, B.W., Nijhuis, J.G., Gravenhorst, J.B., and Buitendijk, S.E. (2009). Perinatal mortality and morbidity in a nationwide cohort of 529,688 low-risk planned home and hospital births. *British Journal of Obstetrics and Gynaecology*, 116(9), pp. 1177–1184.

de Jonge, A., Mesman, J.A., Manniën, J., Zwart, J.J., van Dillen, J., and van Roosmalen, J. (2013). Severe adverse maternal outcomes among low-risk women with planned home versus hospital births in the Netherlands: Nationwide cohort study. *The BMJ*, 346, p. f3263.

de Jonge, A., Geerts, C.C., Van Der Goes, B.Y., Mol, B.W., Buitendijk, S.E., and Nijhuis, J.G. (2015). Perinatal mortality and morbidity up to 28 days after birth among 743,070 low-risk planned home and hospital births: A cohort study based on three merged national perinatal databases. *British Journal of Obstetrics and Gynaecology*, 122(5), pp. 720–728.

de Jonge, A., Peters, L., Geerts, C.C., Van Roosmalen, J.J., Twisk, J.W., Brocklehurst, P., and Hollowell, J. (2017). Mode of birth and medical interventions among women at low risk of complications: A cross-national comparison of birth settings in England and the Netherlands. *PLOS One*, 12(7), p. e0180846.

de Sousa Soares, R., Albuquerque, A., Anjos, U.U., Vianna, R.P.T., Gomes, L.B., Freitas, W.D.M.F., Araújo, J.S.S., Sampaio, J., Palhano, D.B., de Rocco Guimarães, A. and Neto, A.J.M. (2016). Analysis on the doula's influence in childbirth care at a maternity. *International Archives of Medicine*, 9.

Declercq, E., and Stotland, N.E. (2017). Planned home birth. *UpToDate*. Available: https://www.uptodate.com/contents/planned-home-birth.

Declercq, E.R., Sakala, C., Corry, M.P., Applebaum, S. (2006). *Listening to Mothers II: Report of the Second National Survey of Women's Childbearing Experiences*. Available: https://www.nationalpartnership.org/our-work/resources/health-care/maternity/listening-to-mothers-ii-2006.pdf.

Declercq, E.R., Sakala, C., Corry, M.P., and Applebaum, S. (2007). Listening to Mothers II: Report of the Second National Survey of Women's Childbearing Experiences. *The Journal of Perinatal Education*, 16(4), p. 9.

Declercq, E.R., Sakala, C., Corry, M.P., Applebaum, S., and Herrlich, A. (2013). *Listening to Mothers III*. Available: http://www.nationalpartnership.org/our-work/resources/health-care/maternity/listening-to-mothers-iii-new-mothers-speak-out-2013.pdf.

Declercq, E., MacDorman, M., Cabral, H., and Stotland, N. (2016). Prepregnancy body mass index and infant mortality in 38 U.S. States, 2012–2013. *Obstetrics and Gynecology*, 127(2), pp. 279–287.

Deering, S., Rosen, M.A., Salas, E., and King, H.B. (2009). Building team and technical competency for obstetric emergencies: the mobile obstetric emergencies simulator (MOES) system. *Simulation in Healthcare*, 4(3), pp. 166–173.

Defense Health Agency. (2019). *Processes and Procedures for Implementation of Standardized Perinatal Training*. Washington, DC: Defense Health Agency.

Deitz, P.J., Bombard, J., Mulready-Ward, C., Gauthier, J., Sackoff, J., Brozicevic, P., Gambatese, M., Nyland-Funke, M., England, L., Harrison, L., and Farr, S. (2015). Validation of selected items on the 2003 U.S. Standard Certificate of Live Birth: New York City and Vermont. *Public Health Reports*, 130(1), pp. 60–70.

Deputy, N.P., Dub, B., and Sharma, A.J. (2018). *Prevalence and Trends in Prepregnancy Normal Weight: 48 States, New York City, and District of Columbia, 2011–2015.* Available: https://www.cdc.gov/mmwr/volumes/66/wr/mm665152a3.htm.

DeSisto, C.L., Kim, S.Y., and Sharma, A.J. (2014). Peer reviewed: Prevalence estimates of gestational diabetes mellitus in the United States, pregnancy risk assessment monitoring system (PRAMS), 2007–2010. *Preventing Chronic Disease, 11.*

Devereaux, Y., and Sullivan, H. (2013). Doula support while laboring: Does it help achieve a more natural birth? *International Journal of Childbirth Education, 28*(2), pp. 54–61.

DiGuiseppe, D.L., Aron, D.C., Ranbom, L., Harper, D.L., and Rosenthal, G.E. (2002). Reliability of birth certificate information: A multi-hospital comparison to medical records information. *Maternal and Child Health Journal, 6*(3), pp. 169–179.

Dominguez, T.P., Dunkel-Schetter, C., Glynn, L.M., Hobel, C., and Sandman, C. A. (2008). Racial differences in birth outcomes: The role of general, pregnancy, and racism stress. *Health Psychology, 27*(2), pp. 194–203.

Dumont, D.M., Wildeman, C., Lee, H., Gjelsvik, A., Valera, P., and Clarke, J.G. (2014). Incarceration, maternal hardship, and perinatal health behaviors. *Maternal and Child Health Journal, 18*(9), pp. 2179–2187.

Dunkel-Schetter, C., and Tanner, L. (2012). Anxiety, depression and stress in pregnancy: Implications for mothers, children, research, and practice. *Current Opinion in Psychiatry, 25*(2), pp. 141–148.

East, C.E., Biro, M.A., Fredericks, S., and Lau, R. (2019). Support during pregnancy for women at increased risk of low birthweight babies. *Cochrane Database of Systematic Reviews, 4.*

Eden, A.R., and Peterson, L.E. (2018). Challenges faced by family physicians providing advanced maternity care. *Maternal and Child Health Journal, 22*(6), pp. 932–940.

Edmonds, J.K., and Jones, E.J. (2013). Intrapartum nurses' perceived influence on delivery mode decisions and outcomes. *Journal of Obstetric, Gynecologic and Neonatal Nursing, 42*(1), pp. 3–11.

Edmonds, J.K., O'Hara, M., Clarke, S.P., and Shah, N.T. (2017). Variation in cesarean birth rates by labor and delivery nurses. *Journal of Obstetric, Gynecologic and Neonatal Nursing, 46*(4), pp. 486–493.

Edwards, R.C., Thullen, M.J., Korfmacher, J., Lantos, J.D., Henson, L.G., and Hans, S.L. (2013). Breastfeeding and complementary food: Randomized trial of community doula home visiting. *Pediatrics, 132*(2), pp. S160–S166.

Ely, D.M., and Driscoll, A.K. (2019). Infant mortality in the United States, 2017: Data from the period linked birth/infant death file. *National Vital Statistics Reports, 68*(10). Available: https://www.cdc.gov/nchs/data/nvsr/nvsr68/nvsr68_10-508.pdf.

Ely, D.M., Driscoll, A.K., and Matthews, T.J. (2017). *Infant Mortality Rates in Rural and Urban Areas in the United States, 2014.* U.S. Department of Health and Human Services, Centers for Disease Control and Prevention, National Center for Health Statistics. Available: https://www.cdc.gov/nchs/data/databriefs/db285.pdf.

Evans, W.N., and Lien, D.S. (2005). The benefits of prenatal care: Evidence from the PAT bus strike. *Journal of Econometrics, 125*(1–2), pp. 207–239.

Evers, A.C., Brouwers, H.A., Hukkelhoven, C.W., Nikkels, P.G., Boon, J., van Egmond-Linden, A., Hillegersberg, J., Snuif, Y.S., Sterken-Hooisma, S., Bruinse, H.W. and Kwee, A. (2010). Perinatal mortality and severe morbidity in low and high-risk term pregnancies in the Netherlands: Prospective cohort study. *The BMJ, 341*, p. c5639.

Fagerlund, K., and Germano, E. (2009). The costs and benefits of nurse-midwifery education: Model and application. *Journal of Midwifery and Women's Health, 54*(5), pp. 341–350.

Ferré, C., Callaghan, W., Olson, C., Sharma, A., and Barfield, W. (2016). Effects of maternal age and age-specific preterm birth rates on overall preterm birth rates—United States, 2007 and 2014. *Morbidity and Mortality Weekly Report*, 65(43), pp. 1181–1184.

Fine, A., and Kotelchuck, M. (2010). Rethinking MCH: The life course model as an organizing framework. *U.S. Department of Health and Human Services, Health Resources and Services Administration, Maternal and Child Health Bureau*, 1–20.

Fingar, K.R., Hambrick, M.M., Heslin, K.C., and Moore, J.E. (2018). Trends and disparities in delivery hospitalizations involving severe maternal morbidity, 2006–2015. *H-CUP Statistical Brief, 243*. Available: https://www.hcup-us.ahrq.gov/reports/statbriefs/sb243-Severe-Maternal-Morbidity-Delivery-Trends-Disparities.jsp.

Firoz, T., Chou, D., von Dadelszen, P., Agrawal, P., Vanderkruik, R., Tunçalp, O., Magee, L.A., van Den Broek, N., and Say, L. (2013). Measuring maternal health: Focus on maternal morbidity. *Bulletin of the World Health Organization*, 91, pp. 794–796.

Fiscella, K., and Sanders, M.R. (2016). Racial and ethnic disparities in the quality of health care. *Annual Review of Public Health*, 37, pp. 375–394.

Fisch, D.M. (2012). Baby steps: The changing relationship between Michigan obstetricians and certified professional midwives. *Marquette Elder's Adviser*, 14, p. 87.

Flay, B.R., Biglan, A., Boruch, R.F., Castro, F.G., Gottfredson, D., Kellam, S., Moscicki, E.K., Schinke, S., Valentine, J.C., and Ji, P. (2005). Standards of evidence: Criteria for efficacy, effectiveness and dissemination. *Prevention Science*, 6(3), pp. 151–175.

Fleming, S.E., Donovan-Batson, C., Burduli, E., Barbosa-Leiker, C., Martin, C.J.H., and Martin, C.R. (2016). Birth satisfaction scale/birth satisfaction scale-revised (BSS/BSS-R): A large scale United States planned home birth and birth centre survey. *Midwifery*, 41, pp. 9–15.

Ford, C.L., Griffith, D.M., Bruce, M.A., and Gilbert, K.L. (2019). *Racism: Science and Tools for the Public Health Professional*. Washington, DC: American Public Health Association Press.

Forray A. (2016). Substance use during pregnancy. *F1000 Research*, 5, F1000 Faculty Rev-887.

Forray, A., and Foster, D. (2015). Substance use in the perinatal period. *Current Psychiatry Reports*, 17(11), p. 91.

Fox, D., Sheehan, A., and Homer, C. (2014). Experiences of women planning a home birth who require intrapartum transfer to hospital: A metasynthesis of the qualitative literature. *International Journal of Childbirth*, 4(2), pp. 103–119.

Fox, D., Sheehan, A., and Homer, C.S. (2018a). Birthplace in Australia: Antenatal preparation for the possibility of transfer from planned home birth. *Midwifery*, 66, pp. 134–140.

Fox, D., Sheehan, A., and Homer, C. (2018b). Birthplace in Australia: Processes and interactions during the intrapartum transfer of women from planned homebirth to hospital. *Midwifery*, 57, pp. 18–25.

Freedman, L.P., and Kruk, M.E. (2014). Disrespect and abuse of women in childbirth: Challenging the global quality and accountability agendas. *The Lancet*, 384(9948), pp. e42–e44.

Frohlich, K.L., and Potvin, L. (2008). Transcending the known in public health practice: The inequality paradox: The population approach and vulnerable populations. *American Journal of Public Health*, 98(2), pp. 216–221.

Fruscalzo, A., Londero, A.P., Salvador, S., Bertozzi, S., Biasioli, A., Della Martina, M., Driul, L., and Marchesoni, D. (2014). New and old predictive factors for breech presentation: Our experience in 14,433 singleton pregnancies and a literature review. *The Journal of Maternal-Fetal and Neonatal Medicine*, 27(2), pp. 167–172.

Fuentes-Afflick, E., Hessol, N.A., Bauer, T., O'Sullivan, M.J., Gomez-Lobo, V., Holman, S., Wilson, T., and Minkoff, H. (2006). Use of prenatal care by Hispanic women after welfare reform. *Obstetrics and Gynecology, 107*(1), pp. 151–160.

Furber, C.M., and McGowan, L. (2011). A qualitative study of the experiences of women who are obese and pregnant in the UK. *Midwifery, 27*(4), pp. 437–444.

Gadson, A., Akpovi, E., and Mehta, P.K. (2017). Exploring the social determinants of racial/ethnic disparities in prenatal care utilization and maternal outcome. *Seminars in Perinatology, 41*(5), pp. 308–317.

Gagnon, A.J., Waghorn, K., and Covell, C. (1997). A randomized trial of one-to-one nurse support of women in labor. *Birth*, 24(2), pp. 71–77.

Gagnon, A.J., Meier, K.M., and Waghorn, K. (2007). Continuity of nursing care and its link to cesarean birth rate. *Birth*, 34(1), pp. 26–31.

Gams, B., Neerland, C., and Kennedy, S. (2019). Reducing primary cesareans: An innovative multipronged approach to supporting physiologic labor and vaginal birth. *The Journal of Perinatal and Neonatal Nursing, 33*(1), pp. 52–60.

Garfield, R., Orgera, K., and Damico, A. (2019). *The Coverage Gap: Uninsured Poor Adults in States That Do Not Expand Medicaid.* Available: https://www.kff.org/medicaid/issue-brief/the-coverage-gap-uninsured-poor-adults-in-states-that-do-not-expand-medicaid.

Geller, S.E., Koch, A., Pellettieri, B., and Carnes, M. (2011). Inclusion, analysis, and reporting of sex and race/ethnicity in clinical trials: Have we made progress? *Journal of Women's Health, 20*(3), pp. 315–320.

Geller, S.E., Koch, A.R., Garland, C.E., MacDonald, E.J., Storey, F., and Lawton, B. (2018). A global view of severe maternal morbidity: Moving beyond maternal mortality. *Reproductive Health, 15*(1), p. 98.

Germano, E., Schorn, M.N., Phillippi, J.C., and Schuiling, K. (2014). Factors that influence midwives to serve as preceptors: An American College of Nurse-Midwives survey. *Journal of Midwifery and Women's Health, 59*(2), pp. 167–175.

Geronimus, A.T. (1992). The weathering hypothesis and the health of African-American women and infants: evidence and speculations. *Ethnicity and Disease, 2*(3), pp. 207–221.

Geronimus, A.T., Hicken, M., Keene, D., and Bound, J. (2006). "Weathering" and age patterns of allostatic load scores among blacks and whites in the United States. *American Journal of Public Health, 96*(5), pp. 826–833.

Giscombé, C.L., and Lobel, M. (2005). Explaining disproportionately high rates of adverse birth outcomes among African Americans: The impact of stress, racism, and related factors in pregnancy. *Psychological Bulletin, 131*(5), pp. 662–683.

Giuntella, O. (2016). The Hispanic health paradox: New evidence from longitudinal data on second and third-generation birth outcomes. *SSM Population Health, 2*, pp. 84–89.

Giurgescu, C., and Misra, D.P. (2018). Psychosocial factors and preterm birth among black mothers and fathers. *MCN: The American Journal of Maternal/Child Nursing, 43*(5), pp. 245–251.

Glantz, J.C. (2012). Obstetric variation, intervention, and outcomes: Doing more but accomplishing less. *Birth*, 39(4), pp. 286–290.

Goldstein, J.T., Hartman, S.G., Meunier, M.R., Panchal, B., Pecci, C.C., Zink, N.M., and Shields, S.G. (2018). Supporting family physician maternity care providers. *Family Medicine, 50*(9), pp. 662–671.

González Burchard, E., Borrell, L.N., Choudhry, S., Naqvi, M., Tsai, H.J., Rodriguez-Santana, J.R., Chapela, R., Rogers, S.D., Mei, R., Rodriguez-Cintron, W. and Arena, J.F., Kittles, R., Perez-Stable. E.J., Ziv, E., and Risch, N. (2005). Latino populations: A unique opportunity for the study of race, genetics, and social environment in epidemiological research. *American Journal of Public Health, 95*(12), pp. 2161–2168.

Goodwin, C. J. (2005). *Research in Psychology Method and Design*. Hoboken, NJ: John Wiley and Son, Inc.

Greene, N.H., Kilcoyne, J., Grey, A., Hawkes, S.G., Edmonds, J.K., and Gregory, K.D. (2019). Nurse-specific cesarean rates: Why and how. *American Journal of Obstetrics and Gynecology*, 220(1), p. S45.

Gregory, K.D., Jackson, S., Korst, L., and Fridman, M. (2012). Cesarean versus vaginal delivery: Whose risks? Whose benefits? *American Journal of Perinatology*, 29(01), pp. 7–18.

Greiner, K.S., Hersh, A.R., Hersh, S.R., Gallagher, A.C., Caughey, A.B., and Tilden, E.L. (2019). Cost-effectiveness of continuous support from a layperson during a woman's first two births. *Journal of Obstetric, Gynecologic and Neonatal Nursing*, 48(5), pp. 538–551.

Griffiths, P., Recio-Saucedo, A., Dall'Ora, C., Briggs, J., Maruotti, A., Meredith, P., Smith, G.B., Ball, J. and Missed Care Study Group. (2018). The association between nurse staffing and omissions in nursing care: A systematic review. *Journal of Advanced Nursing*, 74(7), pp. 1474–1487.

Grigg, C.P., Tracy, S.K., Tracy, M., Daellenbach, R., Kensington, M., Monk, A., and Schmied, V. (2017). Evaluating maternity units: A prospective cohort study of freestanding midwife-led primary maternity units in New Zealand—Clinical outcomes. *The BMJ Open*, 7(8), p. e016288.

Grimshaw, J., Campbell, M., Eccles, M., and Steen, N. (2000). Experimental and quasi-experimental designs for evaluating guideline implementation strategies. *Family Practice*, 17(1), pp. S11–S16.

Grote, N.K., Bridge, J.A., Gavin, A.R., Melville, J.L., Iyengar, S., and Katon, W.J. (2010). A meta-analysis of depression during pregnancy and the risk of preterm birth, low birth weight, and intrauterine growth restriction. *Archives of General Psychiatry*, 67(10), pp. 1012–1024.

Gruber, K.J., Cupito, S.H., and Dobson, C.F. (2013). Impact of doulas on healthy birth outcomes. *The Journal of Perinatal Education*, 22(1), pp. 49–58.

Grünebaum, A., McCullough, L.B., Sapra, K.J., Brent, R.L., Levene, M.I., Arabin, B., and Chervenak, F.A. (2013). Apgar score of 0 at 5 minutes and neonatal seizures or serious neurologic dysfunction in relation to birth setting. *American Journal of Obstetrics and Gynecology*, 209(4), pp. 323–e1.

Grünebaum, A., McCullough, L.B., Sapra, K.J., Brent, R.L., Levene, M.I., Arabin, B., and Chervenak, F.A. (2014). Early and total neonatal mortality in relation to birth setting in the United States, 2006–2009. *American Journal of Obstetrics and Gynecology*, 211(4), pp. 390–e1.

Grünebaum, A., McCullough, L.B., Brent, R.L., Arabin, B., Levene, M.I., and Chervenak, F.A. (2015a). Justified skepticism about Apgar scoring in out-of-hospital birth settings. *Journal of Perinatal Medicine*, 43(4), pp. 455–460.

Grünebaum, A., McCullough, L.B., Brent, R.L., Arabin, B., Levene, M.I., and Chervenak, F.A. (2015b). Perinatal risks of planned home births in the United States. *American Journal of Obstetrics and Gynecology*, 212(3), pp. 350–e1.

Grünebaum, A., McCullough, L.B., Arabin, B., Brent, R.L., Levene, M.I., and Chervenak, F.A. (2016). Neonatal mortality of planned home birth in the United States in relation to professional certification of birth attendants. *PLOS One*, 11(5), p. e0155721.

Grünebaum, A., McCullough, L.B., Sapra, K.J., Arabin, B., and Chervenak, F.A. (2017a). Planned home births: The need for additional contraindications. *American Journal of Obstetrics and Gynecology*, 216(4), pp. 401–e1.

Grünebaum, A., McCullough, L.B., Arabin, B., Dudenhausen, J., Orosz, B., and Chervenak, F.A. (2017b). Underlying causes of neonatal deaths in term singleton pregnancies: Home births versus hospital births in the United States. *Journal of Perinatal Medicine, 45*(3), pp. 349–357.

Grzybowski, S., Stoll, K., and Kornelsen, J. (2011). Distance matters: A population-based study examining access to maternity services for rural women. *BMC Health Services Research, 11*, p. 147.

Guise, J.M., and Segel, S. (2008). Teamwork in obstetric critical care. *Best Practice and Research: Clinical Obstetrics and Gynaecology, 22*(5), pp. 937–951.

Gurny, P., Hirsch, M.B., and Gondek, K. (1995). *Chapter 11: A Description of Medicaid-Covered Services.* Available: https://www.cms.gov/Research-Statistics-Data-and-Systems/Research/HealthCareFinancingReview/Downloads/CMS1191224dl.pdf.

Guyatt, G.H., Oxman, A.D., Vist, G.E., Kunz, R., Falck-Ytter, Y., Alonso-Coello, P., and Schünemann, H.J. (2008). GRADE: An emerging consensus on rating quality of evidence and strength of recommendations. *The BMJ, 336*, pp. 924–926.

Haight, S.C., Ko, J.Y., Tong, V.T., Bohm, M.K., and Callaghan, W.M. (2018). Opioid use disorder documented at delivery hospitalization—United States, 1999–2014. *Morbidity and Mortality Weekly Report, 67*(31), pp. 845–849.

Halbreich, U., and Karkun, S. (2006). Cross-cultural and social diversity of prevalence of postpartum depression and depressive symptoms. *Journal of Affective Disorders, 91*(2–3), pp. 97–111.

Hale, R.W. (2006). Legal issues impacting women's access to care in the United States: The malpractice insurance crisis. *International Journal of Gynecology and Obstetrics, 94*(3), pp. 382–385.

Hales, C.M., Carroll, M.D., Fryar, C.D., and Ogden, C.L. (2017). Prevalence of obesity among adults and youth: United States, 2015–2016. *National Center for Health Statistics Data Brief, 288*.

Halfon, N., Forrest, C.B., Lerner, R.M., and Faustman, E.M. (2018). *Health Disparities: A Life Course Health Development Perspective and Future Research Directions—Handbook of Life Course Health Development.* Cham, Switzerland: Springer Press.

Hall, J., Hundley, V., Collins, B., and Ireland, J. (2018). Dignity and respect during pregnancy and childbirth: A survey of the experience of disabled women. *BMC Pregnancy and Childbirth, 18*(1), p. 328.

Hamilton, B.E., Rossen, L.M., and Branum, A.M. (2016). Teen birth rates for urban and rural areas in the United States, 2007–2015. *National Center for Health Statistics Data Brief, 264*, 1–8.

Hamilton, B.E., Martin, J.A, Osterman, M.J.K., and Rossen, L.M. (2019). *Births: Provisional Data for 2018.* Available: https://www.cdc.gov/nchs/data/vsrr/vsrr-007-508.pdf.

Han, Z., Mulla, S., Beyene, J., Liao, G., and McDonald, S.D. (2011). Maternal underweight and the risk of preterm birth and low birth weight: A systematic review and meta-analyses. *International Journal of Epidemiology, 40*(1), pp. 65–101.

Haney, K. (2017). *Medicaid Coverage During Pregnancy, Labor, and Delivery.* Available: https://www.growingfamilybenefits.com/medicaid-coverage-during-pregnancy.

Hannah, M.E., Hannah, W.J., Hewson, S.A., Hodnett, E.D., Saigal, S., Willan, A.R., and Collaborative, T.B.T. (2000). Planned caesarean section versus planned vaginal birth for breech presentation at term: A randomised multicentre trial. *The Lancet, 356*(9239), pp. 1375–1383.

Hanson, M.A., and Gluckman, P.D. (2014). Early developmental conditional of later health and disease: Physiology or pathophysiology? *Physiological Reviews, 94*(4), pp. 1027–1076.

Hardeman, R.R., and Kozhimannil, K.B. (2016). Motivations for entering the doula profession: Perspectives from women of color. *Journal of Midwifery and Women's Health*, *61*(6), pp. 773–780.

Hardeman, R.R., Murphy, K.A., Karbeah, J M., and Kozhimannil, K.B. (2018). Naming institutionalized racism in the public health literature: A systematic literature review. *Public Health Reports*, *133*(3), pp. 240–249.

Hardeman, R.R., Karbeah, J., Almanza, J., and Kozhimannil, K.B. (2019). *Roots Community Birth Center: A Culturally-Centered Care Model for Improving Value and Equity in Childbirth*. Available: https://doi.org/10.1016/j.hjdsi.2019.100367.

Hardin, A.M., and Buckner, E.B. (2004). Characteristics of a positive experience for women who have unmedicated childbirth. *The Journal of Perinatal Education*, *13*(4), pp. 10–16.

Harris, A.D., McGregor, J.C., Perencevich, E.N., Furuno, J.P., Zhu, J., Peterson, D.E., and Finkelstein, J. (2006). The use and interpretation of quasi-experimental studies in medical informatics. *Journal of the American Medical Informatics Association*, *13*(1), pp. 16–23.

Health Care Payment Learning and Action Network. (n.d.). *Maternity Episode Payment Model Online Resource Bank*. Available: https://hcp-lan.org/maternity-resource-bank.

Health Care Payment Learning and Action Network. (2016). Maternity care. *Accelerating and aligning clinical episode payment models: Maternity care*. MITRE Corporation. Available: https://hcp-lan.org/clinical-episode-payment.

Health Management Associates. (2007). *Midwifery Licensure and Discipline Program in Washington State: Economic Costs and Benefits*. Available: https://www.nacpm.org/documents/Midwifery_Cost_Study_10-31-07.pdf.

Health Resources and Services Administration. (2016). *National and Regional Projections of Supply and Demand for Women's Health Service Providers: 2013–2025*. Available: https://bhw.hrsa.gov/sites/default/files/bhw/health-workforce-analysis/research/projections/womens-health-report.pdf

Health Resources and Services Administration. (2018). *Collaborative Improvement and Innovation Networks (CoIINs)*. Available: https://mchb.hrsa.gov/maternal-child-health-initiatives/collaborative-improvement-innovation-networks-coiins.

Healy, S., Humphreys, E., and Kennedy, C. (2016). Midwives' and obstetricians' perceptions of risk and its impact on clinical practice and decision-making in labour: An integrative review. *Women and Birth*, *29*(2), pp. 107–116.

Heaman, M.I., Sword, W., Elliott, L., Moffatt, M., Helewa, M. E., Morris, H., Gregory, P., Tjaden, L., and Cook, C. (2015). Barriers and facilitators related to use of prenatal care by inner-city women: Perceptions of health care providers. *BMC Pregnancy and Childbirth*, *15*(1), p. 2.

Henderson, Z.T., Ernst, K., Simpson, K.R., Berns, S., Suchdev, D.B., Main, E., McCaffrey, M., Lee, K., Rouse, T.B., and Olson, C.K. (2018). The national network of state perinatal quality collaboratives: A growing movement to improve maternal and infant health. *Journal of Women's Health*, *27*(3), pp. 221–226

Hendrix, M., Van Horck, M., Moreta, D., Nieman, F., Nieuwenhuijze, M., Severens, J., and Nijhuis, J. (2009). Why women do not accept randomisation for place of birth: Feasibility of an RCT in the Netherlands. *British Journal of Obstetrics and Gynaecology*, *116*(4), pp. 537–544.

Hennegan, J., Redshaw, M., and Miller, Y. (2014). Born in another country: Women's experience of labour and birth in Queensland, Australia. *Women and Birth*, *27*(2), pp. 91–97.

Hermus, M.A., Hitzert, M., Boesveld, I.C., van den Akker-van, M.E., van Dommelen, P., Franx, A., de Graaf, J.P., van Lith, J.M., Luurssen-Masurel, N., Steegers, E.A., and Wiegers, T.A. (2017). Differences in optimality index between planned place of birth in a birth centre and alternative planned places of birth: A nationwide prospective cohort study in The Netherlands: Results of the Dutch Birth Centre Study. *BMJ Open*, *7*(11), p. e016958.

Hickman, A. (2009). Born (not so) free: Legal limits on the practice of unassisted childbirth or freebirthing in the United States. *Minnesota Law Review, 94*, p. 1651.

Hill, I., Dubay, L., Courtot, B., Benatar, S., Garrett, B., Blavin, F., Howell, E., Johnston, E., Allen, E., Thornburgh, S., Markell, J., Morgan, J., Silow-Carroll, S., Bitterman, J., Rodin, D., Odendahl, R., Paez, K., Thompson, L., Lucado, J., Firminger, K., Sinnarajah, B., Paquin, L., and Rouse, M. (2018). *Strong Start for Mothers and Newborns Evaluation: Year 5 Project Synthesis, Vol 1.* Available: https://downloads.cms.gov/files/cmmi/strongstart-prenatal-finalevalrpt-v1.pdf.

Hodnett, E.D. (2002). Pain and women's satisfaction with the experience of childbirth: A systematic review. *American Journal of Obstetrics and Gynecology, 186*(5), pp. S160–S172.

Hodnett, E.D., Lowe, N.K., Hannah, M.E., Willan, A.R., Stevens, B., Weston, J.A., Ohlsson, A., Gafni, A., Muir, H.A., Myhr, T.L, and Stremler, R. (2002). Effectiveness of nurses as providers of birth labor support in North American hospitals: A randomized controlled trial. *Journal of the American Medical Association, 288*(11), pp. 1373–1381.

Hodnett, E.D., Gates, S., Hofmeyr, G.J., and Sakala, C. (2013). Continuous support for women during childbirth. *Cochrane Database of Systematic Reviews 2017, 7.*

Hogue, C.J., and Bremner, J.D. (2005). Stress model for research into preterm delivery among black women. *American Journal of Obstetrics and Gynecology, 192*(5), pp. S47–S55.

Holgash, K., and Heberlein, M. (2019). *Physician Acceptance of New Medicaid Patients.* Available: https://www.macpac.gov/wp-contet/uploads/2019/01/Physician-Acceptance-of-New-Medicaid-Patients.pdf.

Hollander, M.H., van Hastenberg, E., van Dillen, J., Van Pampus, M.G., de Miranda, E., and Stramrood, C.A.I. (2017). Preventing traumatic childbirth experiences: 2192 women's perceptions and views. *Archives of Women's Mental Health, 20*(4), pp. 515–523.

Hollowell, J., Li, Y., Bunch, K., and Brocklehurst, P. (2017). A comparison of intrapartum interventions and adverse outcomes by parity in planned freestanding midwifery unit and alongside midwifery unit births: Secondary analysis of "low risk" births in the Birthplace in England cohort. *BMC Pregnancy and Childbirth, 17*(1), p. 95.

Holten, L., and de Miranda, E. (2016). Women's motivations for having unassisted childbirth or high-risk homebirth: An exploration of the literature on "birthing outside the system." *Midwifery, 38*, pp. 55–62.

Holzman, C., Eyster, J., Kleyn, M., Messer, L.C., Kaufman, J.S., Laraia, B.A., O'Campo, P., Burke, J.G., Culhane, J. and Elo, I.T. (2009). Maternal weathering and risk of preterm delivery. *American Journal of Public Health, 99*(10), pp. 1864–1871.

Home Birth Summit. (n.d.). *Best Practice Guidelines: Transfer from Planned Home Birth to Hospital.* Available: https://www.homebirthsummit.org/wp-content/uploads/2014/03/HomeBirthSummit_BestPracticeTransferGuidelines.pdf.

Homer, C.S., Thornton, C., Scarf, V.L., Ellwood, D.A., Oats, J.J., Foureur, M.J., Sibbritt, D., McLachlan, H.L., Forster, D.A. and Dahlen, H.G. (2014). Birthplace in New South Wales, Australia: An analysis of perinatal outcomes using routinely collected data. *BMC Pregnancy and Childbirth, 14*(1), p. 206.

Horbar, J.D., Edwards, E.M., Greenberg, L.M., Morrow, K.A., Soll, R.F., Buus-Frank, M.E., and Buzas, J.S. (2017). Variation in performance of neonatal intensive care units in the United States. *JAMA Pediatrics, 171*(3). doi:10.1001/jamapediatrics.2016.4396.

Howell, E.A. (2018). Reducing disparities in severe maternal morbidity and mortality. *Clinical Obstetrics and Gynecology, 61*(2), pp. 387–399.

Howell, E., Palmer, A., Benatar, S., and Garrett, B. (2014). Potential Medicaid cost savings from maternity care based at a freestanding birth center. *Medicare and Medicaid Research Review, 4*(3).

Howell, E.A., Egorova, N., Balbierz, A., Zeitlin, J., and Hebert, P.L. (2016). Black-white differences in severe maternal morbidity and site of care. *American Journal of Obstetrics and Gynecology, 214*(1), pp. 122–e1.

Howell, E.A., and Zeitlin, J. (2017). Quality of care and disparities in obstetrics. *Obstetrics and Gynecology Clinics, 44*(1), pp. 13–25.

Hung, P., Kozhimannil, K.B., Casey, M.M., and Moscovice, I.S. (2016). Why are obstetric units in rural hospitals closing their doors? *Health Services Research, 51*(4), pp. 1546–1560.

Hutton, E.K., Reitsma, A.H., and Kaufman, K. (2009). Outcomes associated with planned home and planned hospital births in low-risk women attended by midwives in Ontario, Canada, 2003–2006: A retrospective cohort study. *Birth, 36*(3), pp. 180–189.

Hutton, E.K., Cappelletti, A., Reitsma, A.H., Simioni, J., Horne, J., McGregor, C., and Ahmed, R.J. (2016). Outcomes associated with planned place of birth among women with low-risk pregnancies. *Canadian Medical Association Journal, 188*(5), pp. e80–90.

Huynh, M. (2014). Provider type and preterm birth in New York City births, 2009–2010. *Journal of Health Care for the Poor and Underserved, 25*(4), pp. 1520–1529.

Ickovics, J.R., Reed, E., Magriples, U., Westdahl, C., Schindler Rising, S., and Kershaw, T.S. (2011). Effects of group prenatal care on psychosocial risk in pregnancy: Results from a randomised controlled trial. *Psychology and Health, 26*(2), pp. 235–250.

Illuzzi, J., Stapleton, S., and Rathbun, L. (2015). Early and total neonatal mortality in relation to birth setting in the United States, 2006–2009. *American Journal of Obstetrics and Gynecology, 212*(2), p. 250.

Institute of Medicine. (1985). *Preventing Low Birth Weight.* Washington, DC: The National Academies Press.

Institute of Medicine. (1988). *Prenatal Care: Reaching Mothers, Reaching Infants* (Vol. 926). Washington, DC: The National Academies Press.

Institute of Medicine. (2003). *Unequal Treatment: Confronting Racial and Ethnic Disparities in Health Care.* Washington, DC: The National Academies Press.

Institute of Medicine. (2004). *In the Nation's Compelling Interest: Ensuring Diversity in the Health-Care Workforce.* Washington, DC: The National Academies Press.

Institute of Medicine. (2007). *Preterm Birth: Causes, Consequences, and Prevention.* Washington, DC: The National Academies Press.

Institute of Medicine. (2008). *Knowing What Works in Health Care: A Roadmap for the Nation.* Washington, DC: The National Academies Press.

Institute of Medicine. (2010). *Bridging the Evidence Gap in Obesity Prevention: A Framework to Inform Decision Making.* Washington, DC: The National Academies Press.

Institute of Medicine. (2011). *The Future of Nursing: Leading Change, Advancing Health.* Washington, DC: National Academies Press.

Institute of Medicine. (2013). *Delivering High-Quality Cancer Care: Charting a New Course for a System in Crisis.* Washington, DC: The National Academies Press.

Institute of Medicine and National Research Council. (1982). *Research Issues in the Assessment of Birth Settings: Report of a Study.* Washington, DC: The National Academies Press.

Institute of Medicine and National Research Council. (2009). *Weight Gain During Pregnancy: Reexamining the Guidelines.* Washington, DC: The National Academies Press.

Institute of Medicine and National Research Council. (2013). *An Update on Research Issues in the Assessment of Birth Settings: Workshop Summary.* Washington, DC: The National Academies Press.

International Confederation of Midwives, White Ribbon Alliance, International Pediatric Association, and World Health Organization. (2015). Mother–baby friendly birthing facilities. *International Journal of Gynecology and Obstetrics, 128*(2), pp. 95–99.

International Federation of Health Plans. (2015). *2015 Comparative Price Report: Variation in Medical and Hospital Prices by Country*. Available: https://fortunedotcom.files.wordpress.com/2018/04/66c7d-2015comparativepricereport09-09-16.pdf.

Ireland, S., Montgomery-Andersen, R., and Geraghty, S. (2019). Indigenous doulas: A literature review exploring their role and practice in western maternity care. *Midwifery, 75*, pp. 52–58.

Isbey. C., and Martin, H. (2017). *Achieving Perinatal Care Certification and Lessons Learned from 2016*. Available: https://www.jointcommission.org/assets/1/6/PNC_03-29-17.pdf.

Ishola, F., Owolabi, O., and Filippi, V. (2017). Disrespect and abuse of women during childbirth in Nigeria: A systematic review. *PLOS One, 12*(3), p. e0174084.

Itkowitz, C. (2017). Closure of two D.C. maternity wards hurts low-income women most. *The Washington Post*, October 28. Available: https://www.washingtonpost.com/local/closure-of-two-dc-maternity-wards-hurts-low-income-women-most/2017/10/28/753e4dee-ad06-11e7-9e58-e6288544af98_story.html?noredirect=on.

Jadad, A.R., and Enkin, M.W. (2008). *Randomized Controlled Trials: Questions, Answers and Musings*. Malden, MA: Blackwell Publishing, Inc.

James, D.C., Simpson, K.R., and Knox, G.E. (2003). How do expert labor nurses view their role? *Journal of Obstetric, Gynecologic, and Neonatal Nursing, 32*(6), pp. 814–823.

Jankowski, J., and Burcher, P. (2015). Home birth of infants with anticipated congenital anomalies: A case study and ethical analysis of careproviders' obligations. *The Journal of Clinical Ethics, 26*(1), pp. 27–35.

Janssen, P.A., Carty, E.A., and Reime, B. (2006). Satisfaction with planned place of birth among midwifery clients in British Columbia. *The Journal of Midwifery and Women's Health, 51*(2), pp. 91–97.

Janssen, P.A., Saxell, L., Page, L.A., Klein, M.C., Liston, R.M., and Lee, S.K. (2009). Outcomes of planned home birth with registered midwife versus planned hospital birth with midwife or physician. *Canadian Medical Association Journal, 181*(6–7), pp. 377–383.

Janssen, P.A., Mitton, C., and Aghajanian, J. (2015). Costs of planned home vs. hospital birth in British Columbia attended by registered midwives and physicians. *PLOS One, 10*(7), p. e0133524.

Jennings, J., Nielsen, P., Buck, M.L., Collins-Fulea, C., Corry, M., Cutler, C., Faucher, M.A., Kendig, S., Kraft, C., McGinnity, J. and Miller, K.P. (2016). Collaboration in practice: Implementing team-based care: Report of the American College of Obstetricians and Gynecologists' Task Force on Collaborative Practice. *Obstetrics and Gynecology, 127*(3), pp. 612–617.

Johnson, K.C., and Daviss, B.A. (2005). Outcomes of planned home births with certified professional midwives: Large prospective study in North America. *The BMJ, 330*(7505), p. 1416.

Johnson, R.B., and Onwuegbuzie, A. J. (2004). Mixed methods research: A research paradigm whose time has come. *Educational Researcher, 33*(7), pp. 14–26.

Jolles, D.R., Langford, R., Stapleton, S., Cesario, S., Koci, A., and Alliman, J. (2017). Outcomes of childbearing Medicaid beneficiaries engaged in care at Strong Start Birth Center sites between 2012 and 2014. *Birth, 44*(4), pp. 298–305.

Kaiser Family Foundation. (2007). *Maternity Care and Consumer-Driven Health Plans*. Available: https://www.kff.org/health-costs/report/maternity-care-and-consumer-driven-health-plans.

Kaiser Family Foundation. (2017). *Medicaid Coverage of Pregnancy and Perinatal Benefits: Results from a State Survey*. Available: http://files.kff.org/attachment/Report-Medicaid-Coverage-of-Pregnancy-and-Perinatal-Benefits.

Kaiser Family Foundation. (2019a). *Status of State Action on the Medicaid Expansion Decision.* Available: https://www.kff.org/medicaid/issue-brief/status-of-state-medicaid-expansion-decisions-interactive-map.

Kaiser Family Foundation. (2019b). *Medicaid Benefits: Freestanding Birth Center Services.* Available: https://www.kff.org/other/state-indicator/medicaid-benefits-freestanding-birth-center-services/?currentTimeframe=0&sortModel=%7B%22colId%22:%22Benefit%20Covered%22,%22sort%22:%22desc%22%7D.

Kaiser Family Foundation. (2019c). *Total Medicaid MCOs.* Available: https://www.kff.org/medicaid/state-indicator/total-medicaid-mcos/?currentTimeframe=0&sortModel=%7B%22colId%22:%22Location%22,%22sort%22:%22asc%22%7D.

Kane, R.L., Shamliyan, T., Mueller, C., Duval, S., and Wilt, T. (2007). Nursing staffing and quality of patient care. *Evidence Report/Technology Assessment, 151*(1), p. 115.

Kaplan, L., Skillman, S.M., Fordyce, M.A., McMenamin, P.D., and Doescher, M.P. (2012). Understanding APRN distribution in the United States using NPI data. *The Journal of Nurse Practitioners, 8*(8), pp. 626–635.

Karbeah, J.M., Hardeman, R., Almanza, J., and Kozhimannil, K.B. (2019). Identifying the key elements of racially concordant care in a freestanding birth center. *Journal of Midwifery and Women's Health.* Available: https://doi.org/10.1111/jmwh.13018.

Kataoka, Y., Eto, H., and Iida, M. (2013). Outcomes of independent midwifery attended births in birth centres and home births: A retrospective cohort study in Japan. *Midwifery, 29*(8), pp. 965–972.

Kennare, R.M., Keirse, M.J., Tucker, G. R., and Chan, A. C. (2010). Planned home and hospital births in South Australia, 1991–2006: Differences in outcomes. *Medical Journal of Australia, 192*(2), pp. 76–80.

Kennedy, H.P., Cheyney, M., Dahlen, H.G., Downe, S., Foureur, M.J., Homer, C.S., Jefford, E., McFadden, A., Michel-Schuldt, M., Sandall, J., and Soltani, H. (2018). Asking different questions: A call to action for research to improve the quality of care for every woman, every child. *Birth, 45*(3), pp. 222–231.

Kennedy, H.P., Balaam, M.C., Dahlen, H., Declercq, E., de Jong, A., Downe, S., Ellwood, D., Homer, C.S.E., Sandall, J., Vedam, S., and Wolfe, I. (2019). *Report for SOW on Assessing Health Outcomes by Birth Settings, and, in Particular, on International Insights for Maternity Care in the United States.* Commissioned by the Committee on Assessing Health Outcomes by Birth Settings. Washington, DC: National Academies of Sciences, Engineering, and Medicine.

Kentoffio, K., Berkowitz, S.A., Atlas, S.J., Oo, S.A., and Percac-Lima, S. (2016). Use of maternal health services: Comparing refugee, immigrant and U.S.-born populations. *Maternal and Child Health Journal, 20*(12), pp. 2494–2501.

Khan, K. (2019). The CROWN Initiative: Journal editors invite researchers to develop core outcomes in women's health. *Best Practice and Research: Clinical Obstetrics and Gynaecology, 57*, pp. e1–e4.

Kim, H., and Xie, B. (2017). Health literacy in the eHealth era: A systematic review of the literature. *Patient Education and Counseling, 100*(6), pp. 1073–1082.

Kim, S.Y., England, L., Wilson, H.G., Bish, C., Satten, G.A., and Dietz, P. (2010). Percentage of gestational diabetes mellitus attributable to overweight and obesity. *American Journal of Public Health, 100*(6), pp. 1047–1052.

Ko, J.Y., Rockhill, K.M., Tong, V.T., and Morrow, B. (2017). Trends in postpartum depressive symptoms: 27 states, 2004, 2008, and 2012. *Morbidity and Mortality Weekly Report, 66*, pp. 153–158.

Koblinsky, M., Moyer, C. A., Calvert, C., Campbell, J., Campbell, O. M., Feigl, A. B., Graham, W.J., Hatt, L., Hodgins. S., Matthews, Z., McDougal, L., Moran, A., Nandakumar, A.K. and McDougall, L. (2016). Quality maternity care for every woman, everywhere: A call to action. *The Lancet, 388*(10057), pp. 2307–2320.

Kontos, E., Blake, K.D., Wen-Ying, S.C., and Prestin, A. (2014). Predictors of ehealth usage: Insights on the digital divide from the health information national trends survey 2012. *Journal of Medical Internet Research, 16*(7), p. e172.

Kornelsen, J., Kotaska, A., Waterfall, P., Willie, L., and Wilson, D. (2010). The geography of belonging: The experience of birthing at home for First Nations women. *Health and Place, 16*(4), pp. 638–645.

Kozhimannil, K. (2014). Rural-urban differences in childbirth care, 2002–2010, and implications for the future. *Medical Care, 52*(1), pp. 4–9.

Kozhimannil, K.B., Pereira, M.A., and Harlow, B.L. (2009). Association between diabetes and perinatal depression among low-income mothers. *Journal of the American Medical Association, 301*(8), pp. 842–847.

Kozhimannil, K.B., Hardeman, R.R., Attanasio, L.B., Blauer-Peterson, C., and O'Brien, M. (2013). Doula care, birth outcomes, and costs among Medicaid beneficiaries. *American Journal of Public Health, 103*(4), pp. e113–e121.

Kozhimannil, K.B., Vogelsang, C.A., and Hardeman, R.R. (2015). Medicaid coverage of doula services in Minnesota: Preliminary findings from the first year. *Interim Report to the Minnesota Department of Human Services.* Available: https://static1.squarespace.com/static/577d7562ff7c5018d6ea200a/t/5840c791cd0f683f8477920a/1480640403710/FullReport.pdf.

Kozhimannil, K.B., Hardeman, R.R., Alarid-Escudero, F., Vogelsang, C.A., Blauer-Peterson, C., and Howell, E.A. (2016). Modeling the cost-effectiveness of doula care associated with reductions in preterm birth and cesarean delivery. *Birth, 43*(1), pp. 20–27.

Kozhimannil, K.B., Hung, P., Henning-Smith, C., Casey, M.M., and Prasad, S. (2018a). Association between loss of hospital-based obstetric services and birth outcomes in rural counties in the United States. *Journal of the American Medical Association, 319*(12), pp. 1239–1247.

Kozhimannil, K.B., Graves, A.J., Ecklund, A.M., Shah, N., Aggarwal, R., and Snowden, J.M. (2018b). Cesarean delivery rates and costs of childbirth in a state Medicaid program after implementation of a blended payment policy. *Medical Care, 56*(8), pp. 658–664.

Kozhimannil, K.B., Muoto, I., Darney, B.G., Caughey, A.B., and Snowden, J.M. (2018c). Early elective delivery disparities between non-Hispanic black and white women after statewide policy implementation. *Women's Health Issues, 28*(3), 224–231.

Krieger, N., Kosheleva, A., Waterman, P.D., Chen, J.T., Beckfield, J., and Kiang, M. V. (2014). 50-year trends in US socioeconomic inequalities in health: U.S.-born Black and White Americans, 1959–2008. *International Journal of Epidemiology, 43*(4), pp. 1294–1313.

Krolikowski-Ulmer, K., Watson, T.J., Westhoff, E.M., Ashmore, S.L., Thompson, P.A., and Landeen, L.B. (2018). The Collaborative Laborist and Midwifery Model: An accepted and sustainable model. *South Dakota Medicine, 71*(12), pp. 534–537.

Kurki, T., Hiilesmaa, V., Raitasalo, R., Mattila, H., and Ylikorkala, O. (2000). Depression and anxiety in early pregnancy and risk for preeclampsia. *Obstetrics and Gynecology, 95*(4), pp. 487–490.

Kushel, M.B., Gupta, R., Gee, L., and Haas, J.S. (2006). Housing instability and food insecurity as barriers to health care among low-income Americans. *Journal of General Internal Medicine, 21*(1), pp. 71–77.

Lagrew, D.C., Kane Low, L., Brennan, R., Corry, M.P., Edmonds, J.K., Gilpin, B.G, Frost, J., Pinger, W., Reisner, D.P. and Jaffer, S. (2018). National Partnership for Maternal Safety: Consensus bundle on safe reduction of primary cesarean births-supporting intended vaginal births. *Journal of Obstetric, Gynecologic and Neonatal Nursing, 47*(2), pp. 214–226.

Lantz, P.M., Low, L.K., Varkey, S., and Watson, R.L. (2005). Doulas as childbirth paraprofessionals: Results from a national survey. *Women's Health Issues, 15*(3), pp. 109–116.

Laura and John Arnold Foundation. (2017). *Social Programs That Work Review: Evidence Summary for the Nurse Family Partnership*. Available: https://evidencebasedprograms. org/document/nurse-family-partnership-nfp-evidence-summary.

Laws, P.J., Xu, F., Welsh, A., Tracy, S.K., and Sullivan, E.A. (2014). Maternal morbidity of women receiving birth center care in New South Wales: A matched-pair analysis using linked health data. *Birth, 41*(3), pp. 268–275.

Leeman, L., Dresang, L.T., and Fontaine, P. (2016). Hypertensive disorders of pregnancy. *American Family Physician, 93*(2).

Leighton, C., Conroy, M., Bilderback, A., Kalocay, W., Henderson, J.K., and Simhan, H.N. (2019). Implementation and impact of a maternal–fetal medicine telemedicine program. *American Journal of Perinatology, 36*(07), pp. 751–758.

Lemelle, A J., Reed, W., and Taylor, S. (Eds.). (2011). *Handbook of African American Health: Social and Behavioral Interventions*. New York: Springer Science and Business Media.

Leone, J., Mostow, J., Hackney, D., Gokhale, P., Janata, J., and Greenfield, M. (2016). Obstetrician attitudes, experience, and knowledge of planned home birth: An exploratory study. *Birth, 43*(3), pp. 220–225.

Li, Q., Jenkins, D.D., and Kinsman, S.L. (2017). Birth settings and the validation of neonatal seizures recorded in birth certificates compared to Medicaid claims and hospital discharge abstracts among live births in South Carolina, 1996–2013. *Maternal and Child Health Journal, 21*(5), pp. 1047–1054.

Likis, F.E., King, T.L., Murphy, P.A., and Swett, B. (2018). Intentional inconsistency as gender-neutral language evolves. *Journal of Midwifery and Women's Health, 63*(2), pp. 155–156.

Lima, S.A.M., El Dib, R.P., Rodrigues, M.R.K., Ferraz, G.A.R., Molina, A.C., Neto, C.A.P., Ferraz de Lima, M.A., and Rudge, M.V.C. (2018). Is the risk of low birth weight or preterm labor greater when maternal stress is experienced during pregnancy? A systematic review and meta-analysis of cohort studies. *PLOS One, 13*(7), p. e0200594.

Lindgren, H., and Erlandsson, K. (2010). Women's experiences of empowerment in a planned home birth: A Swedish population-based study. *Birth, 37*(4), pp. 309–317.

Lindgren, H.E., Rådestad, I.J., Christensson, K., and Hildingsson, I.M. (2008). Outcome of planned home births compared to hospital births in Sweden between 1992 and 2004: A population-based register study. *Acta Obstetricia et Gynecologica Scandinavica, 87*(7), pp. 751–759.

Lipkind, H.S., Zuckerwise, L.C., Bragan Turner, E., Collins, J.J., Campbell, K.H., Reddy, U.M., Illuzi, J.L., and Merriam, A.A. (2019). Severe maternal morbidity during delivery hospitalization in a large international administrative database, 2008–2013: A retrospective cohort. *British Journal of Obstetrics and Gynaecology, 126*(10), pp. 1223–1230.

Little, M., Shah, R., Vermeulen, M.J., Gorman, A., Dzendoletas, D., and Ray, J.G. (2005). Adverse perinatal outcomes associated with homelessness and substance use in pregnancy. *Canadian Medical Association Journal, 173*(6), pp. 615–618.

Livingston, G. (2016). *Births Outside Marriage Decline for Immigrant Women*. Pew Research Center. Available: https://www.pewsocialtrends.org/2016/10/26/births-outside-of-marriage-decline-for-immigrant-women.

Lobel, M., Dunkel-Schetter, C., and Scrimshaw, S.C. (1992). Prenatal maternal stress and prematurity: A prospective study of socioeconomically disadvantaged women. *Health Psychology, 11*(1), p. 32.

Lothian, J.A. (2013). Being safe: making the decision to have a planned home birth in the United States. *The Journal of Clinical Ethics, 24*(3), 266–275.

Lu, M.C., and Halfon, N. (2003). Racial and ethnic disparities in birth outcomes: A life-course perspective. *Maternal and Child Health Journal, 7*(1), pp. 13–30.

Lucero, R.J., Lake, E.T., and Aiken, L.H. (2010). Nursing care quality and adverse events in U.S. hospitals. *Journal of Clinical Nursing, 19*(15–16), pp. 2185–2195.

Lundeen, E.A., Park, S., Pan, L., O'Toole, T., Matthews, K., and Blanck, H.M. (2018). Obesity prevalence among adults living in metropolitan and nonmetropolitan counties—United States, 2016. *Morbidity and Mortality Weekly Report, 67*, pp. 653–658.

Lundsberg, L.S., Illuzzi, J.L., Gariepy, A.M., Sheth, S.S., Pettker, C.M., Lee, H.C., Lipkind, H.S., and Xu, X. (2017). Variation in hospital intrapartum practices and association with cesarean rate. *Journal of Obstetric, Gynecologic and Neonatal Nursing, 46*(1), pp. 5–17.

Luntz, F. (2007). *Words That Work: It's Not What You Say, It's What People Hear.* New York: Hyperion Books.

Lyerly, A. (2013). *A Good Birth: Finding the Positive and Profound in Your Childbirth Experience.* New York, NY: Penguin Random House.

Lyndon, A., Johnson, M.C., Bingham, D., Napolitano, P.G., Joseph, G., Maxfield, D.G., and O'Keeffe, D.F. (2015). Transforming communication and safety culture in intrapartum care: A multi-organization blueprint. *Journal of Obstetric, Gynecologic and Neonatal Nursing, 44*(3), pp. 341–349.

Lyndon, A., Simpson, K.R., and Spetz, J. (2017). Thematic analysis of U.S. stakeholder views on the influence of labour nurses' care on birth outcomes. *BMJ Quality and Safety, 26*(10), pp. 824–831.

Lyndon, A., Malana, J., Hedli, L. C., Sherman, J., and Lee, H. C. (2018). Thematic analysis of women's perspectives on the meaning of safety during hospital-based birth. *Journal of Obstetric, Gynecologic and Neonatal Nursing, 47*(3), pp. 324–332.

MacDorman, M.F., and Declercq, E. (2016). Trends and characteristics of United States out-of-hospital births 2004–2014: New information on risk status and access to care. *Birth, 43*(2), pp. 116–24.

MacDorman, M.F., and Declercq, E. (2019). Trends and state variations in out-of-hospital births in the United States, 2004–2017. *Birth, 46*(2), pp. 279–288.

MacKinnon, D.P. (2008). *An Introduction to Statistical Mediation Analysis.* New York: Lawrence Erlbaum Associates.

Macpherson, I., Roqué-Sánchez, M.V., Legget, F.O., Fuertes, F., and Segarra, I. (2016). A systematic review of the relationship factor between women and health professionals within the multivariant analysis of maternal satisfaction. *Midwifery, 41*, pp. 68–78.

Main, E.K., Morton, C.H., Hopkins, D., Giuliani, G., Melsop, K., and Gould, J.B. (2011). Cesarean deliveries, outcomes, and opportunities for change in California: Toward a public agenda for maternity care safety and quality. *California Medical Quality Care Collaborative White Paper.* Available: https://www.cmqcc.org/resource/cesarean-deliveries-outcomes-and-opportunities-change-california-toward-public-agenda.

Main, E.K., Cape, V., Abreo, A., Vasher, J., Woods, A., Carpenter, A., and Gould, J.B. (2017). Reduction of severe maternal morbidity from hemorrhage using a state perinatal quality collaborative. *American Journal of Obstetrics and Gynecology, 216*(3), pp. 298–e1.

Main, E.K., Markow, C., and Gould, J. (2018). Addressing maternal mortality and morbidity in California through public-private partnerships. *Health Affairs, 37*(9), pp. 1484–1493.

Main, E.K., Chang, S.C., Cape, V., Sakowski, C., Smith, H., and Vasher, J. (2019). Safety assessment of a large-scale improvement collaborative to reduce nulliparous cesarean delivery rates. *Obstetrics and Gynecology, 133*(4), pp. 613–623.

Malloy, M.H. (2010). Infant outcomes of certified nurse midwife attended home births: United States 2000 to 2004. *Journal of Perinatology, 30*(9), pp. 622–627.

Manojlovich, M., Kerr, M., Davies, B., Squires, J., Mallick, R., and Rodger, G.L. (2014). Achieving a climate for patient safety by focusing on relationships. *International Journal for Quality in Health Care, 26*(6), pp. 579–584.

Maqbool, N., Ault, M., and Viveiros, J. (2015). *The Impacts of Affordable Housing on Health: A Research Summary.* Center for Housing Policy. Available: https://www.rupco.org/wp-content/uploads/pdfs/The-Impacts-of-Affordable-Housing-on-Health-CenterforHousingPolicy-Maqbool.etal.pdf.

March of Dimes. (2018a). *Nowhere to Go: Maternity Care Deserts Across the U.S.* Available: https://www.marchofdimes.org/materials/Nowhere_to_Go_Final.pdf.

March of Dimes. (2018b). *Low Birthweight.* Available: https://www.marchofdimes.org/complications/low-birthweight.aspx.

Markow, C., and Main, E.K. (2019). Creating change at scale: Quality improvement strategies used by the California Maternal Quality Care Collaborative. *Obstetrics and Gynecology Clinics, 46*(2), pp. 317–328.

Marmot, M., Allen, J., and Goldblatt, P. (2010). A social movement, based on evidence, to reduce inequalities in health. *Social Science and Medicine, 71*(7), pp. 1254–1258.

Martin, J.A., Wilson, E.C., Osterman, M.J., Saadi, E.W., Sutton, S.R., and Hamilton, B.E. (2013). Assessing the quality of medical and health data from the 2003 birth certificate revision: Results from two states. *National Vital Statistics Reports, 62*(3).

Martin, J.A., Hamilton, B.E., Osterman, M.J., Driscoll, A.K., and Drake, P. (2018a). Births: Final data for 2016. *National Vital Statistics Reports, 67*(1). Available: https://www.cdc.gov/nchs/data/nvsr/nvsr67/nvsr67_01.pdf.

Martin, J.A., Hamilton, B.E., Osterman, M.J., and Driscoll, A.K. (2018b). Births: Final data for 2017. *National Vital Statistics Reports, 67*(8). Available: https://www.cdc.gov/nchs/data/nvsr/nvsr67/nvsr67_08-508.pdf.

Martin, J.A., Hamilton, B.E., Osterman, M.J., and Driscoll, A.K. (2019). Births: Final data for 2018. *National Vital Statistics Reports, 68*(13). Available: https://www.cdc.gov/nchs/data/nvsr/nvsr68/nvsr68_13-508.pdf.

Mathews, T.J., and Hamilton, B.E. (2016). Mean age of mothers is on the rise: United States, 2000–2014. *National Center for Health Statistics Data Brief, 232.*

Matthews, R., and Callister, L.C. (2004). Childbearing women's perceptions of nursing care that promotes dignity. *Journal of Obstetric, Gynecologic, and Neonatal Nursing, 33*(4), pp. 498–507.

Mazul, M.C., Ward, T.C.S., and Ngui, E.M. (2017). Anatomy of good prenatal care: Perspectives of low income African-American women on barriers and facilitators to prenatal care. *Journal of Racial and Ethnic Health Disparities, 4*(1), pp. 79–86.

McCormack, S.A., and Best, B.M. (2014). Obstetric pharmacokinetic dosing studies are urgently needed. *Frontiers in Pediatrics, 2,* p. 9.

McCullough, L.B., and Chervenak, F.A. (1994). *Ethics in Obstetrics and Gynecology.* New York: Oxford University Press, Inc.

McEwen, B.S., and Seeman, T. (1999). Protective and damaging effects of mediators of stress: Elaborating and testing the concepts of allostasis and allostatic load. *Annals of the New York Academy of Sciences, 896*(1), pp. 30–47.

McLaren, L. (2007). Socioeconomic status and obesity. *Epidemiologic Reviews, 29*(1), pp. 29–48.

McLemore, M.R. (2019). *To Prevent Women from Dying in Childbirth, First Stop Blaming Them*. Available: https://www.scientificamerican.com/article/to-prevent-women-from-dying-in-childbirth-first-stop-blaming-them.

McLemore, M.R., Altman, M.R., Cooper, N., Williams, S., Rand, L., and Franck, L. (2018). Health care experiences of pregnant, birthing and postnatal women of color at risk for preterm birth. *Social Science and Medicine (1982)*, 201, pp. 127–135.

Meader, N., King, K., Llewellyn, A., Norman, G., Brown, J., Rodgers, M., Moe-Byrne, T., Higgins, J.P., Snowden, A., and Stewart, G. (2014). A checklist designed to aid consistency and reproducibility of GRADE assessments: Development and pilot validation. *Systematic Review*, 3(82)

Menard, M.K., Main, E.K., and Currigan, S.M. (2014). Executive summary of the reVITALize initiative: Standardizing obstetric data definitions. *Obstetrics and Gynecology*, 124(1), p. 150–153.

Menard, M.K., Kilpatrick, S., Saade, G., Hollier, L.M., Joseph Jr, G.F., Barfield, W., Callaghan, W., Jennings, J., Conry, J. and American College of Obstetricians and Gynecologists. (2015). Levels of maternal care. *American Journal of Obstetrics and Gynecology*, 212(3), p. 259–271.

Mercer, S. L., DeVinney, B.J., Fine, L.J., Green, L.W., and Dougherty, D. (2007). Study designs for effectiveness and translation research: Identifying trade-offs. *American Journal of Preventive Medicine*, 33(2), pp. 139–154.

Meyerson, C. (2019). Every Black Woman Deserves a Doula. *New York Intelligencer, March 5*. Available: https://nymag.com/intelligencer/2019/03/new-yorks-medicaid-reimbursement-plan-for-doulas.html.

Midwifery Education Accreditation Council. (2019). *School Directory*. Available: http://meacschools.org/member-school-directory.

Miller, A.C., and Shriver, T.E. (2012). Women's childbirth preferences and practices in the United States. *Social Science and Medicine*, 75(4), pp. 709–716.

Miller, S., and Lalonde, A. (2015). The global epidemic of abuse and disrespect during childbirth: History, evidence, interventions, and FIGO's mother–baby friendly birthing facilities initiative. *International Journal of Gynecology and Obstetrics*, 131, pp. S49–S52.

Miller, S., Abalos, E., Chamillard, M., Ciapponi, A., Colaci, D., Comandé, D., Diaz, V., Geller, S., Hanson, C., Langer, A. and Manuelli, V. (2016). Beyond too little, too late and too much, too soon: A pathway towards evidence-based, respectful maternity care worldwide. *The Lancet*, 388(10056), pp. 2176–2192.

Milliman, Inc. (2019). *Patient-Centered Medical Home: Developing the Business Case from a Practice Perspective*. Available: https://www.ncqa.org/wp-content/uploads/2019/06/06142019_WhitePaper_Milliman_BusinessCasePCMH_Final.pdf.

Moaddab, A., Dildy, G.A., Brown, H.L., Bateni, Z.H., Belfort, M.A., Sangi-Haghpeykar, H., and Clark, S.L. (2018). Health care disparity and pregnancy-related mortality in the United States, 2005–2014. *Obstetrics and Gynecology*, 131(4), pp. 707–712.

Montagne, R. (2018). *For Every Woman Who Dies in Childbirth in the U.S., 70 More Come Close*. Available: https://www.npr.org/2018/05/10/607782992/for-every-woman-who-dies-in-childbirth-in-the-u-s-70-more-come-close.

Morris, T., and Schulman, M. (2014). Race inequality in epidural use and regional anesthesia failure in labor and birth: An examination of women's experience. *Sexual and Reproductive Healthcare*, 5(4), pp. 188–194.

Mueller, N.T., Bakacs, E., Combellick, J., Grigoryan, Z., and Dominguez-Bello, M.G. (2015). The infant microbiome development: Mom matters. *Trends in Molecular Medicine*, 21(2), pp. 109–117.

Mulherin, K., Miller, Y.D., Barlow, F.K., Diedrichs, P.C., and Thompson, R. (2013). Weight stigma in maternity care: Women's experiences and care providers' attitudes. *BMC Pregnancy and Childbirth, 13*, p. 19.

Mullings, L., and Wali, A. (2001). *Stress and Resilience: The Social Context of Reproduction in Central Harlem.* New York: Springer Science and Business Media.

National Academies of Sciences, Engineering, and Medicine. (2015). *Health Literacy: Past, Present, and Future: Workshop Summary.* Washington, DC: The National Academies Press. https://doi.org/10.17226/21714.

National Academies of Sciences, Engineering, and Medicine. (2017). *Communities in Action: Pathways to Health Equity.* Washington, DC: The National Academies Press. https://doi.org/10.17226/24624.

National Academies of Sciences, Engineering, and Medicine. (2018). *Advancing Obesity Solutions Through Investments in the Built Environment: Proceedings of a Workshop.* Washington, DC: The National Academies Press. https://doi.org/10.17226/25074.

National Academies of Sciences, Engineering, and Medicine. (2019). *Vibrant and Healthy Kids: Aligning Science, Practice, and Policy to Advance Health Equity.* Washington, DC: The National Academies Press. https://doi.org/10.17226/25466.

National Association of Certified Professional Midwives. (2014). *Who are CPMs.* Available: https://nacpm.org/about-cpms/who-are-cpms.

National Association of Certified Professional Midwives. (2019). *Legal Recognition of CPMs.* Available: https://nacpm.org/about-cpms/who-are-cpms/legal-recognition-of-cpms.

National Committee for Quality Assurance. (2019). *How NCQA Patient-Centered Medical Homes Address Disparities.* Available: https://www.ncqa.org/white-papers/how-ncqa-patient-centered-medical-homes-address-disparities.

National Immigration Law Center. (2010*). Facts about Federal Funding for States to Provide Health to Immigrant Children and Pregnant Women.* Available: https://www.nilc.org/issues/health-care/federal-funding-for-states-to-provide-health-coverage.

National Institute for Health and Care Excellence. (2017). *Intrapartum Care for Healthy Women and Babies.* Available: https://www.nice.org.uk/guidance/cg190.

National Institute of Diabetes and Digestive and Kidney Diseases. (2016). *Risk Factors for Type 2 Diabetes.* Available: https://www.niddk.nih.gov/health-information/diabetes/overview/risk-factors-type-2-diabetes.

National Institute of Diabetes and Digestive and Kidney Diseases. (2017). *Type 1 Diabetes.* Available: https://www.niddk.nih.gov/health-information/diabetes/overview/what-is-diabetes/type-1-diabetes.

National Institute on Drug Abuse. (2018). *Substance Use While Pregnant and Breastfeeding.* Available: https://www.drugabuse.gov/publications/substance-use-in-women/substance-use-while-pregnant-breastfeeding.

National Institutes of Health. (n.d.). *Sex and Gender.* Available: https://orwh.od.nih.gov/sex-gender.

National Institutes of Health. (2019). *Genetics Home Reference: Preeclampsia.* Available: https://ghr.nlm.nih.gov/condition/preeclampsia#sourcesforpage.

National Institutes of Health Consensus Development Conference Panel (2010). Vaginal birth after cesarean: New insights March 8–10, 2010. *Obstetrics and Gynecology, 115*(6), pp. 1279–1295.

National Partnership for Women & Families. (2018a). *Raising Expectations: A State-by-State Analysis of Laws That Help Working Family Caregivers.* Available: https://www.nationalpartnership.org/our-work/resources/economic-justice/raising-expectations-2018.pdf.

National Partnership for Women & Families. (2018b). *Meeting the Promise of Paid Leave: Best Practices in State Paid Leave Implementation.* Available: https://www. nationalpartnership.org/our-work/resources/economic-justice/paid-leave/new-and-expanded-employer-paid-family-leave-policies.pdfhttps://www.nationalpartnership.org/our-work/resources/economic-justice/paid-leave/meeting-the-promise-of-paid-leave.pdf.

National Partnership for Women & Families. (2018c). *Paid Family and Medical Leave: A Racial Justice Issue—And Opportunity.* Available: https://www.nationalpartnership.org/our-work/resources/economic-justice/paid-leave/paid-family-and-medical-leave-racial-justice-issue-and-opportunity.pdf.

National Partnership for Women & Families. (2019a). *Tackling Maternal Health Disparities: A Look at Four Local Organizations with Innovative Approaches.* Available: http://www. nationalpartnership.org/our-work/resources/health-care/maternity/tackling-maternal-health-disparities-a-look-at-four-local-organizations-with-innovative-approaches.pdf.

National Partnership for Women & Families. (2019b). *America's Women and the Wage Gap.* Available: https://www.nationalpartnership.org/our-work/resources/economic-justice/fair-pay/americas-women-and-the-wage-gap.pdf.

National Research Council. (2006). *Letter Report to Sir Michael Marmot on the Social Determinants of Health.* Washington, DC: The National Academies Press.

National Research Council. (2014). *The Growth of Incarceration in the United States: Exploring Causes and Consequences.* Washington, DC: The National Academies Press.

Neal, J.L., Carlson, N.S., Phillippi, J.C., Tilden, E.L., Smith, D.C., Breman, R.B., Dietrich, M.S. and Lowe, N.K. (2019). Midwifery presence in United States medical centers and labor care and birth outcomes among low-risk nulliparous women: A Consortium on Safe Labor study. *Birth*, 46(3), pp. 475–486.

Nebraska Legislature. (2007). *Nebraska Revised Statute 38-613.* Available: https://nebraskalegislature.gov/laws/statutes.php?statute=38-613.

New York State. (2019). *New York State Doula Pilot Program.* Available: https://www.health.ny.gov/health_care/medicaid/redesign/doulapilot/pilot.htm#enrollment.

National Heart, Lung, and Blood Institute. (n.d.). *Classification of Overweight and Obesity by BMI, Waist Circumference, and Associated Disease Risks.* Available: https://www.nhlbi.nih.gov/health/educational/lose_wt/BMI/bmi_dis.htm.

Nielsen-Bohlman, L., Panzer, A.M., Kindig, D.A., Scrimshaw, S.C. (2018). Cultural influences: The bottom line. *Teaching Strategies for Health Education and Health Promotion: The Art of Teaching Patients, Families and Communities.* Sudbury, MA: Jones and Bartlett.

Nijagal, M.A., Shah, N.T., and Levin-Scherz, J. (2018). Both patients and maternity care providers can benefit from payment reform: Four steps to prepare. *American Journal of Obstetrics and Gynecology*, 218(4), pp. 411–e1.

North American Registry of Midwives. (n.d.). *History of the Development of the CPM.* Available: http://narm.org/certification/history-of-the- development-of-the-cpm.

North American Registry of Midwives. (2019). *Certified Professional Midwife (CPM): Candidate Information Booklet (CIB).* Available: http://narm.org/pdffiles/CIB.pdf.

Notah Begay III Foundation. (2015). *Native Strong: The Social Determinants of Health of Type 2 Diabetes and Obesity.* Available: http://www.nb3foundation.org/assets/docs/2015-10-20-SDOH%20Full%20Summary%20FINAL.pdf.

Novak, N.L., Geronimus, A.T., and Martinez-Cardoso, A.M. (2017). Change in birth outcomes among infants born to Latina mothers after a major immigration raid. *International Journal of Epidemiology*, 46(3), pp. 839–849.

Nurse-Family Partnership. (2019). *Nurse-Family Partnership: Reduces Maternal and Child Mortality.* Available: https://www.nursefamilypartnership.org/wp-content/uploads/2019/01/Maternal-and-Child-Mortality.pdf.

Nuru-Jeter, A., Williams, C.T., and LaVeist, T.A. (2008). A methodological note on modeling the effects of race: The case of psychological distress. *Stress and Health: Journal of the International Society for the Investigation of Stress*, 24(5), pp. 337–350.

O'Cathian, A. (2009). Mixed methods research in the health sciences: A quiet revolution. *Journal of Mixed Methods Research*, 3(1), pp. 3–6.

O'Connor, A. (2001). Using patient decision aids to promote evidence-based decision making. *BMJ Evidence-Based Medicine*, 6(4), pp.100–102.

O'Connor, A.M., Rostom, A., Fiset, V., Tetroe, J., Entwistle, V., Llewellyn-Thomas, H., Holmes-Rovner, M., Barry, M., and Jones, J. (1999). Decision aids for patients facing health treatment or screening decisions: Systematic review. *The BMJ*, 319(7212), pp. 731–734.

Office for National Statistics. (2019). *Live Births and Stillbirths by Area of Usual Residence of Mother, Numbers, Total Fertility Rates and Stillbirths Rates, 2017*. Available: https://www.ons.gov.uk/peoplepopulationandcommunity/birthsdeathsandmarriages/livebirths/bulletins/birthcharacteristicsinenglandandwales/2017.

Office of Disease Prevention and Health Promotion. (2019). *MICH-7: Reduce Cesarean Births among Low-Risk Women with No Prior Cesarean Births*. Available: https://www.healthypeople.gov/2020/topics-objectives/topic/maternal-infant-and-child-health/objectives.

Office of the Assistant Secretary for Planning and Evaluation. (2014). *Work-Family Supports for Low-Income Families: Key Research Findings and Policy Trends*. Available: https://aspe.hhs.gov/pdf-report/work-family-supports-low-income-families-key-research-findings-and-policy-trends.

Office of the Secretary of Defense. (2019). *Maternal and Infant Mortality Rates in the Military Health System*. Requested by: Conference Report 115-874, Page 861 to Accompany the John S. McCain National Defense Authorization Act for Fiscal Year 2019 (Public Law 115-232).

Ogburn, J.A.T., Espey, F., Pierce-Bulger, M., Waxman, A., Allee, L., Haffner, W.H., and Howe, J. (2012). Midwives and obstetrician-gynecologists collaborating for Native American women's health. *Obstetrics and Gynecology Clinics*, 39(3), pp. 359–366.

Øian, P., Askeland, O.M., Engelund, I.E., Roland, B., and Ebbing, M. (2018). Births in Norwegian midwife-led birth units 2008–10: A population-based study. *Tidsskrift for den Norske Laegeforening: Tidsskrift for Praktisk Medicin, Ny Raekke*, 138(10).

Okafor, I.I., Ugwu, E.O., and Obi, S.N. (2015). Disrespect and abuse during facility-based childbirth in a low-income country. *International Journal of Gynecology and Obstetrics*, 128(2), pp. 110–113.

Oliveira, F.C., Surita, F.G., e Silva, J.L.P., Cecatti, J.G., Parpinelli, M.A., Haddad, S.M., Costa, M.L., Pacagnella, R.C., Sousa, M.H., and Souza, J.P. (2014). Severe maternal morbidity and maternal near miss in the extremes of reproductive age: results from a national cross-sectional multicenter study. *BMC Pregnancy and Childbirth*, 14(1), p. 77.

Olson, R., Garite, T.J., Fishman, A., and Andress, I.F. (2012). Obstetrician/gynecologist hospitalists: Can we improve safety and outcomes for patients and hospitals and improve lifestyle for physicians? *American Journal of Obstetrics and Gynecology*, 207(2), pp. 81–86.

Oparah, J.C., and Bonaparte, A.D. (Eds.). (2015) *Birthing Justice: Black Women, Pregnancy, and Childbirth*. New York: Routledge.

Oparah, J.C., Arega, H., Hudson, D., Jones, L., Of Black Women Birthing Justice, and Oseguera, T. (2018). *Battling over Birth: Black Women and the Maternal Health Care Crisis*. Available: DOI: 10.1891/2158-0782.9.3.150.

Organisation for Economic Co-operation and Development. (2018). *Spending on Health: Latest Trends*. Available: http://www.oecd.org/health/health-systems/Health-Spending-Latest-Trends-Brief.pdf.

Organisation for Economic Co-Operation and Development. (2019). *OECD Data*. Available: https://stats.oecd.org.

Oregon Health Authority. (2015). *Coverage Guidance: Planned Out-of-Hospital Birth*. Available: https://www.oregon.gov/oha/HPA/DSI-HERC/EvidenceBasedReports/Planned-out-of-hospital-birth-11-12-15.pdf.

Ozimek, J.A., Eddins, R.M., Greene, N., Karagyozyan, D., Pak, S., Wong, M., Aakowski, M., and Kilpatrick, S.J. (2015). Opportunities for improvement in care among women with severe maternal morbidity. *American Journal of Obstetrics and Gynecology*, 215(4), pp. 509.e1–509.e6.

Pacific Business Group on Health. (2015). *Case Study: Maternity Payment and Care Redesign Pilot*. Available: http://www.pbgh.org/storage/documents/TMC_Case_Study_Oct_2015.pdf.

Patterson, J., Foureur, M., and Skinner, J. (2017). Remote rural women's choice of birthplace and transfer experiences in rural Otago and Southland New Zealand. *Midwifery*, 52, pp. 49–56.

Pearlstein, T. (2015). Depression during pregnancy: Best practice and research. *Clinical Obstetrics and Gynaecology*, 29(5), pp. 754–764.

Perined. (2019). *Perinatal Care in the Netherlands 2017*. Available: http://www.perinatreg-data.nl/JB2017/Jaarboek2017.html.

Petersen, E.E., Davis, N.L., Goodman, D., Cox, S., Mayes, N., Johnston, E., Syverson, C., Seed, K., Shapiro-Mendoza, C.K., Callaghan, W.M. and Barfield, W. (2019). Vital signs: Pregnancy-related deaths, United States, 2011–2015, and strategies for prevention, 13 States, 2013–2017. *Morbidity and Mortality Weekly Report*, 68(18), p. 423.

Petrou, S. (2019). Health economic aspects of late preterm and early term birth. *Seminars in Fetal and Neonatal Medicine*, 24(1), pp. 18–26.

Petrou, S., Yiu, H.H., and Kwon, J. (2019). Economic consequences of preterm birth: A systematic review of the recent literature (2009–2017). *Archives of Disease in Childhood*, 104(5), pp. 456–465.

Phelan, S.M., Puhl, R.M., Burke, S.E., Hardeman, R., Dovidio, J. F., Nelson, D. B., Przedworski, J., Burges, D.J., Yeazel, M.W., and van Ryn, M. (2015). The mixed impact of medical school on medical students' implicit and explicit weight bias. *Medical Education*, 49(10), pp. 983–992.

Phillippi, J.C., Danhausen, K., Alliman, J., and Phillippi, D. (2018) Neonatal outcomes in the birth center setting: A systematic review. *Journal of Midwifery and Women's Health*, 63(1), pp. 68–89.

Podulka, J., Stranges, E., and Steiner, C. (2011). Hospitalizations related to childbirth, 2008. *H-CUP Statistical Brief, 110*. Available: https://www.hcup-us.ahrq.gov/reports/statbriefs/sb110.jsp.

Ponce, N.A., Lucia, L., and Shimada, T. (2018). *Proposed Changes to Immigration Rules Would Cost California Jobs, Harm Public Health*. Available: https://healthpolicy.ucla.edu/publications/search/pages/detail.aspx?PubID=1789.

Pont, S. J., Puhl, R., Cook, S.R., and Slusser, W. (2017). Stigma experienced by children and adolescents with obesity. *Pediatrics*, 140(6), p. e20173034.

Popova, S., Lange, S., Probst, C., Gmel, G., and Rehm, J. (2017). Estimation of national, regional, and global prevalence of alcohol use during pregnancy and fetal alcohol syndrome: A systematic review and meta-analysis. *The Lancet*, 5(3), pp. e290–e299.

Porter, M., Van Teijlingen, E., Chi Ying Yip, L., and Bhattacharya, S. (2007). Satisfaction with cesarean section: Qualitative analysis of open-ended questions in a large postal survey. *Birth*, 34(2), pp. 148–154.

Porter, M.E., and Kaplan, R.S. (2016). How to pay for health care. *Harvard Business Review*, 94(7–8), pp. 88–98.

Prather, C., Fuller, T.R., Marshall, K.J., and Jeffries IV, W.L. (2016). The impact of racism on the sexual and reproductive health of African American women. *Journal of Women's Health*, 25(7), pp. 664–671.

Prather, C., Fuller, T.R., Jeffries IV, W.L., Marshall, K.J, Howell, A.V., Belyue-Umole, A., and King, W. (2018). Racism, African American women, and their sexual and reproductive health: A review of historical and contemporary evidence and implications for health equity. *Health Equity*, 2(1), pp. 249–259.

Presser, H.B. (2003). Race-ethnic and gender differences in nonstandard work shifts. *Work and Occupations*, 30(4), pp. 412–439.

Provenzi, L., Guida, E., and Montirosso, R. (2018). Preterm behavioral epigenetics: A systematic review. *Neuroscience and Biobehavioral Reviews*, 84, pp. 262–271.

Puhl, R., and Brownell, K.D. (2001). Bias, discrimination, and obesity. *Obesity Research*, 9(12), pp. 788–805.

Puhl, R., and Latner, J. (2008). Weight bias: New science on an significant social problem. *Obesity*, 16(S2), p. S1.

Quinn, M. (2018). *To Reduce Fatal Pregnancies, Some States Look to Doulas*. Available: https://www.governing.com/topics/health-human-services/gov-doula-medicaid-new-york-2019-pregnant.html.

Radin, T.G., Harmon, J.S., and Hanson, D.A. (1993). Nurses' care during labor: Its effect on the cesarean birth rate of healthy, nulliparous women. *Birth*, 20(1), pp. 14–21.

Rainey, E., Simonsen, S., Stanford, J., Shoaf, K., and Baayd, J. (2017). Utah obstetricians' opinions of planned home birth and conflicting NICE/ACOG guidelines: A qualitative study. *Birth*, 44(2), pp. 137–144.

Raisler, J., and Kennedy, H. (2005). Midwifery care of poor and vulnerable women, 1925–2003. *Journal of Midwifery and Women's Health*, 50(2), pp. 113–121.

Rakover, J. (2016). *The Maternity Medical Home: The Chassis for a More Holistic Model of Pregnancy Care?* Available: http://www.ihi.org/communities/blogs/_layouts/15/ihi/community/blog/itemview.aspx?List=7d1126ec-8f63-4a3b-9926-c44ea3036813&ID=222.

Ramraj, C., Pulver, A., and Siddiqi, A. (2015). Intergenerational transmission of the healthy immigrant effect (HIE) through birth weight: A systematic review and meta-analysis. *Social Science and Medicine*, 146, pp. 29–40.

Ranji, U., Gomez, I., and Salgonicoff, A. (2019). *Expanding Postpartum Medicaid Coverage: Issue Brief*. San Francisco: Henry J. Kaiser Family Foundation. Available: https://www.kff.org/womens-health-policy/issue-brief/expanding-postpartum-medicaid-coverage.

Ranjit, A., Jiang, W., Zhan, T., Kimsey, L., Staat, B., Witkop, C.T., Little, S.E., Haider, A.H. and Robinson, J.N. (2017). Intrapartum obstetric care in the United States military: Comparison of military and civilian care systems within TRICARE. *Birth*, 44(4), pp. 337–344.

Rathke, L. (2011). *Home Births to Be Insured in Vermont*. Available: http://www.nbcnews.com/id/43094589/ns/health-health_care/t/home-births-be-insured-vermont/#.XXppAy5KiHt.

Rayburn, W.F. (2017). *The Obstetrician-Gynecologist Workforce in the United States*. Washington DC: American Congress of Obstetricians and Gynecologists.

Rayburn, W.F., Petterson, S.M., and Phillips, R.L. (2014). Trends in family physicians performing deliveries, 2003–2010. *Birth*, 41(1), pp. 26–32.

Recio-Saucedo, A., Dall'Ora, C., Maruotti, A., Ball, J., Briggs, J., Meredith, P., Redfern, O.C., Kovacs, C., Prytherch, D., Smith, G.B., and Griffiths, P. (2018). What impact does nursing care left undone have on patient outcomes? Review of the literature. *Journal of Clinical Nursing*, 27(11–12), pp. 2248–2259.

Reed, R., Sharman, R., and Inglis, C. (2017). Women's descriptions of childbirth trauma relating to care provider actions and interactions. *BMC Pregnancy and Childbirth*, 17(1), p. 21.

Reszel, J., Sidney, D., Peterson, W.E., Darling, E.K., Van Wagner, V., Soderstrom, B., Rogers, J., Graves, E., Khan, B. and Sprague, A.E. (2018). The integration of Ontario birth centers into existing maternal-newborn services: Health care provider experiences. *Journal of Midwifery and Women's Health, 63*(5), pp. 541–549.

Review to Action. (2018). *Report from Nine Maternal Mortality Review Committees.* Available: http://reviewtoaction.org/sites/default/files/national-portal-material/Reportpercent-20frompercent20Ninepercent20MMRCspercent20final_0.pdf.

Richards, R., Merrill, R.M., and Baksh, L. (2011). Health behaviors and infant health outcomes in homeless pregnant women in the United States. *Pediatrics, 128*(3), pp. 438–446.

Rickert, J. (2012). *Patient-Centered Care: What It Means and How to Get There.* Available: https://www.healthaffairs.org/do/10.1377/hblog20120124.016506/full.

Roberts, J.M., August, P.A., Bakris, G., Barton, J.R., Bernstein, I.M., Druzin, M., Gaiser, R.R., Granger, J.P., Jeyabalan, A., Johnson, D.D., Karumanchi, S.A., Lindheimer, M., Owents, M.Y., Saade, G.R., Sibai, B.M., Spong, C.Y., Tsigas, E., Joseph, O'Reilly, N., Politzer, A., Son, S., and Ngaiza, K. (2013). Hypertension in pregnancy: Executive summary. *Obstetrics and Gynecology, 122*(5), pp. 1122–1131.

Romero, L. (2016). Reduced disparities in birth rates among teens aged 15–19 years—United States, 2006–2007 and 2013–2014. *Morbidity and Mortality Weekly Report, 65.*

Roome, S., Hartz, D., Tracy, S., and Welsh, A.W. (2016). Why such differing stances? A review of position statements on home birth from professional colleges. *British Journal of Obstetrics and Gynaecology, 123*(3), pp. 376–382.

Rosenthal, E. (2013). American way of birth, costliest in the world. *The New York Times.* Available: https://www.nytimes.com/2013/07/01/health/american-way-of-birth-costliest-in-the-world.html.

Ross, L., and Solinger, R. (2017). *Reproductive Justice: An Introduction (Vol. 1).* Oakland: University of California Press.

Ross, L.J. (2017). Reproductive justice as intersectional feminist activism. *Souls, 19*(3), pp. 286–314.

Roth, C., Dent, S.A., Parfitt, S.E., Hering, S.L., and Bay, R.C. (2016). Randomized controlled trial of use of the peanut ball during labor. *The American Journal of Maternal/Child Nursing, 41*(3), pp. 140–146.

Rowe, R.E., Kurinczuk, J.J., Locock, L., and Fitzpatrick, R. (2012). Women's experience of transfer from midwifery unit to hospital obstetric unit during labour: A qualitative interview study. *BMC Pregnancy and Childbirth, 12*(1), p. 129.

Royal College of Obstetricians and Gynaecologists. (2017). Management of breech presentation. *British Journal of Obstetrics and Gynaecology, 124*(7), pp. e151–e177.

Rubin, L.P. (2016). Maternal and pediatric health and disease: Integrating biopsychosocial models and epigenetics. *Pediatric Research, 79*(1–2), pp. 127–135.

Sadler, M., Santos, M.J., Ruiz-Berdún, D., Rojas, G.L., Skoko, E., Gillen, P., and Clausen, J.A. (2016). Moving beyond disrespect and abuse: Addressing the structural dimensions of obstetric violence. *Reproductive Health Matters, 24*(47), pp. 47–55.

Sakala, C., Yang, Y.T., and Corry, M.P. (2013). Maternity care and liability: Pressing problems, substantive solutions. *Women's Health Issues, 23*(1), pp. e7–e13.

Sakala, C., Declercq, E., Turon, J.M., and Corry, M.P. (2018). *Listening to Mothers in California: A Population-Based Survey of Women's Childbearing Experiences, Full Survey Report.* Available: https://www.chcf.org/wp-content/uploads/2018/09/ListeningMothersCAFullSurveyReport2018.pdf.

Sandall, J., Devane, D., Soltani, H., Hatem, M., and Gates, S. (2010). Improving quality and safety in maternity care: The contribution of midwife-led care. *The Journal of Midwifery and Women's Health, 55*(3), pp. 255–261.

Sando, D., Ratcliffe, H., McDonald, K., Spiegelman, D., Lyatuu, G., Mwanyika-Sando, M., Emil, F., Wegner, M.N., Chalamilla, G., and Langer, A. (2016). The prevalence of disrespect and abuse during facility-based childbirth in urban Tanzania. *BMC Pregnancy and Childbirth*, 16(1), p. 236.

Scarf, V., Catling, C., Viney, R., and Homer, C. (2016). Costing alternative birth settings for women at low risk of complications: A systematic review. *PLOS One*, 11(2), p. e0149463.

Scarf, V. L., Rossiter, C., Vedam, S., Dahlen, H. G., Ellwood, D., Forster, D., Foureur, M.J., McLachlan, H., Oats, J., Sibbritt, D., Thornton, C., and Homer, C.S.E. (2018). Maternal and perinatal outcomes by planned place of birth among women with low-risk pregnancies in high-income countries: A systematic review and meta-analysis. *Midwifery*, 62, pp. 240–255.

Scheufele, D.A. (1999). Framing as a theory of media effects. *Journal of Communication*, 49(1), pp. 103–122.

Scheufele, D.A., and Tewksbury, D. (2006). Framing, agenda setting, and priming: The evolution of three media effects models. *Journal of Communication*, 57(1), pp. 9–20.

Schneider, P.D., Sabol, B.A., King, P.A.L., Caughey, A.B., and Borders, A.E. (2017). The hard work of improving outcomes for mothers and babies: Obstetric and perinatal quality improvement initiatives make a difference at the hospital, state, and national levels. *Clinics in Perinatology*, 44(3), pp. 511–528.

Schoendorf, K.C., and Branum, A.M. (2006). The use of United States vital statistics in perinatal and obstetric research. *American Journal of Obstetrics and Gynecology*, 194(4), pp. 911–915.

Schroeder, E., Petrou, S., Patel, N., Hollowell, J., Puddicombe, D., Redshaw, M., and Brocklehurst, P. (2012). Cost effectiveness of alternative planned places of birth in woman at low risk of complications: Evidence from the Birthplace in England National Prospective Cohort study. *The BMJ*, 344, p. e2292.

Schroeder, L., Patel, N., Keeler, M., Rocca-Ihenacho, L., and Macfarlane, A. (2017). The economic costs of intrapartum care in Tower Hamlets: A comparison between the cost of birth in a freestanding midwifery unit and hospital for women at low risk of obstetric complications. *Midwifery*, 45, pp. 28–35.

Schuit, E., Hukkelhoven, C.W.M., van der Goes, B.Y., Overbeeke, I., Moons, K.G., Mol, B.W., Groenwold, R.H., and Kwee, A. (2016). Risk indicators for referral during labor from community midwife to gynecologist: A prospective cohort study. *The Journal of Maternal-Fetal and Neonatal Medicine*, 29(20), pp. 3304–3311.

Schummers, L., Hutcheon, J.A., Bodnar, L.M., Lieberman, E., and Himes, K.P. (2015). Risk of adverse pregnancy outcomes by prepregnancy body mass index: A population-based study to inform prepregnancy weight loss counseling. *Obstetrics and Gynecology*, 125(1), pp. 133–143.

Schünemann, H. (Ed.). (2013). *The GRADE Handbook*. Cochrane Collaboration. Available: https://gdt.gradepro.org/app/handbook/handbook.html.

Scrimshaw, S.C. (2019). Science, health and cultural literacy in a rapidly changing communications landscape. *Proceedings of the National Academy of Sciences* 116 (16), pp. 7650–7655.

Seeman, T.E., Singer, B.H., Rowe, J.W., Horwitz, R.I., and McEwen, B.S. (1997). Price of adaptation—Allostatic load and its health consequences: MacArthur studies of successful aging. *Archives of Internal Medicine*, 157(19), pp. 2259–2268.

Seng, J.S., Oakley, D.J., Sampselle, C.M., Killion, C., Graham-Bermann, S., and Liberzon, I. (2001). Posttraumatic stress disorder and pregnancy complications. *Obstetrics and Gynecology*, 97(1), pp. 17–22.

Seng, J.S., Low, L.K., Sperlich, M., Ronis, D.L., and Liberzon, I. (2011). Post-traumatic stress disorder, child abuse history, birthweight and gestational age: A prospective cohort study. *British Journal of Obstetrics and Gynaecology, 118*(11), pp. 1329–1339.

Shah, N. (2015). A NICE Delivery—The cross-Atlantic divide over treatment intensity in childbirth. *New England Journal of Medicine, 372*(23), pp. 2181–2183.

Shah, N. (2018). Eroding access and quality of childbirth care in rural U.S. counties. *Journal of the American Medical Association, 319*(12), pp. 1203–1204.

Shakibazadeh, E., Namadian, M., Bohren, M.A., Vogel, J.P., Rashidian, A., Nogueira Pileggi, V., Madeira, S., Leathersich, S., Tunçalp, Ö., Oladapo, O.T. and Souza, J.P., and Gülmezoglu, A.M. (2018). Respectful care during childbirth in health facilities globally: A qualitative evidence synthesis. *British Journal of Obstetrics and Gynaecology, 125*(8), pp. 932–942.

Shaw, D., Guise, J.M., Shah, N., Gemzell-Danielsson, K., Joseph, K.S., Levy, B., Wong, F., Woodd, S., and Main, E.K. (2016). Drivers of maternity care in high-income countries: Can health systems support woman-centered care? *The Lancet, 388*(10057), pp. 2282–2295.

Sheppard, V.B., Zambrana, R.E., and O'Malley, A.S. (2004). Providing health care to low-income women: A matter of trust. *Family Practice, 21*(5), pp. 484–491.

Sigurdson, K., Morton, C., Mitchell, B., and Profit, J. (2018). Disparities in NICU quality of care: A qualitative study of family and clinician accounts. *Journal of Perinatology, 38*(5), p. 600.

Simpson, K.R., and Lyndon, A. (2017a). Labor nurses' views of their influence on cesarean birth. *The American Journal of Maternal/Child Nursing, 42*(2), pp. 81–87.

Simpson, K.R., and Lyndon, A. (2017b). Consequences of delayed, unfinished, or missed nursing care during labor and birth. *The Journal of Perinatal and Neonatal Nursing, 31*(1), pp. 3240.

Simpson, K.R., James, D.C., and Knox, G.E. (2006). Nurse-physician communication during labor and birth: Implications for patient safety. *Journal of Obstetric, Gynecologic and Neonatal Nursing, 35*(4), pp. 547–556.

Simpson, K.R., Lyndon, A., Wilson, J., and Ruhl, C. (2012). Nurses' perceptions of critical issues requiring consideration in the development of guidelines for professional registered nurse staffing for perinatal units. *Journal of Obstetric, Gynecologic and Neonatal Nursing, 41*(4), pp. 474–482.

Simpson, K.R., Lyndon, A., and Ruhl, C. (2016). Consequences of inadequate staffing include missed care, potential failure to rescue, and job stress and dissatisfaction. *Journal of Obstetric, Gynecologic and Neonatal Nursing, 45*(4), pp. 481–490.

Simpson, K.R., Lyndon, A., Spetz, J., Gay, C.L., and Landstrom, G.L. (2019). Adherence to the AWHONN staffing guidelines as perceived by labor nurses. *Nursing for Women's Health, 23*(3), pp. 217–223.

Simpson, M., and Catling, C. (2016). Understanding psychological traumatic birth experiences: A literature review. *Women and Birth, 29*(3), pp. 203–207.

Singh, G.K., and DiBari, J.N. (2019). Marked disparities in pre-pregnancy obesity and overweight prevalence among U.S. women by race/ethnicity, nativity/immigrant status, and sociodemographic characteristics, 2012–2014. *Journal of Obesity*, in-press. Available: https://www.ncbi.nlm.nih.gov/pubmed/30881701.

Sister Song. (n.d.). *Reproductive Justice*. Available: https://www.sistersong.net/reproductive-justice.

Slaughter-Acey, J.C., Sneed, D., Parker, L., Keith, V.M., Lee, N.L., and Misra, D.P. (2019). Skin tone matters: Racial microaggressions and delayed prenatal care. *American Journal of Preventive Medicine, 57*(3), pp. 321–329.

Sleutel, M., Schultz, S., and Wyble, K. (2007). Nurses' views of factors that help and hinder their intrapartum care. *Journal of Obstetric, Gynecologic, and Neonatal Nursing, 36*(3), pp. 203–211.

Smith, A., and Anderson, M. (2018). *Social Media Use in 2018.* Available: https://www.pewinternet.org/2018/03/01/social-media-use-in-2018.

Smith, D.J., Bono, R.C., and Slinger, B.J. (2017). Transforming the military health system. *Journal of the American Medical Association, 318*(24), pp. 2427–2428.

Snowden, J.M., Tilden, E.L., Snyder, J., Quigley, B., Caughey, A.B., and Cheng, Y.W. (2015). Planned out-of-hospital birth and birth outcomes. *New England Journal of Medicine, 373*(27), pp. 2642–2653.

Snowden, J.M., Tilden, E.L., and Odden, M.C. (2018). Formulating and answering high-impact causal questions in physiologic childbirth science: Concepts and assumptions. *Journal of Midwifery and Women's Health, 63*(6), pp. 721–730.

Snyder, C.C., Wolfe, K.B., Loftin, R.W., Tabbah, S., Lewis, D.F., and Defranco, E.A. (2011). The influence of hospital type on induction of labor and mode of delivery. *American Journal of Obstetrics and Gynecology, 205*(4), pp. 346–e1.

Society for Maternal and Fetal Medicine. (2014). *Advanced Maternal Age and the Risk of Antepartum Stillbirth.* Available: https://www.smfm.org/publications/81-advanced-maternal-age-and-the-risk-of-antepartum-stillbirth.

Song, J.W., and Chung, K.C. (2010). Observational studies: Cohort and case-control studies. *Plastic and Reconstructive Surgery, 126*(6), pp. 2234–2242.

Southwell, B.G., Thorson, E.A., and Sheble, L. (Eds.). (2018). *Misinformation and Mass Audiences.* Austin, TX: University of Texas Press.

Sperlich, M., Gabriel, C., and Seng, J. (2017). Where do you feel safest? Demographic factors and place of birth. *Journal of Midwifery and Women's Health, 62*(1), pp. 88–92.

Spetz, J., Blash, L., Jura, M., and Chu, L. (2018). *2017 Survey of Nurse Practitioners and Certified Nurse Midwives.* Available: https://healthforce.ucsf.edu/sites/healthforce.ucsf.edu/files/publication-pdf/survey2017npcnm-final.pdf.

Sprague, A.E., Sidney, D., Darling, E.K., Van Wagner, V., Soderstrom, B., Rogers, J., Graves, E., Coyle, D., Sumner, A., Holmberg, V., and Khan, B. (2018). Outcomes for the first year of Ontario's Birth Center Demonstration Project. *Journal of Midwifery and Women's Health, 63*(5), pp. 532–540.

Srinivas, S., Durnwald, C., Line, L., Patti, M., Bucher, M., Cunningham, S., and Riis, V. (2019). "Safe Start": A community health worker program that improves perinatal outcomes in high risk women. *American Journal of Obstetrics and Gynecology, 220*(1).

Stacey, D., Légaré, F., Lewis, K., Barry, M.J., Bennett, C.L., Eden, K.B., Holmes-Rovner, M., Llewellyn-Thomas, H., Lyddiatt, A., Thomson, R., and Trevena, L. (2017). Decision aids for people facing health treatment or screening decisions. *Cochrane Database of Systematic Reviews, 4.*

Stahlman, S., Witkop, C., Clark, L., and Taubman, S.B. (2017). Pregnancies and live births, active component service women, U.S. Armed Forces, 2012–2016. *Medical Surveillance Monthly Report, 24*(11), pp. 2–9.

Stanley, D., Sata, N., Oparah, J.C., and McLemore, M.R. (2015). Evaluation of the East Bay Community Birth Support Project, a community-based program to decrease recidivism in previously incarcerated women. *Journal of Obstetric, Gynecologic and Neonatal Nursing, 44*(6), pp. 743–750.

Stapleton, S.R. (2011). Validation of an online data registry for midwifery practices: A pilot project. *The Journal of Midwifery and Women's Health, 56*(5), pp. 452–460.

Stapleton, S.R., Osborne, C., and Illuzzi, J. (2013). Outcomes of care in birth centers: Demonstration of a durable model. *Journal Midwifery and Women's Health, 58*(1), pp. 3–14.

Statistics Canada. (2019). *Live Births and Fetal Deaths (Stillbirths), By Place of Birth (Hospital or Non-hospital)*. Available: https://www150.statcan.gc.ca/t1/tbl1/en/tv.action?pid=1310042901.

Stephenson-Famy, A., Masarie, K.S., Lewis, A., and Schiff, M.A. (2018). What are the risk factors associated with hospital birth among women planning to give birth in a birth center in Washington State? *Birth, 45*(2), pp. 130–136.

Sun, R., Karaca, Z., and Wong, H.S. (2018). Trends in hospital inpatients stays by age and payer, 2000–2015. *H-CUP Statistical Brief, 235*. Available: https://www.hcup-us.ahrq.gov/reports/statbriefs/sb235-Inpatient-Stays-Age-Payer-Trends.jsp.

Suto, M., Takehara, K., Misago, C., and Matsui, M. (2015). Prevalence of perineal lacerations in women giving birth at midwife-led birth centers in Japan: A retrospective descriptive study. *Journal of Midwifery and Women's Health, 60*(4), pp. 419–427.

Swartz, J.J., Hainmueller, J., Lawrence, D., and Rodriguez, M.I. (2017). Expanding prenatal care to unauthorized immigrant women and the effects on infant health. *Obstetrics and Gynecology, 130*(5), pp. 938–945.

Swendsen, J., Conway, K.P., Degenhardt, L., Glantz, M., Jin, R., Merikangas, K.R., Sampson, N., and Kessler, R. C. (2010). Mental disorders as risk factors for substance use, abuse and dependence: Results from the 10-year follow-up of the National Comorbidity Survey. *Addiction, 105*(6), pp. 1117–1128.

Tani, F., and Castagna, V. (2017). Maternal social support, quality of birth experience, and post-partum depression in primiparous women. *The Journal of Maternal-Fetal and Neonatal Medicine, 30*(6), pp. 689–692.

Teune, M.J., van Wassenaer, A.G., Malin, G.L., Asztalos, E., Alfirevic, A., Mol, B.W., and Opmeer, B.C. (2013). Long-term child follow-up after large obstetric randomized controlled trials for the evaluation of perinatal interventions: A systematic review of the literature. *British Journal of Obstetrics and Gyaenocology, 120*(1), pp. 15–22.

Texas Department of State Health Services. (2019). *CHW Certification Requirements*. Available: https://www.dshs.texas.gov/mch/chw/chwdocs.aspx.

The City of Columbus. (2019). *Prenatal Trip Assistance*. Available: https://smart.columbus.gov/projects/prenatal-trip-assistance.

The Editorial Board. (2014). *Are Midwives Safer Than Doctors?* Available: https://www.nytimes.com/2014/12/15/opinion/are-midwives-safer-than-doctors.html.

The General Court of New Hampshire. (n.d.). *Chapter Mid 500: Scope of Midwifery Practice*. Available: http://www.gencourt.state.nh.us/rules/state_agencies/mid500.html.

The Joint Commission. (2004). *Sentinel Event Alert, Issue 30: Preventing Infant Death and Injury During Delivery*. Available: https://www.jointcommission.org/sentinel_event_alert_issue_30_preventing_infant_death_and_injury_during_delivery.

The Joint Commission. (2010). *Preventing Maternal Death*. Available: http://www.jointcommission.org/assets/1/18/sea_44.pdf.

The Joint Commission. (2018). *Facts about Hospital Accreditation*. Available: https://www.jointcommission.org/facts_about_hospital_accreditation.

The Medicaid and CHIP Payment and Access Commission. (2014). *Issues in Pregnancy Coverage under Medicaid and Exchange Plans*. Available: https://www.macpac.gov/publication/ch-3-issues-in-pregnancy-coverage-under-medicaid-and-exchange-plans.

The Medicaid and CHIP Payment and Access Commission. (2017). *Federal Requirements and State Options: Eligibility*. Available: https://www.macpac.gov/wp-content/uploads/2017/03/Federal-Requirements-and-State-Options-Eligibility.pdf.

The Midwifery Center Healthcare. (2019). *Frequently Asked Questions*. Available: https://www.tmcaz.com/tmc-for-women/maternity/the-midwifery-center/frequently-asked-questions.

The World Bank. (2019). *DataBank: Birth Rate, Crude (per 1,000 people).* Available: https://databank.worldbank.org/reports.aspx?source=2&series=SP.DYN.CBRT.IN&country=#.

Thomas, M.P., Ammann, G., Brazier, E., Noyes, P., and Maybank, A. (2017). Doula services within a healthy start program: Increasing access for an underserved population. *Maternal and Child Health Journal*, 21(1), pp. 59–64.

Thornton, P., McFarlin, B.L., Park, C., Rankin, K., Schorn, M., Finnegan, L., and Stapleton, S. (2017). Cesarean outcomes in U.S. birth centers and collaborating hospitals: A cohort comparison. *Journal of Midwifery and Women's Health*, 62(1), pp. 40–48.

Thurston, L.A.F., Abrams, D., Dreher, A., Ostrowski, S.R., and Wright, J.C. (2019). Improving birth and breastfeeding outcomes among low resource women in Alabama by including doulas in the interprofessional birth care team. *Journal of Interprofessional Education and Practice*, 17, p. 100278.

Tilden, E.L., Cheyney, M., Guise, J.M., Emeis, C., Lapidus, J., Biel, F.M., Wiedrick, J., and Snowden, J.M. (2017). Vaginal birth after cesarean: Neonatal outcomes and United States birth setting. *American Journal of Obstetrics and Gynecology*, 216(4), pp. 403.e1–403.e8.

Tjaden, P., and Thoennes, N. (2000). *Findings from the National Violence Against Women Survey.* Washington, DC: Department of Justice. Available: https://www.ncjrs.gov/pdffiles1/nij/183781.pdf.

Tong, S.T., Makaroff, L.A., Xierali, I.M., Parhat, P., Puffer, J.C., Newton, W.P., and Bazemore, A.W. (2012). Proportion of family physicians providing maternity care continues to decline. *Journal of the American Board of Family Medicine*, 25(3), pp. 270–271.

Triebwasser, J.E., Kamdar, N., Moniz, M.H., Langen, E.S., Journal of the American Medical Association, J., Smith, R.D., and Morgan, D.M. (2018). Hospital contribution to variation in rates of vaginal birth after cesarean: A Michigan Value Collaborative study. *American Journal of Obstetrics and Gynecology*, 218(1), pp. S351–S352.

Trotter, C., Wolman, W.L., Hofmeyr, J., Nikodem, C., and Turton, R. (1992). The effect of social support during labour on postpartum depression. *South African Journal of Psychology*, 22(3), pp. 134–139.

Truven Health Analytics. (2013). *The Cost of Having a Baby in the United States.* Available: http://www.nationalpartnership.org/our-work/resources/health-care/maternity/archive/the-cost-of-having-a-baby-in-the-us.pdf.

Tumblin, A., and Simkin, P. (2001). Pregnant women's perceptions of their nurse's role during labor and delivery. *Birth*, 28(1), pp. 52–56.

Tussey, C.M., Botsios, E., Gerkin, R.D., Kelly, L.A., Gamez, J., and Mensik, J. (2015). Reducing length of labor and cesarean surgery rate using a peanut ball for women laboring with an epidural. *The Journal of Perinatal Education*, 24(1), p. 16.

United Nations Population Fund. (2006). *State of World Population 2006: A Passage to Hope: Women and International Migration.* Available: https://www.unfpa.org/sites/default/files/pub-pdf/sowp06-en.pdf.

United States Committee for Refugees and Immigrants. (n.d.). *Study of Domestic Capacity to Provide Medical Care for Vulnerable Refugees.* Available: https://refugees.org/wp-content/uploads/2015/12/Study-of-Domestic-Capacity-to-Provide-Medical-Care-for-Vulnerable-Refugees-Quick-View.pdf.

U.S. Census Bureau. (2017). *Fertility of Women in the United States: 2016.* Available: https://www.census.gov/data/tables/2016/demo/fertility/women-fertility.html#par_list_58.

U.S. Census Bureau. (2018). *Foreign-Born Population by Sex, Age, and Year of Entry: 2018.* Available: https://www.census.gov/data/tables/2018/demo/foreign-born/cps-2018.html.

U.S. Census Bureau. (2019). *About Foreign Born.* Available: https://www.census.gov/topics/population/foreign-born/about.html.

U.S. Midwifery Education, Regulation, and Association Professional Regulation Committee. (2015a). *Principles for Model U.S. Midwifery Legislation and Regulation.* Available: http://www.usmera.org/wp-content/uploads/2015/11/US-MERALegislativeStatement2015.pdf.

U.S. Midwifery Education, Regulation, and Association Professional Regulation Committee. (2015b). *Statement on the Licensure of Certified Professional Midwives (CPM).* Available: http://www.usmera.org/index.php/2015/07/01/statement-on-the-licensure-of-certified-professional-midwives-cpm.

U.S. Preventive Services Task Force. (2017). Screening for preeclampsia: U.S. Preventive Services Task Force recommendation statement. *Journal of the American Medical Association,* *317*(16), pp. 1661–1667.

van der Kooy, J., Poeran, J., de Graaf, J.P., Birnie, E., Denktas, S., Steegers, E.A., and Bonsel, G.J. (2011). Planned home compared with planned hospital births in the Netherlands: Intrapartum and early neonatal death in low-risk pregnancies. *Obstetrics and Gynecology,* *118*(5), pp. 1037–1046.

Vanderbilt University Medical Center. (2019). *Department of Obstetrics and Gynecology: Residency Program.* Available: https://www.vumc.org/obgyn/person/residency-program.

Vanderbilt University School of Nursing. (2019). Available: https://www.vanderbiltnursemidwives.org/cnm-ourpractice.html.

Vedam, S., Leeman, L., Cheyney, M., Fisher, T.J., Myers, S., Low, L.K. and Ruhl, C. (2014a). Transfer from planned home birth to hospital: Improving interprofessional collaboration. *Journal of Midwifery and Women's Health,* *59*(6), pp. 624–634.

Vedam, S., Stoll, K., Schummers, L., Fairbrother, N., Klein, M.C., Thordarson, D., Kornelsen, J., Dharamsi, S., Rogers, J., Liston, R., and Kaczorowski, J. (2014b). The Canadian Birth Place study: Examining maternity care provider attitudes and interprofessional conflict around planned home birth. *BMC Pregnancy and Childbirth,* *14*(1), p. 353.

Vedam, S., Rossiter, C., Homer, C.S., Stoll, K., and Scarf, V.L. (2017). The ResQu Index: A new instrument to appraise the quality of research on birth place. *PLOS One,* *12*(8), p. e0182991.

Vedam, S., Stoll, K., MacDorman, M.F., Declercq, E., Cramer, R., Cheyney, M., Fisher, T., Butt, E., Yang, Y.T., and Kennedy, H.P. (2018). Mapping integration of midwives across the United States: Impact on access, equity, and outcomes. *PLOS One,* *13*(2), p. e0192523.

Vedam, S., Stoll, K., Khemet Taiwo, T., Rubashkin, N., Cheyney, M., Strauss, N., McLemore, M., Cadena, M., Nethery, E., Ruston, E., Schummers, L., Declercq, E., and the GVtM-UA Steering Council. (2019). The Giving Voice to Mothers study: Inequity and mistreatment during pregnancy and childbirth in the United States. *Reproductive Health,* *16*(1), p. 77.

Veterans Affairs/DoD Management of Pregnancy Work Group. (2018). *VA/DoD Clinical Practice Guideline for the Management of Pregnancy.* Washington, DC. Available: https://www.healthquality.va.gov/guidelines/WH/up/VADoDPregnancyCPG4102018.pdf.

Vinikoor, L.D., Messer, L.D., Laraia, B.A., and Kaufman, J.S. (2010). Reliability of variables on the North Carolina birth certificate: A comparison with directly queried values from a cohort study. *Pediatric and Perinatal Epidemiology,* *24*(1), pp. 102–112.

Virginia Law. (2013). *18VAC85-130-80. General Disclosure Requirements.* Available: https://law.lis.virginia.gov/admincode/title18/agency85/chapter130/section80.

Vogel, L. (2011). "Do it yourself" births prompt alarm. *Canadian Medical Association Journal,* *183*(6), pp. 648–650.

Wallace, M.E., and Harville, W.W. (2013). Allostatic load and birth outcomes among white and black women in New Orleans. *Maternal and Child Health Journal,* *17*(6), pp. 1025–1029.

Walsh, D., Spiby, H., Grigg, C.P., Dodwell, M., McCourt, C., Culley, L., Bishop, S., Wilkinson, J., Coleby, D., Pacanowski, L., and Thornton, J. (2018). Mapping midwifery and obstetric units in England. *Midwifery*, 56, pp. 9–16.

Wasden, S.W., Chasen, S.T., Perlman, J.M., Illuzzi, J.L., Chervenak, F.A., Grünebaum, A., and Lipkind, H.S. (2017). Planned home birth and the association with neonatal hypoxic ischemic encephalopathy. *Journal of Perinatal Medicine*, 45(9), pp. 1055–1060.

Watterberg, K.L. (2013). Policy statement on planned home birth: Upholding the best interests of children and families. *Pediatrics*, 132(5), pp. 924–926.

Wax, J.R., Lucas, F.L., Lamont, M., Pinette, M.G., Cartin, A., and Blackstone, J. (2010). Maternal and newborn outcomes in planned home birth vs. planned hospital births: A meta-analysis. *American Journal of Obstetrics and Gynecology*, 203(3), pp. 243–e1.

West, S.G., Duan, N., Pequegnat, W., Gaist, P., Des Jarlais, D.C., Holtgrave, D., Szapocznik, J., Fishbein, M., Rapkin, B., Clatts, M., and Mullen, P.D., 2008. Alternatives to the randomized controlled trial. *American Journal of Public Health*, 98(8), pp. 1359–1366.

White VanGompel, E., Perez, S., Wang, C., Datta, A., Cape, V., and Main, E. (2019). Measuring labor and delivery unit culture and clinicians' attitudes toward birth: Revision and validation of the Labor Culture Survey. *Birth*, 46(2), pp. 300–310.

Wiegerinck, M.M., Van Der Goes, B.Y., Ravelli, A.C., Van Der Post, J.A., Buist, F.C., Tamminga, P., and Mol, B.W. (2018). Intrapartum and neonatal mortality among low-risk women in midwife-led versus obstetrician-led care in the Amsterdam region of the Netherlands: A propensity score matched study. *BMJ Open*, 8(1), p. e018845.

Wier, L.M., and Andrews, R.M. (2011). *The National Hospital Bill: The Most Expensive Conditions by Payer, 2008*. Available: https://www.hcup-us.ahrq.gov/reports/statbriefs/sb107.pdf.

Wildeman, C. (2012). Imprisonment and infant mortality. *Social Problems*, 59(2), pp. 228–257.

Wint, K., Elias, T.I., Mendez, G., Mendez, D.D., and Gary-Webb, T.L. (2019). Experiences of community doulas working with low-income, African American mothers. *Health Equity*, 3(1), pp. 109–116.

Wisdom, J.P., Cavaleri, M.A., Onwuegbuzie, A.J., and Green, C.A. (2012). Methodological reporting in qualitative, quantitative, and mixed methods health services research articles. *Health Services Research*, 47(2), pp. 721–745.

World Health Organization. (2014). *The Prevention and Elimination of Disrespect and Abuse During Facility-Based Childbirth*. Available: https://apps.who.int/iris/bitstream/handle/10665/134588/WHO_RHR_14.23_eng.pdf;jsessionid=A4E8D847C6366097051BEDCF76776AD8?sequence=1.

World Health Organization. (2015). *WHO Statement on Caesarean Section Rates*. Available: https://apps.who.int/iris/bitstream/handle/10665/161442/WHO_RHR_15.02_eng.pdf;jsessionid=8F2C265B420604B6FD35FA593767F1CE?sequence=1%20And%20https://www.BMJ.com/content/360/BMJ.k55.

World Health Organization. (2018). *WHO Recommendations: Intrapartum Care for a Positive Childbirth Experience*. Available: https://apps.who.int/iris/bitstream/handle/10665/260178/9789241550215-eng.pdf.

World Health Organization. (2019). *Maternal Mortality Ratio (per 100,000 Live Births)*. Available: https://www.who.int/healthinfo/statistics/indmaternalmortality/en.

Wu, Y., Kataria, Y., Wang, Z., Ming, W.K., and Ellervik, C. (2019). Factors associated with successful vaginal birth after a cesarean section: A systematic review and meta-analysis. *BMC Pregnancy and Childbirth*, 19(1), p. 360.

Xu, X., Gariepy, A., Lundsberg, L.S., Sheth, S.S., Pettker, C.M., Krumholz, H.M., and Illuzzi, J.L. (2015). Wide variation found in hospital facility costs for maternity stays involving low-risk childbirth. *Health Affairs*, 34(7), pp. 1212–1219.

Xu, X., Lee, H.C., Lin, H., Lundsberg, L.S., Pettker, C.M., Lipkind, H.S., and Illuzzi, J.L. (2018). Hospital variation in cost of childbirth and contributing factors: A cross-sectional study. *British Journal of Obstetrics and Gynaecology, 125*(7), pp. 829–839.

Xue, Y., and Brewer, C. (2014). Racial and ethnic diversity of the U.S. national nurse workforce 1988–2013. *Policy, Politics, and Nursing Practice, 15*(3–4), pp. 102–110.

Yang, Y.T., L.B. Attanasio, and K.B. Kozhimannil. (2016). State scope of practice laws, nurse-midwifery workforce, and childbirth procedures and outcomes. *Women's Health Issues, 26*(3), pp. 262–267.

Yoder, H., and Hardy, L.R. (2018). Midwifery and antenatal care for black women: A narrative review. *SAGE Open, 8*(1).

Young, R.A. (2017). Maternity care services provided by family physicians in rural hospitals. *The Journal of the American Board of Family Medicine, 30*(1), pp. 71–77.

Young, R.K. (2009). *AMA Manual of Style: A Guide for Authors and Editors (10th edition).* Available: https://www.amamanualofstyle.com/view/10.1093/Journal of the American Medical Association/9780195176339.001.0001/med-9780195176339-div2-350.

Zambrana, R.E., Dunkel-Schetter, C., Collins, N.L., and Scrimshaw, S.C. (1999). Mediators of ethnic-associated differences in infant birth weight. *Journal of Urban Health, 76*(1), pp. 102–116.

Zhang, X., Joseph, K.S., and Kramer, M.S. (2010). Decreased term and postterm birthweight in the United States: impact of labor induction. *American Journal of Obstetrics and Gynecology, 203*(2), pp. 124–e1.

Zielinski, R., Ackerson, K., and Kane Low, L. (2015). Planned home birth: Benefits, risks, and opportunities. *International Journal of Women's Health, 7*, pp. 361–377.

Zollinger, T.W., Przybylski, M.J., and Gamache, R.E. (2006). Reliability of Indiana birth certificate data compared to medical records. *Annuals of Epidemiology, 16*(1), pp. 1–10.

Appendix

Biographical Sketches of Committee Members and Staff

SUSAN C. SCRIMSHAW (*Chair*) recently retired as president of The Sage Colleges. Previously, she was president of Simmons College and, at the University of Illinois at Chicago, she served as dean of the School of Public Health and professor of community health sciences and of anthropology. Her research includes community participatory research methods, addressing health disparities, improving pregnancy outcomes, violence prevention, health literacy, and culturally appropriate delivery of health care. She is a member of the National Academy of Medicine and a fellow of the American Association for the Advancement of Science, the American Anthropological Association, the Society for Applied Anthropology, and the Institute of Medicine of Chicago. She is a past president of the board of directors of the U.S.-Mexico Foundation for Science, former chair of the Association of Schools of Public Health, and past president of the Society for Medical Anthropology. Her honors and awards include the Margaret Mead Award, a Hero of Public Health gold medal awarded by President Vicente Fox of Mexico, the Adam Yarmolinsky Medal awarded by the National Academy of Medicine, the Chicago Community Clinic Visionary Award, and the Career Achievement Award of the Society for Medical Anthropology. She has an M.A. and a Ph.D. in anthropology from Columbia University.

JILL ALLIMAN is a member on the faculty of Frontier Nursing University, where she teaches master's and doctoral nursing students. She is also program director of the Strong Start project of the American Association of Birth Centers (AABC), which collects data in 45 birth centers on the impact of enhanced prenatal care. Previously, as a birth center midwife in rural

345

Appalachia, she worked to improve access to care for some of the most underserved women in the United States. She is past president of AABC and currently serves as chair of its Government Affairs Committee, where she assisted with a successful effort to add birth center facility coverage to Medicaid covered services. Her current focus is on extending the birth center model of care to a wider group of women. She has a doctorate in nursing practice from Frontier Nursing University with a concentration in nursing practice.

EMILY P. BACKES (*Study Director*) is a program officer with the Board on Children, Youth, and Families (BCYF) in the Division of Behavioral, Social Sciences, and Education at the National Academies of Sciences, Engineering, and Medicine. She previously served as director for BCYF studies on adolescence and the financing of early care and education and provided analytical and editorial support to other projects covering a wide range of topics, including juvenile justice, policing and illicit markets, education and literacy, science communication, and human rights. She has a B.A. and an M.A. in history from the University of Missouri, specializing in U.S. human rights policy, and a J.D. from the University of the District of Columbia, where she represented clients as a student attorney with the Low-Income Taxpayer Clinic and the Juvenile and Special Education Law Clinic.

MELISSA CHEYNEY is associate professor of clinical medical anthropology at Oregon State University (OSU) with additional appointments in global health and in women's, gender, and sexuality studies. She is also a licensed midwife in active practice. Dr. Cheyney directs the International Reproductive Health Laboratory at OSU, where she serves as the Primary Investigator on more than 20 maternal and infant health-related research projects, including the Community Doula Project. She is the author of an ethnography, *Born at Home*, along with dozens of peer-reviewed articles that examine the cultural beliefs and clinical outcomes associated with midwife-led births at home and in birth centers in the United States. She is the mother of a daughter born at home on International Day of the Midwife in 2009. She has a Ph.D. in medical anthropology from the University of Oregon.

MICHELLE R. COLLINS is a professor and associate dean of academic affairs at Rush University College of Nursing. She has a widely diverse clinical practice that includes initiating a successful waterbirth service at that site in Marion, Illinois, where she was the first certified nurse-midwife. She is active in the Vanderbilt nurse-midwifery practice, having a special interest in cervical dysplasia diagnosis and treatment. She has received awards for teaching and expertise in working with the media. Her work focuses not only on clinical practice, but also on teaching the next generation of certified nurse-midwives, with the goal of helping students develop their passion in caring for women through every stage of their lives. She has published in a variety of journals, such as the *Journal for Nurse Practitioners*, *Journal of Midwifery & Women's Health*, *Reviews in Obstetrics & Gynecology*, and *Nursing for Women's Health*. She is a fellow of the American College of Nurse-Midwives and the American Academy of Nursing. She has an M.S. in nursing from Marquette University and a Ph.D. from the University of Tennessee Health Science Center.

BROWNSYNE TUCKER EDMONDS is an obstetrician-gynecologist and health services researcher at the Indiana University School of Medicine, where she is also an associate professor of obstetrics and gynecology and serves as an assistant dean for faculty affairs, professional development, and diversity. Her work focuses on disparities, shared decision making, and periviable care, with the goals of eliminating health disparities, advancing social justice, and promoting professionalism and humanism in the care of underserved populations. In the Office of Diversity Affairs, she focuses on faculty development for populations underrepresented in medicine and developing programming to help junior faculty of color advance professionally in the Indiana University School of Medicine community. She was a Norman F. Grant/American Board of Obstetrics and Gynecology fellow at the National Academy of Medicine. She has a B.A. from Brown University, an M.A. in public health from the Harvard School of Public Health, an M.A. in health policy research from the University of Pennsylvania, and an M.D. from Brown University.

MARY GHITELMAN (*Senior Program Assistant*) is on the staff of the Board on Children, Youth, and Families and the Committee on Population in the Division of Behavioral and Social Sciences and Education at the National Academies of Sciences, Engineering, and Medicine. She has been with the Academies since April 2015, working on reports including *The Integration of Immigrants into American Society*; *Valuing Climate Damages: Updating Estimation of the Social Cost of Carbon Dioxide*; *Transforming the Financing of Early Care and Education*; and *The Promise of Adolescence: Realizing Opportunity for All Youth*. She received her B.A. in psychology from Beloit College and studied abroad in Copenhagen, Denmark, with a focus in cross-cultural psychology.

WENDY GORDON is an associate professor and chair of the Department of Midwifery at Bastyr University, and she has an active practice as a licensed midwife at the Center for Birth Midwives in Seattle. Her teaching and research interests include the provision of midwifery care in home and birth center settings; the role of racism in perinatal health disparities; and the ability to translate and evaluate research. She serves as the president of the board of directors of the Association of Midwifery Educators, is active in the Midwives Association of Washington State as a member of the Data Committee, and is also a member of the Practice Committee Workgroup for the National Association of Certified Professional Midwives. She has a B.S. in chemical engineering, an M.P.H. from Oregon Health & Sciences University with a focus in health disparities, and a doctorate in midwifery from Jefferson University.

ERIN HAMMERS FORSTAG is a science writer and public health lawyer. She has contributed to the National Academies of Sciences, Engineering, and Medicine reports on topics as varied as the Ebola epidemic, mitochondrial replacement techniques, and the financing of early childhood education. Her interests include the intersection between public health and the First Amendment, bioethics, and issues relating to women and children. Prior to her career in science writing, she worked in political advocacy and as a Peace Corps volunteer in rural Uzbekistan. She holds an M.P.H. from Columbia University and her juris doctorate from Georgetown University.

ELIZABETH S. HOWE-HUIST (*Associate Program Officer*) is on the staff of the Board on Children, Youth, and Families in the Division of Behavioral and Social Sciences and Education at the National Academies of Sciences, Engineering, and Medicine. She has a B.A. in psychology from Wright State University, with additional training in marriage and family counseling, and an M.A. in sociology from the University of Mississippi. She is currently completing a Ph.D. in sociology at Bowling Green State University in Ohio, where she has engaged in demographic research on family processes and how these family relationships affect youth and young adults.

BRIDGET B. KELLY (*Consultant*) specializes in research and evaluation, policy analysis, strategy development, stakeholder engagement, and meeting design and facilitation. Previously, at the National Academies of Sciences, Engineering, and Medicine, she oversaw a portfolio of projects that included early childhood, mental health, chronic diseases, HIV, and evaluation science. More recently, she cofounded the nonprofit Bridging Health & Community, with the mission of helping the health sector work more effectively with communities. Trained in medicine and developmental neurobiology, she has a B.A. from Williams College and an M.D. and a Ph.D. from Duke University.

MARIAN FRANCES MACDORMAN is a research professor at the Maryland Population Research Center at the University of Maryland, College Park. She is also editor-in-chief of the journal *Birth: Issues in Peri-*

natal Care. Her research focuses on reproductive health issues, including maternal, fetal, infant and perinatal morbidity and mortality, preterm birth, out-of-hospital births, and cesarean deliveries. Previously, she was on the staff at the National Center for Health Statistics of the Centers for Disease Control and Prevention, conducting research and producing national data sets on reproductive and child health issues. She has a Ph.D. in demography from Australian National University.

M. KATHRYN MENARD is distinguished professor and vice chair of the Department of Obstetrics and Gynecology at the University of North Carolina School of Medicine, where she also serves as director of the Center for Maternal Infant Health and director of the Division of Maternal Fetal Medicine. She also serves as medical director of the pregnancy medical home model through Community Care of North Carolina, a statewide program designed to enhance access to high-quality prenatal care and improve birth outcomes for pregnant women with Medicaid coverage. Her work is focused at the intersect between public health and the everyday challenges of clinical obstetric care. She recently served as president of the Society for Maternal Fetal Medicine, and she currently serves on the executive committee for the Alliance for Innovation on Maternal Health and on the Patient Quality and Safety Committee of the American College of Obstetricians and Gynecologists. She has an M.P.H. from the University of North Carolina and an M.D. from the University of Medicine and Dentistry of New Jersey, and she completed her medical residency at the University of Pennsylvania.

KAREN MILGATE is a health care policy consultant whose specialty is Medicare and Medicaid policies, programs, operations, and data. Most recently, she was the deputy director of the Center for Strategic Planning in the Centers for Medicare & Medicaid Services (CMS) in the U.S. Department of Health and Human Services, where she led strategic planning efforts, helped build analytical tools, coordinated interagency initiatives, and helped build the data infrastructure to enable CMS to better manage and direct its programs. Previously, she was a research director for the Medicare Payment Advisory Commission and senior associate director for policy development for the American Hospital Association, and she served as the executive director for a nonprofit organization focused on education around women's reproductive health. She has a B.A. in economics and a B.A. in international studies from American University and an M.A. in public policy from the University of Maryland.

JOCHEN PROFIT is the chief quality officer at the California Perinatal Quality Care Collaborative and an associate professor of pediatrics at

Stanford University. He also practices as a neonatologist. Previously, he was an assistant professor of pediatrics at Baylor College of Medicine. His research concentrates on measuring and improving the quality of neonatal and pediatric health care delivery, with a focus on enhancing organizational effectiveness. He developed a composite indicator quality of care provided to very low-birthweight infants in a neonatal intensive care unit (NICU), which has been used to benchmark quality of care delivery in California's NICUs. His research has also focused on organizational determinants of excellence, including patient safety culture, high reliability, and caregiver resilience. He has served as an advisor to a variety of national quality of care and safety organizations and is a standing scientific reviewer for the National Institutes of Health. He has a medical degree from the Albert-Ludwigs-University in Freiburg, Germany, and he completed pediatric residency training at Tufts University.

CAROL SAKALA leads maternal health and maternity care programming at the National Partnership for Women & Families. She works as a maternity care advocate, educator, researcher, author, and policy analyst, with a continuous focus on meeting the needs and interests of childbearing women and their families. Previously, she served as director of programs at Childbirth Connection, which became a core program of the National Partnership for Women & Families in 2014. She has been an investigator on all national *Listening to Mothers* surveys and was principal investigator of the most recent *Listening to Mothers in California* survey. She has contributed to creating or commissioning foundational resources for the field on such topics as the cost of having a baby, maternity care and liability, evidence-based maternity care, effectiveness of labor support, hormonal physiology of childbearing, and performance of the nation's maternity care system. She has an M.A. from the University of Chicago, an M.S. in public health from the University of Utah, and a Ph.D. in health policy from Boston University.

NEEL SHAH is an assistant professor of obstetrics, gynecology, and reproductive biology at Harvard Medical School and director of the Delivery Decisions Initiative at Ariadne Labs. He also holds appointments in health policy and management at the Harvard Chan School of Public Health and in health law policy at Harvard Law School. In his academic work, he designs and tests health system innovations that aim to improve the well-being of mothers in the United States and globally. In collaboration with professional colleagues in obstetrics, midwifery, and nursing, he has published extensively on the design of maternal health systems in leading journals, including the *New England Journal of Medicine* and *JAMA*. He is also an obstetrician-gynecologist at Beth Israel Deaconess Medical Center in Boston. Earlier, he founded Costs of Care, a global nongovernmental organization that curates insights from clinicians to help delivery systems provide better care, and he cofounded the March for Moms Association, a coalition of 40 leading organizations, to increase public and private investment in the well-being of mothers. He has an M.D. from Brown Medical School.

DARA SHEFSKA (*Associate Program Officer*) is on the staff of the Board on Children, Youth, and Families (BCYF) in the Division of Behavioral and Social Sciences and Education at the National Academies of Sciences, Engineering, and Medicine. Previously, she provided research and analytic support to two BCYF reports, *A Roadmap to Reducing Child Poverty* and *The Promise of Adolescence: Realizing Opportunity for All Youth*. She also previously worked on the staff of the Food and Nutrition Board. She is a graduate of McGill University and is currently pursuing a master's degree at the University of Maryland School of Public Policy.

KATHLEEN RICE SIMPSON is a perinatal clinical nurse specialist in St. Louis, Missouri. She is the editor-in-chief of *MCN: The American Journal of Maternal/Child Nursing*. As principal investigator, she has conducted research on such topics as fetal well-being during labor, uterine activity during labor, fetal monitoring, labor induction, and nurse staffing, among others. She was the principal investigator of the Michigan Hospital Association's Keystone OB Patient Safety Project, and is currently serving as chair of the March of Dimes National Advisory Committee. She has been a member of the Joint Commission Perinatal Technical Advisory Panel, the National Quality Forum Steering Committee on National Voluntary Consensus Standards for the Perinatal Care, the National Priorities Partnership Maternity Action Team of the National Quality Forum, and the National Institute of Child Health and Human Development Expert Panel for Electronic Fetal Heart Rate Monitoring. She also provides consultation to hospitals and health care systems to promote safe care for mothers and babies. She has a nursing degree from Loyola University Chicago and a Ph.D. in nursing from Saint Louis University.

LORI TREGO (*Nurse Scholar in Residence*) is a certified nurse midwife and associate professor at the University of Colorado Denver Anschutz Medical Campus College of Nursing, where she teaches in the veteran and military health care graduate program. Previously, she retired from service in the military as a U.S. Army Nurse Corps officer, where she provided leadership over a wide range of obstetric practices. She has extensive experience in inpatient and outpatient obstetrical/gynecological care as a registered nurse, as the director of obstetric and well woman clinics, and in full-scope midwifery practice. She has done extensive work on military women's health and sex- and gender-specific health needs, and, more generally, improving the health of military women across the life course. Her current research investigates women's perceptions of the care afforded to them by the Veterans Administration.

RUTH ENID ZAMBRANA is professor and interim chair in the Department of Women's Studies and director of the Consortium on Race, Gender and Ethnicity at the University of Maryland, College Park. She is also an adjunct professor of family medicine at the University of Maryland, Baltimore, School of Medicine. Her work applies a critical intersectional lens to structural inequality and racial, Hispanic ethnicity, and gender inequities in population health and higher education trajectories. She has published extensively and serves on many social science and public health journal editorial boards. She is the recipient of numerous awards, including the Julian Samora Distinguished Career Award by the Latino/as Section of the American Sociological Association for her contributions to the sociology of Latinos and immigrant studies, teaching, and mentoring, and the 2013 American Public Health Association Latino Caucus Founding Member Award for Vision and Leadership. She has a B.A. from Queens College of the City University of New York, an M.A. from the University of Pennsylvania, and a Ph.D. from Boston University.

BOARD ON CHILDREN, YOUTH, AND FAMILIES